Case-Control Studies

MONOGRAPHS IN EPIDEMIOLOGY AND BIOSTATISTICS

Case-Control Studies
Design, Conduct, Analysis

James J. Schlesselman, Ph.D.
with contributions by
Paul D. Stolley, M.D., M.P.H.

New York   Oxford
OXFORD UNIVERSITY PRESS
1982

Copyright © 1982 by Oxford University Press, Inc.

Library of Congress Cataloging in Publication Data

Schlesselman, James J.
    Case-control studies.

    (Monographs in epidemiology and biostatistics)
    Bibliography: p.
    Includes index.
    1. Epidemiology—Statistical methods.   2. Experimental
design.   I. Stolley, Paul D.   II. Title.   III. Series.
RA652.2.M3S34   614.4'0723   81-1517
ISBN 0-19-502933-X   AACR2

Printing (last digit): 20 19 18 17 16 15 14 13

Printed in the United States of America

For Sarah

Preface

Case-control studies, often called "retrospective" studies, provide a research method for investigating factors that may prevent or cause disease. Basically the method involves the comparison of patients (cases) with a group of controls that consists of persons who are free of the disease under study. The comparison is aimed at discovering factors that may differ in the two groups and explain the occurrence of disease in the patients. The underlying factors may either elevate or reduce the risk of disease, and a case-control study can quantify the alteration in risk associated with each factor individually and in combination. The case-control approach is commonly used to assess the risk of cancer from environmental and industrial exposures, to conduct postmarketing surveillance of adverse or beneficial drug effects, and to discover factors that cause or prevent disease in humans. Thus, the relation of toxic shock syndrome to the use of tampons, the discovery of the link between vaginal cancer in young women and a maternal exposure to DES (diethylstilbestrol), the establishment of the effect of cigarette smoking on the development of lung cancer, the finding of a reduced risk of fractures with the use of estrogens, and the investigation of various cancers suspected to be associated with asbestos, radiation, and artificial sweeteners, have all been approached by the case-control method.

My impetus for writing a book on case-control studies arose in 1976 from the questions asked by my wife, Sarah, and by a colleague, Bruce V. Stadel. They were collaborating with others on the development of a case-control study (Women's Health Study) of various gynecologic disorders and the use of intrauterine devices. Their inquiries emphasized that no discussion of the case-control method had yet been written that was sufficiently detailed to provide a comprehensive guide to the design, conduct, and analysis of case-control studies. The relevant epidemiologic and statistical literature was scattered across numerous journals. Contradictory advice and opinion were rife; terminology was inconsistently used, and the burden of sorting fact from fiction was a daunting prospect to anyone first contemplating the exercise. Given this situation, the utility of a thorough treatment of the topic was self-evident.

This work is intended to provide the key epidemiologic and statistical techniques pertinent to the design, conduct, analysis, and interpretation of case-control studies. It reviews the strengths and limitations of the case-control method and indicates the scope of problems that are suited to this investigational approach. The reader is provided with a guide to the design of study protocols, shown how to plan the size of an investigation, and how to prepare for field operations. The proper use of matching and the likely sources of bias that may be encountered in a case-control study are discussed in detail. Basic and advanced methods of statistical analysis are presented along with their application to case-control studies appearing in the recent medical and epidemiologic literature.

The reader who has a background knowledge at the level of first courses in epidemiology and statistics should be adequately prepared to read most of the text, with the exception of the last chapter which discusses multivariate methods of analysis. A familiarity with the use of regression analysis and the ability to follow simple algebraic arguments are necessary for a full comprehension of this material. Even the unprepared reader, however, may find that perusal of some of this chapter is worthwhile.

When used to refer generally to a connection between a disease and some factor under study, the term "association" should be understood to mean that the factor may be associated with either an *elevation* in the risk of disease (positive association) or a *reduction* in risk (negative association), the direction being unspecified. For convenience of expression, I have used the term "exposure" to refer not only to external factors that may impinge upon an individual and alter risk, but also to personal attributes such as age, sex, race, serum cholesterol, or HLA type, for example.

Technical details that one may want to ignore at a first reading and extended examples which may break the flow of argument in the main text are distinguished by small type. Conditional probability is denoted in standard fashion. Thus, if D denotes "disease" and E denotes "exposure," $P(D\,|\,E)$ represents the "probability of disease occurring within some period of time, *given that an individual is exposed*." An algebraic expression such as $a + b/c$ should be read as $a + (b/c)$ and *not* as $(a + b)/c$.

Computations for the statistical methods given in Chapters 6 and 7 can often be done on a programmable calculator. Rothman and Boice (1979) have published a number of programs, some of which correspond to the techniques presented here. Recently, Breslow and Day (1980) wrote a monograph which discusses the analysis of case-control studies and their application to cancer research.

Although the experimental method is unquestionably the most incisive approach to a scientific problem, ethical or logistic considerations often prevent its application to the study of disease in humans. Even though laboratory investigations may suggest that certain environmental, genetic, or behavioral factors alter the risk of disease, an observational study is often necessary, not only to establish the connection beyond reasonable doubt, but also to quantify the magnitude of the risk involved. In this regard, the case-control method is an important technique of epidemiologic investigation. My hope is that this book will further the understanding and proper application of it.

Bethesda   J. J. S.
September 1981

Acknowledgments

I have had the singular good fortune of receiving Dr. Paul D. Stolley's collaboration on this project. Dr. Stolley, who is Professor of Medicine and Co-Director of the Clinical Epidemiology Unit at the University of Pennsylvania School of Medicine, contributed numerous ideas to the development of this work. He shared generously from his broad knowledge of clinical epidemiology and medicine, practical experience in conducting studies, and perception of investigators' and students' needs in regard to the level and content of material. He contributed to the writing of the chapters on research strategies and sources of bias, and assumed major responsibility for the chapter on planning and conducting case-control studies. He was ably assisted in his work by Ms. Rita Schinnar and Ms. Elizabeth Hepler-Smith, who conducted literature reviews and provided technical and editorial support.

Dr. James B. Sidbury, Jr., Scientific Director of the National Institute of Child Health and Human Development (NICHD), gave initial encouragement and strong administrative support to my work on this project. This was furthered by Dr. Norman Kretchmer, Director of the NICHD, and by Dr. Heinz W. Berendes, Director of the Epidemiology and Biometry Research Program, NICHD. Dr. Llewellyn J. Legters, Chairman of the Department of Preventive Medicine and Biometrics at the Uniformed Services University of the Health Sciences, continued to support my work through its final stages.

A number of colleagues reviewed chapters of the text, giving wise advice and discerning comment. In this regard, I am indebted to Dr. Mitchell H. Gail and Dr. Jay H. Lubin of the National Cancer Institute, Dr. Sonja M. McKinlay of The Memorial Hospital, Pawtucket, Rhode Island, and Dr. Bruce V. Stadel and Dr. James L. Mills of the National

Institute of Child Health and Human Development. Professor Nathan Mantel of the George Washington University Biostatistics Center shared his insight into case-control studies in numerous conversations and by his permission to read some of his personal correspondence on the topic.

An exceptionally perceptive critique and review of the entire manuscript was made by Dr. Sander Greenland, Division of Epidemiology, University of California School of Public Health, Los Angeles. His advice led to numerous major and minor revisions throughout the text, forced the removal of obscurities and error, and markedly improved the discussions of matching and measures of risk.

Dr. Charles C. Brown of the National Cancer Institute kindly made available matched and unmatched versions of his logistic regression programs, and patiently answered questions about their use. Dr. Stephen D. Walter, Yale University, and Dr. Bernard S. Pasternack and Dr. Roy E. Shore, New York University Medical Center, gave approval for the use of their sample size tables, which appear as Appendices C and D. The reproduction of these tables is made with the permission of the American Journal of Epidemiology.

My writing received outstanding technical support from the staff of the Biometry Branch, NICHD. Mr. Daniel W. Denman performed the statistical computing for all of the major analyses, checked a multitude of derivations and reexpressions of equations, assisted in the literature review, and laboriously proofed and edited the text through all of its drafts. Ms. Erica Brittain suggested revisions for the final draft, checked many of the computations, and helped edit the text. Ms. Gwendolyn Artis and Ms. Dorothy M. Day provided excellent secretarial support, using a computerized text-editor for the typing of countless revisions.

Finally, I wish to thank my wife, Sarah, who shared her experience from the Women's Health Study, and who was patient with my use of time for writing that might otherwise have been spent with her.

Contents

Prologue   3

1. Research Strategies   7
James J. Schlesselman and Paul D. Stolley

  1.0   Introduction   7
  1.1   Experimental Studies   7
  1.2   Observational Studies   10
  1.3   Choosing Among Research Strategies   17
  1.4   Causation   20
  1.5   History of Case-Control Studies   25

2. Basic Concepts in the Assessment of Risk   27

  2.0   Introduction   27
  2.1   Disease Occurrence   27
  2.2   Relative Measures of Disease Occurrence   32
  2.3   Cohort and Case-Control Sampling Schemes   34
  2.4   Risk of Disease Attributable to Exposure   40
  2.5   Exposure   45
  2.6   Interpretation of Relative Risk (Data Example)   49
  2.7   Cumulative Risk of Disease   52
  2.8   Association and Testing for Significance   53
  2.9   Relative Risk as a Measure of the Strength of Association   56
  2.10 Confounding   58
  2.11 Interaction   63
  2.12 Summary   68

3. Planning and Conducting a Study   69
Paul D. Stolley and James J. Schlesselman

  3.0   Introduction   69
  3.1   Stating the Research Question   69

3.2 Definition of Cases   71
3.3 Defining a Control Group   76
3.4 Methods of Selecting Cases and Controls   80
3.5 Developing the Research Instrument   86
3.6 Informed Consent and Confidentiality   92
3.7 Pilot Testing   94
3.8 Preparing for and Conducting Field Operations   97
3.9 Preparation for Data Analysis   99
3.10 Checklist for Protocol Development   101

4. Matching   105

4.0 Introduction   105
4.1 Criteria for Matching   107
4.2 Overmatching   109
4.3 Alternatives to Matching   111
4.4 Effectiveness of Matching and Its Alternatives   115
4.5 Expected Number of Matches   117
4.6 How Closely Should One Match?   118
4.7 Advantages and Disadvantages of Matching   120
4.8 Summary   122

5. Sources of Bias   124
James J. Schlesselman and Paul D. Stolley

5.0 Introduction   124
5.1 Ascertainment and Selection Bias   124
5.2 Bias in the Estimation of Exposure   135
5.3 Misclassification   137
5.4 Other Sources of Error   140
5.5 Summary   143

6. Sample Size   144

6.0 Introduction   144
6.1 Sample Size and Power for Unmatched Studies   145
6.2 Sample Size and Power with Multiple Controls per Case   150
6.3 Smallest Detectable Relative Risk   152
6.4 Optimal Allocation   154
6.5 Adjustment for Confounding   159
6.6 Sample Size and Power for Pair-Matched Studies   160
6.7 Sequential Case-Control Studies   163
6.8 Further Considerations in Estimating Sample Size   165
6.9 Summary   170

7. Basic Methods of Analysis   171

7.0   Introduction   171
7.1   Unmatched Analysis of a Single 2 × 2 Table   174
7.2   Adjustment for Confounding   181
7.3   Assessment of Individual and Joint Effects
      of Two or More Variables   196
7.4   Test for Dose Response   200
7.5   Test-Based Confidence Limits   206
7.6   Matched Analysis with One Control per Case   207
7.7   Matched Analysis with Two Controls per Case   213
7.8   Matched Analysis with Three or More Controls per Case   216
7.9   Estimation of the Etiologic Fraction   220

8. Multivariate Analysis   227

8.0   Introduction   227
8.1   Interpretation of Logistic Parameters   230
8.2   Logistic Regression for Case-Control Studies   235
8.3   Indicator Variables   241
8.4   Estimation of Logistic Parameters   244
8.5   Discussion of Logistic Models   250
8.6   Application of Logistic Regression   254
8.7   Further Topics in Logistic Regression   263
8.8   Matched Analysis   269
8.9   Confounder Score   275
8.10 Loglinear Models   280

Epilogue   291

Appendices   293

A. Case-Control Sample Size   293
B. Cumulative Normal Frequency Distribution   315
C. Largest and Smallest Detectable Relative Risks   319
D. Sample Size for Group Sequential Case-Control Studies   324

References   325

Index   344

Prologue

On April 22, 1971, a study with startling and profound implications appeared in the *New England Journal of Medicine* (Herbst, Ulfelder, and Poskanzer 1971). Three physicians from the Vincent Memorial Hospital in Boston made the first report of a striking association between the use of diethylstilbestrol (DES) during the first trimester of pregnancy and the development, fifteen to twenty years later, of vaginal cancer in daughters born of these pregnancies. Although cancer of the vagina rarely occurs in women under 50 years of age, between 1966 and 1969 these investigators diagnosed clear-cell adenocarcinoma of the vagina in seven young women 15 to 22 years old. Prior to 1966, this condition had not been seen in patients treated at Vincent Memorial Hospital.

Because of the apparent clustering of cases, seven occurring within four years, the investigators first attempted to find similarities among them. This proved unsuccessful. The young women did not uniformly use any vaginal irritant, douches, or tampons. Only one patient had had sexual intercourse, and none had used birth control pills prior to her illness. The physicians then decided to conduct a study that would systematically compare these patients (cases) and their families with an appropriate comparison group (controls) in order to identify factors that might be associated with the sudden appearance of the tumors. Four matched controls, consisting of young women who were free of vaginal cancer, were selected for each patient. An eighth case of adenocarcinoma of the vagina occurred in 1969 in a 20-year-old patient who was treated at another Boston hospital. This patient and her family were available for study and consequently were included with the initial group of seven cases.

The controls were identified from the birth records of the hospital in which each case was born. Females born within five days and on the same type of service (ward or private) were first identified. Births occurring closest in time to each patient were selected as controls. A personal interview of mothers of cases and controls was made by a trained interviewer using a standard questionnaire.

A variety of factors were compared between cases and controls. Those factors showing no significant differences between the two groups were occupation and education of parents, maternal age at the time of pregnancy, intrauterine X-ray exposure, maternal smoking and alcohol consumption, complications and outcome of the study pregnancy, breast feeding, use of cosmetics in mothers and daughters, presence of household pets, noteworthy illnesses and childhood ingestions, and age at onset of menses in daughters. Three factors, all related to the maternal use of estrogens during pregnancy, showed marked differences. In particular, mothers of seven of the eight cases had taken estrogens during the first trimester of pregnancy. Among the 32 controls, however, none of the mothers had such a history of estrogen use. Apart from the maternal use of estrogens, cases and controls did not differ with respect to other medications taken by their mothers.

One of the eight mothers whose daughter had vaginal cancer had not taken estrogens during her pregnancy. This, in addition to the fact that clear-cell adenocarcinoma of the vagina was known to occur, though rarely, in women born before the availability of oral estrogens, indicated that other factors were also involved in the development of the disease. Furthermore, all *in utero* exposures to DES did not lead to the development of vaginal cancer. In this study, among four of the eight families with a cancer patient, there were five female siblings, ranging in age from 18 to 22 years, who were also exposed *in utero* to DES. At the time of the 1971 report, a vaginal tumor had not been diagnosed in any of these women.

Reflecting upon possible mechanisms by which DES might contribute to increasing the risk of cancer, the investigators suggested that diethylstilbestrol might alter fetal vaginal cells *in utero* with changes that do not become evident as a malignancy until years later. Animal experiments were proposed to further assess this conjecture.

Given the suspicion that DES might be a cause of vaginal cancer in female offspring, there would have been no ethical or feasible way to study this issue experimentally in humans. One could not have administered DES in good conscience to pregnant women in hopes of confirming or refuting this hypothesis. Although animal studies might be conducted, the application of their findings to humans usually leaves room for conflicting interpretations. Despite the absence of direct experimental evidence, the investigators concluded that maternal ingestion of diethylstilbestrol during early pregnancy increased the risk of vaginal adenocarcinoma developing years later in the exposed offspring.

This investigation provides an excellent example of the *case-control study* and its application to the discovery of a previously unrecognized cause of disease. The tactic of working from effect (vaginal cancer) to cause (*in utero* exposure to DES) arose naturally from the observation of a time clustering of patients at a single hospital, and the question of what might differ in the daughters who developed cancer as compared with those who were cancer free. The study was *exploratory* in the sense that no single hypothesis had been advanced for the cause of these cancers. However, even if *in utero* exposure to DES had been suspected prior to this study as the most likely cause, the case-control design would have been one of two study methods of choice. [A historical cohort study would have provided an alternative approach (Chapter 1).]

1 Research Strategies

James J. Schlesselman
Paul D. Stolley

1.0 INTRODUCTION

Generally speaking, one may take either an experimental or an observational approach to the study of disease. Whereas an observational (nonexperimental) study is one in which no deliberate human intervention is made, an experiment involves planned intervention on factors suspected of altering the phenomenon under study. Apart from a purely descriptive function of certain observational studies such as surveys, the objective of both observational and experimental studies is the elucidation of cause-and-effect relationships.

1.1 EXPERIMENTAL STUDIES

In discussing the role of experimentation, Cornfield (1954) noted that "we all have a vague feeling that if we can make an event occur, we understand it better than if we simply observe it passively." In an experiment that allows control over important disturbing variables, one is inclined to believe that the intervention itself has produced the observed effect. With simple observation, potentially important variables are not under the direct control of the investigator, thereby engendering skepticism. Even with direct experimentation, however, one can never be certain that all important variables have been controlled. A notable example is the experiment conducted by the distinguished hygienist and chemist, Prof. Max von Pettenkofer of Munich, who tried to demonstrate that the cholera *Vibrio* did not cause cholera. He was skeptical of person-to-per·son transmission through contaminated water supplies, believing that th organism required a phase in dry soil to acquire some factor of virulence. To prove his point, von Pettenkofer conducted his *experimentum crucium* in 1880, in which he swallowed 1 cc of freshly grown broth culture from a case of cholera. He suffered no ill effects, despite excreting large amounts of cholera *Vibrio,* thereby confirming his hypothesis. However, the dose was probably too small, since it is now known that a large inoculation is required for the organism to survive the stomach's acidity and produce acute symptoms (Susser 1973, Evans 1976).

Advantages of Experimentation

A fundamental advantage of the experimental method is that it permits one to disentangle a complex causal problem by proceeding in stepwise fashion. The investigator can break the main problem into subproblems and explore each by a series of separate experiments with comparatively simple causal assumptions. In this regard, Benzer (1973) gives a fascinating discussion of experiments with fruit flies designed to identify those behavioral patterns that are under genetic control, to determine the actual site at which the gene influences behavior, and to discover the mechanism of genetic regulation.

In an experiment, one may choose which factors are varied, either singly, in combination, or in sequence. One may vary their quantitative, temporal, or qualitative features, as, for example, in choosing a particular dose, schedule, and route of administration for a new vaccine. Experiments permit one to elaborate causal chains, which in turn allows opportunities for control or intervention at any one of the points in the sequence.

An experiment provides a variety of methods for removing the effects of disturbing variables (those that influence the response, but are not under investigation). One method is direct control, such as using an inbred strain of animals to remove genetic variability in response, or by feeding a standard diet. A second approach, which can remove the effects of disturbing variables not under direct experimental control, including some whose presence is unknown to the investigator, is the use of randomization and replication (Wold 1956, Cochran 1965).

A study that exemplifies some of the strengths of the experimental method is that of Yoon, Austin, Onodera, and Notkins (1979), who reported the isolation of a virus from the pancreas of a ten-year-old child who had died of diabetic ketoacidosis. Neutralization data showed that the virus was related to a diabetogenic variant derived from Coxsackie virus B4, and the investigators demonstrated that the virus could produce diabetes in mice. Through a series of clinical studies in the patient and experiments in animals, the investigators concluded that the patient's diabetes was virus-induced.

First, 130 male SJL mice were inoculated with the human isolate, which was derived from pancreatic tissue at autopsy. Using serum glucose levels in 20 uninfected animals as a standard of reference, over 50 percent of the inoculated animals became hyperglycemic within five days. To determine whether the hyperglycemia was secondary to beta-cell damage, SJL mice were killed at different times after infection with the human isolate and their pancreata were examined under a light microscope. Inflammation seen in the islets of Langerhans was similar to that seen in the patient's pancreas.

Next, sections of the pancreata of the infected SJL mice were specially stained to determine whether the human isolate had actually infected cells in the islets of Langerhans. Four days after infection, viral antigens were clearly seen in the cytoplasm of the beta cells. To demonstrate susceptibility of human beta cells to the viral isolate, cultures enriched with human beta cells were inoculated with the human isolate. At 60 hours after infection, approximately 37 percent of the insulin-containing cells showed viral antigens.

Before death, the rise in antibody in the child's serum provided evidence that the isolate from the pancreas was not an inadvertent contaminant. Studies with encephalomyocarditis virus showed that the rise in antibody in the patient's serum was not a nonspecific toxic effect.

Disadvantages of Experimentation

An experimental approach may not be feasible for certain problems. Limitations of human or material resources may prevent the resolution of a question by direct experiment. An example is the requirement for exceptionally large numbers of animals to detect a possible increased risk of malignant tumors resulting from low-dose ionizing radiation. If a tumor occurs spontaneously at the rate of one per 100,000 animals per year, then an experiment designed to give one a 90 percent chance of detecting a true tenfold increase in the tumor rate would require one year's follow up of more than 142,000 animals in both an experimental and a control group in order to find a significant (α = 0.05 two-sided) difference.

The sample size required in each of an experimental and a control group is given by

$$N \simeq 2\bar{p}\bar{q}(z_\alpha + z_\beta)^2/(p_1 - p_2)^2. \qquad (1.1)$$

The terms z_α and z_β are values from the unit normal distribution corresponding to α and β (Chapter 6); p_1 and p_2 are estimates of the event rates in the control and the experimental group respectively; $\bar{p}$ = $\frac{1}{2}(p_1 + p_2)$ and $\bar{q}$ = $1 - \bar{p}$. Equation (1.1) approximates an alternative formula given by Fleiss [1981, equation (3.14)].

For the problem concerning tumor induction by low-dose ionizing radiation, one has z_α = 1.96, z_β = 1.64, p_1 = 1/100,000 and p_2 = 10/100,000. Hence, $N \simeq 142,560$. [See Land (1980) for a general discussion of estimating cancer risks from low-dose ionizing radiation.]

Experiments are often hampered by the duration of study required to address certain questions. For example, a randomized clinical trial of surgical versus medical intervention in the treatment of coronary disease, taking five-year mortality as an endpoint, may require eight to ten years to complete, considering study planning, patient recruitment, follow-up, analysis, and reporting. Surgical or medical practice may be rapidly changing in the interim, so that one's findings may become primarily of historical interest. Similarly difficult to conduct would be human studies of agents thought to prevent cancers, some of which may have a twenty-year latency between initial exposure to a carcinogen and the development of clinical symptoms. Ethical considerations may also restrict human experimentation, since interventions that may harm rather than benefit individuals are generally proscribed. A further difficulty may arise in the study of phenomena that are beyond the current capacity of experimental control. Examples include studies in humans of an association between early age at menarche and an increased risk of breast cancer, and an association between elevated levels of alpha-fetoprotein in amniotic fluid and the occurrence of anencephaly in offspring.

1.2 OBSERVATIONAL STUDIES

Cohort Studies

There are two basic approaches to investigating the causes of disease. One is to work from cause to effect; the other is to proceed from effect to cause. The observational paradigm that proceeds in the same direction as an experiment, working from a postulated cause to effect, is the *cohort study*. (*Prospective study* and *follow-up study* are terms commonly used as synonyms.) In a cohort study, individuals are selected for observation and followed over time. Selection may depend on the presence or absence of certain characteristics that are thought to influence the development of disease, or it may be at random within some target population, effectively yielding a sample of individuals who vary in exposure to one or more factors of interest. To study associations with the development of disease, persons are classified on the basis of their characteristics before its development. The groups so defined are compared in terms of their subsequent morbidity or mortality rates.

The interim report of a cohort study of oral contraceptives and health, conducted by the Royal College of General Practitioners in England (1974), provides a good example of the design and analysis of a cohort study. This example is discussed in some detail in order to acquaint the reader with some considerations pertaining to the method of subject selection, problems of discontinuation or change in exposure-status over time, and the need to adjust comparisons for baseline inequalities. The full report should be consulted for an in-depth discussion.

Initiated in 1968 after two years of planning, the Royal College study brought under observation a total of 23,000 *users* of oral contraceptives, together with a similar number of *never-users* who served as a comparison (control) group. The observations of the study subjects were made by 1400 general practitioners throughout the United Kingdom. Subjects were selected for study in the following way. Each doctor was instructed to report as eligible the first two women in each calendar month for whom he or she wrote a prescription for oral contraceptives. This could be either a first prescription or a renewal. A control subject was recruited for each user. Starting with a user's record, returned to its correct place in the doctor's file, each subsequent record was examined in alphabetical order until the next record was found for a woman whose year of birth was within three years of the user's. If this woman had never used oral contraceptives, she was recruited as a control.

The simple design of the study at recruitment, comparing users with never-users, rapidly and predictably became complicated by users who discontinued and non-users who initiated oral contraceptive use. Thus, the investigators compared the experience for three groups of subjects: *user, ex-user,* and *control* (never-user). The data in the user group included the experience of all women who had remained on the Pill continuously since recruitment. If a control, who must have never used oral contraceptives, began to take the Pill, her experience was included in the user group from the start of the month in which she began to use the Pill. When a user stopped the Pill, her experience was included in the ex-user category from the following calendar month. Some ex-users restarted the Pill. Their experience, from the start of the calendar month in which they resumed the use of oral contraceptives, was excluded from the interim report.

A morbidity rate was calculated for each contraceptive group by expressing the number of episodes per thousand woman-years of experience for that group. At the time of recruitment, users and non-users differed to some extent in characteristics related to the development of disease. Therefore, adjustment was made for age, parity, social class, and cigarette consumption by indirect standardization of the morbidity rates (Fleiss 1981), taking as a standard the experience of the entire study population.

Oral contraceptive use was found to adversely affect the risk of conditions such as urinary tract infection, eczematous conditions, hypertension, superficial and deep-vein thrombosis of the leg, gallbladder disease, and cerebrovascular accidents. Beneficial effects of oral contraceptive use were related to menstrual disorders, iron deficiency anemia, premenstrual syndrome, benign breast neoplasia, ovarian cyst, acne, and sebaceous cyst.

Taking as a specific example benign neoplasms of the breast, for which current oral contraceptive use showed a protective effect, Table 1.1 reports the observed number of episodes and the standardized rates for each of the three study groups. The diagnoses of fibro-adenoma, chronic cystic disease, and mastitis were based on clinical rather than histological examinations. Among clinicians the terms are used virtually synonymously, so that the three categories have been combined to form the category fibro-adenosis. Table 1.1 shows that users had a 20 percent reduction in the risk of fibro-adenosis compared with controls. A dose response was observed in relation to the progestogen

Table 1.1. Benign Neoplasms of the Breast

ICD Category[1]	Users		Ex-Users		Controls		Ratio of rates	
	obs no.	std rate[2]	obs no.	std rate	obs no.	std rate	users/ control	ex-user/ control
217	43	1.31	11	1.20	60	1.33	0.99	0.90
610	103	3.00	40	4.42	189	4.34	0.69[3]	1.02
6110	144	4.20	55	5.78	214	4.96	0.85	1.17
Combined	290	8.51	106	11.40	463	10.63	0.80[3]	1.07

1. ICD categories: fibroadenoma (217), chronic cystic diseases of the breast (610), mastitis (6110), combined (217 + 610 + 6110) — fibroadenosis.
2. Standardized rate per thousand woman years.
3. $p < 0.01$.

Source: Royal College of General Practitioners 1974.

Table 1.2. Benign Neoplasms of the Breast in Relation to Duration of Oral Contraceptive Use

	Duration of use (yrs)					
	0	1	2	3	4	5
Observed number	450	101	85	48	27	29
Observed rate/TWY[1]	10.6	9.6	9.8	7.9	6.8	5.4
Ratio of rates	1.0[2]	.91	.92	.75	.64	.51

1. TWY: Thousand woman years.
2. Reference group.

Source: Royal College of General Practitioners 1974.

component of the pill. Among women taking pills containing less than 3 mg of progestogen, the frequency of benign neoplasms of the breast was 9.95 per thousand woman-years of use. The corresponding rate for women using 3 mg preparations was 5.82, and the rate for those using pills containing more than 3 mg was 3.75.

Further evidence of a protective effect was derived from a decrease in risk with increasing duration of use, as shown in Table 1.2. The reduction in risk becomes apparent only after two years of continuous usage.

Historical vs. Current Cohort Studies

Cohort studies may be distinguished on the basis of the time of occurrence of disease in relation to the time at which the investigation is initiated. A *current* cohort study is one in which the outcomes (disease, death, etc.) occur after the investigation begins, the aforementioned study of oral contraceptives and health (Royal College of General Practitioners 1974) being an example. A *historical* cohort study is a cohort study in which the outcomes have all occurred before the start of the investigation, cohorts being established and their experience assessed from existing records (MacMahon and Pugh 1970).

An investigation of the effect of fetal monitoring on neonatal death rates provides an example of a historical cohort study (Neutra et al. 1978). Between January 1, 1969, and December 31, 1975, a total of 17,080 babies were born at the Beth Israel Hospital in Boston, Massachusetts. Of these infants, 46.7 percent (7,961) were subjected to electronic fetal monitoring during labor. This involved the insertion of an intrauterine catheter to assess the pattern of uterine contractions and the placement of an electrode on the fetus to obtain instantaneous fetal heart rate. (Fetal heart rates of less than 100 or more than 160 beats per minute suggest fetal distress and the possibility of impending intrapartum death or the risk of neurologic damage from hypoxia.)

Several exclusions were applied to the study population. For comparability with other studies, babies of gestational age less than 28 weeks were excluded, as were infant deaths resulting from congenital abnormalities incompatible with life. Neither group would be expected to derive benefit from monitoring. Babies delivered by cesarean section before labor were also excluded, since this precluded the use of intrapartum monitoring. An additional 117 intrauterine deaths (most occurring before labor) and 234 subjects with incomplete information were also excluded. The group remaining for study consisted of 15,846 live births.

A number of potentially confounding variables were controlled in the data analysis. These included: gestational age, race, maternal age, and parity, and complications of pregnancy and delivery. Using neonatal death (0-28 days) as the outcome, a risk score for each infant was estimated as a function of the confounding variables by means of multiple linear regression. The deliveries were stratified into five categories from lowest to highest risk, and the neonatal death rates in monitored and unmonitored labors were compared within these strata.

Table 1.3 summarizes the neonatal death rates for monitored and unmonitored infants in the five risk categories. The crude neonatal death rate was 1.7 times higher in unmonitored infants. Adjusting for the slight difference in the distribution of monitored and unmonitored infants across the five categories of risk, a summary relative risk was estimated to be 1.44, with an approximate 95 percent confidence interval of (0.85, 2.45).

Although the stratum-specific relative risks were found not to differ significantly from the summary estimate 1.44, one sees a systematic decline in the death rate difference, from 109 deaths per thousand in the high-risk group to -0.6 per thousand in the lowest-risk group. Interpreting the stratum-specific difference in death rates as "lives saved per thousand babies monitored," the investigators estimated that most of the benefit of monitoring occurs in high-risk deliveries.

This example points out the use of exclusion criteria to obtain a more precise and valid treatment comparison, and it shows the application of adjustment for baseline inequalities by making treatment comparisons within subgroups of equal risk. Finally, Table 1.3 indicates the difference of perspective obtained by an examination of relative risk as compared with differences in risk. Even though the relative risk may be constant

Table 1.3. Effect of Fetal Monitoring on Neonatal Death Rates Within Strata of Risk

Risk score category	Monitored	Number of infants	Death rate[1]	Death rate difference	Relative risk[2]
Highest	No	79	303.8	108.7	1.6
	Yes	41	195.1		
High	No	62	80.7	43.0	2.1
	Yes	53	37.7		
Medium	No	338	20.7	5.9	1.4
	Yes	271	14.8		
Low	No	1722	5.2	2.7	2.1
	Yes	1225	2.5		
Lowest	No	6463	0.5	−0.6	0.4
	Yes	5592	1.1		
Total	No	8664	5.5	2.3	1.7
(crude)	Yes	7182	3.2		

1. Death rate per 1000 infants.
2. Within each category of risk, the ratio of the death rate in unmonitored as compared with monitored infants (e.g., 1.6 = 303.8/195.1).

Source: Neutra et al. 1978.

across subgroups, the difference in risk may vary. A simple algebraic argument corroborates this fact. Consider the rates of disease or death, p_1 and p_2, for two groups. Suppose that the rate p_2 for the second group depends on some variable x, $p_2 = f(x)$. If the *relative risk* (p_1/p_2) is constant, then $p_1/p_2 = c$. By substitution, the *risk difference* $(p_1 - p_2)$ can then be written $p_1 - p_2 = (c - 1) f(x)$, which indicates a dependence on x, provided that $c \neq 1$.

Case-Control Studies

The *case-control study*, also commonly called a *retrospective study*, follows a paradigm that proceeds from effect to cause. In a case-control study, individuals with a particular condition or disease (the *cases*) are selected for comparison with a series of individuals in whom the condition or disease is absent (the *controls*). Cases and controls are compared with respect to existing or past attributes or exposures thought to be relevant to the development of the condition or disease under study.

The requirement for a control group should be self-evident. For example, returning to the case-control study of vaginal cancer discussed in the Prologue, the finding that seven of eight cancer patients had an *in utero* exposure to DES immediately raises the question whether ⅞ is higher than "expected." The control series provides an estimate of the frequency of exposure expected among individuals free of the disease. Although one might like to know the incidence rate of vaginal cancer in young women exposed *in utero* to DES, one cannot determine this rate solely from a case-control study. One can, however, estimate the ratio of the incidence rates in exposed women compared with unexposed women. This ratio, called the *relative risk*, is discussed more fully in Chapter 2.

Even case-history studies, commonly used by clinicians, have implicit control groups. The symptoms of a particular disease, such as myocardial infarction, are supplemented in reaching a diagnosis by a physical examination, laboratory tests, and personal history. In reaching a judgment about a particular symptom or historical feature being characteristic of the disease, the clinician relies on the recollection of patients he or she has seen with other diseases, or who were free from the disease in question (Mantel and Haenszel 1959, Sartwell 1974).

The major difference between the cohort and the case-control methods is in the selection of study subjects. A cohort study selects subjects who are initially free of disease and, at least conceptually, follows them over time to determine the rates of disease in the presence or absence of exposure. By contrast, the case-control method selects subjects on the basis of the presence or absence of the disease under study. Both methods allow one to estimate the effect of exposure on the risk of disease in terms of the relative risk parameter (Chapter 2).

At times a distinction is made between the sources from which cases and controls are selected. In a *population-based* case-control study, all cases of the study disease occurring within a defined geographic area during a specified period of time are ascertained, often through a disease registry or hospital network. The entire case series or a random sample of it is selected for study. Controls are selected by taking a probability sample of individuals free of the study disease in the geographic area from which the cases arose. In a *hospital-based* case-control study, all cases of the study disease admitted to a single hospital or network of hospitals are ascertained during a specified period of time. The entire case series or a random sample of it is selected for study. In the hospitals from which the cases arose, controls are selected from persons admitted for conditions other than the study disease.

Exploratory vs. Analytic Studies

Had a specific hypothesis of an association between DES and vaginal cancer been advanced at the outset of the case-control study by Herbst,

Ulfelder, and Poskanzer (1971), a historical cohort study could have provided an alternative approach to an investigation of the problem. In principle, one could have searched hospital records for women who were given DES during pregnancy fifteen to twenty-five years before the diagnoses of the initial cases. Selecting for comparison an appropriate group of women who were not given DES, one could have attempted follow-up on the daughters in two groups, exposed vs. unexposed, to determine whether their rates of vaginal cancer differed.

The case-control method of investigation is often the research strategy of choice, however, particularly when initiating an exploratory study of disease etiology or investigating a rare disease (Mantel and Haenszel 1959, Sartwell 1974). An *exploratory* study, colloquially called a "fishing expedition," is one in which multiple hypotheses are proposed for investigation. The purpose of such studies is to learn enough about possible causes of the disease in question so that a specific hypothesis may be suggested and be sufficiently supported to justify a detailed investigation.

An example of an exploratory case-control study, in addition to the previously discussed study of vaginal cancer, is one conducted by Martin-Bouyer and his colleagues in 1972, after the sudden appearance of a new and peculiar neurologic disease among newborn children residing in certain provinces in France (Martin-Bouyer et al. 1982). At the start of this investigation, epidemiologists did not know if this disease was infectious or caused by a toxic agent. Historical information was collected from mothers of the affected infants, and environmental investigations were conducted in their homes. A similar inquiry was made for "control" or unaffected infants. A specific hypothesis emerged from the finding that exposure to a certain baby talc powder was universal among the affected infants, but was much less common among the controls. This totally unexpected result was followed up by an investigation designed to examine specifically this association.

Irrespective of the terminology employed, the characteristics of exploratory case-control studies are similar: (1) data concerning the distribution of potentially important characteristics among cases and controls are unavailable, and knowledge of the natural history of the disease is insufficient to justify study of a specific hypothesis; (2) an attempt is made to gather data concerning possible differences on a variety of factors among the cases as compared with the controls in the hope that etiologic clues worthy of further study will emerge.

While certain investigators have disparaged exploratory studies, they are often the logical first step to understanding disease etiology and are to be favored over a study restricted to a specific hypothesis that is speculative or weakly supported. For example, the outbreak of Legionnaire's Disease in Philadelphia in 1976 was investigated by means of a large descriptive study that finally helped solve the epidemic. However, a small group of scientists were urging an analytic study to test the conjecture that the disease was due to nickel carbonyl toxicity, a hypothesis weakly supported by fact, though strongly advocated. Such a study would have been premature and would have diverted energies from the completion of a comprehensive descriptive investigation. Eventually an infectious organism was isolated and analytic studies showed this to be the causal agent (Fraser and McDade 1979).

An *analytic* study is an investigation designed to test a specific hypothesis concerning the cause of the disease in question. The hypothesis must be stated in a way that permits definitive assessment. "Cigarette smoking causes lung cancer" is a hypothesis of a different degree of clarity than a hypothesis stated as follows: "Cigarette smoking is associated with lung cancer. Compared with individuals who are free of this tumor, patients with lung cancer will have smoked cigarettes with more tars, will have inhaled more deeply, and will have smoked more cigarettes per day and for longer periods of time."

1.3 CHOOSING AMONG RESEARCH STRATEGIES

While the experimental method is universally acknowledged to be the most powerful explanatory method, it is often not available to the medical investigator because of ethical or logistic considerations. As a consequence, the choice of a research strategy often is limited to the cohort or the case-control approach. Tables 1.4 and 1.5 provide summaries of some of the advantages and disadvantages of these two methods.

The case-control method is especially useful for the study of rare diseases. In this situation, a cohort study is inefficient, because virtually all of the effort is devoted to follow-up of individuals who remain free of the study disease. For example, suppose that one wanted to determine whether maternal exposure to estrogens around the time of conception resulted in an increased risk of congenital heart defects among offspring. Assuming a rate of eight heart defects per 1000 births among unexposed women, a cohort study would require observation of the pregnancy outcomes of approximately 3889 exposed women and 3889 unexposed women in order to detect a potential twofold increase in risk. [Application of equation (1.1) with $\alpha = .05$ (two-sided), $\beta = .10$, $p_1 = \frac{8}{1000}$ and $p_2 = \frac{16}{1000}$ gives $N \simeq 3889$.] A case-control study would require only 188

Table 1.4   Advantages and Disadvantages of the Case-Control Method

Advantages
1. Well suited to the study of rare diseases or those with long latency.
2. Relatively quick to mount and conduct.
3. Relatively inexpensive.
4. Requires comparatively few subjects.
5. Existing records can occasionally be used.
6. No risk to subjects.
7. Allows study of multiple potential causes of a disease.

Disadvantages
1. Relies on recall or records for information on past exposures.
2. Validation of information is difficult or sometimes impossible.
3. Control of extraneous variables may be incomplete.
4. Selection of an appropriate comparison group may be difficult.
5. Rates of disease in exposed and unexposed individuals cannot be determined.
6. Method relatively unfamiliar to medical community and difficult to explain.
7. Detailed study of mechanism is rarely possible.

Table 1.5   Advantages and Disadvantages of the Cohort Method

Advantages
1. In principle, provides a complete description of experience subsequent to exposure, including rates of progression, staging of disease, and natural history.
2. Allows study of multiple potential effects of a given exposure, thereby obtaining information on potential benefits as well as risks.
3. Allows for the calculation of rates of disease in exposed and unexposed individuals.
4. Permits flexibility in choosing variables to be systematically recorded.
5. Allows for thorough quality control in measurement of study variables.

Disadvantages
1. Large numbers of subjects are required to study rare diseases.
2. Potentially long duration for follow-up.
3. Current practice, usage, or exposure to study factors may change, making findings irrelevant.
4. Relatively expensive to conduct.
5. Maintaining follow-up is difficult.
6. Control of extraneous variables may be incomplete.
7. Detailed study of mechanism is rarely possible.

cases and 188 controls, assuming that approximately 30 percent of women are exposed to estrogens around the time of conception. (Chapter 6 provides the details of this analysis.) A cohort study would thus require approximately twenty times as many subjects as would a case-control approach. If one were interested in a specific heart defect, such as cono-truncal malformations, which occur at a rate of 2 cases per 1000 births, one would need follow-up on cohorts of approximately 15,700 exposed and 15,700 non-exposed women in order to detect a potential twofold increase in risk. A case-control study would still require only 188 cases and 188 controls (Schlesselman 1974).

The case-control method is also most appropriate for studying diseases with long latency. An investigator using the case-control method studies persons who have already developed the disease of interest, so that there is no need to wait for time to elapse between an exposure and the manifestation of disease. One can begin the search for cases immediately. A historical cohort study provides a similar opportunity, although the determination of exposed and unexposed groups from existing records may be impractical or infeasible. Thus, for example, the question of whether the risk of bladder cancer in humans is increased by the consumption of saccharin is best answered by the case-control approach.

The search for cases and the choice of and search for a suitable control or comparison group can pose difficulties that often affect the design of a case-control study. If the disease under investigation is exceedingly rare, as is myocardial infarction in young women, then the search for cases may have to extend into several cities and backward in time. Conducting a study in several different cities may be a formidable managerial task. Methods of searching for and selecting cases and controls, the establishment of interview and abstract procedures, and the search for documentation must be standardized, and personnel supervised uniformly, all in different geographic locations and often simultaneously. Nevertheless, a case-control study will almost invariably be less costly and less difficult to mount and complete than a current cohort investigation. The speed with which the case-control study can be accomplished and its smaller required sample size also permit a reduction in costs for personnel and data processing.

Although an advantage of the case-control method may lie in the availability of existing records pertinent to the hypothesis under study, sufficiently accurate information may not be available from either records or interviews. Information on the dose, duration of use, and the taking of a drug in relation to important life events, such as past pregnancies, menarche, or menopause may be inadequately recorded and imperfectly recalled. A person's past biochemical or nutritional status can often be only crudely assessed. The absence of accurate data weakens a study's ability to detect underlying associations and at times may preclude the use of the case-control method. Thus, one must state precisely the questions to be researched and assess whether crucial data can be gathered by personal interview, physical exam, or from existing records.

Another consideration relates to the investigation of drugs, chemicals, or other factors suspected of increasing the risk of disease. At times it may be prudent to restrict or discontinue the use of a substance while further investigating its potential dangers. Since the cases have acquired the disease of interest, the investigation merely collects information on past exposures. There is no need to continue exposure and thereby perpetuate a potential risk, a point that applies equally to a historical cohort study.

At times a case-control study may encounter the problem of intruding into sensitive areas of an individual's past. Thus, a study of determinants of the decision to seek an abortion, taking as cases women undergoing an induced abortion, and taking controls from women who deliver, may be regarded by some as infringing upon a woman's "right to privacy." There is also the possibility that legal restrictions on epidemiologic studies may create the peculiar situation in which informed consent is required before an individual may participate in a study, but various laws enacted to protect individual privacy prohibit access to information necessary to identify study subjects and obtain informed consent (Gordis and Gold 1980).

The case-control method is not suited to the evalution of therapy or prophylaxis of disease. Compared with nondiseased individuals, cases of the study disease would necessarily be expected to have a higher rate of exposure to drugs or other factors that are used for treatment. In this situation, one should use experimental trials (Sartwell 1974).

1.4 CAUSATION

Observational and experimental studies in medicine and public health are designed to identify factors that cause or prevent the occurrence of disease. The ultimate goal of such studies is intervention on these factors to alter the frequency or severity with which disease occurs, or to retard the rate at which it progresses. From this perspective, if an alteration in a factor is followed by a change in the frequency or character of disease, one may regard the factor to be a cause (MacMahon and Pugh 1970). There are two elements in this definition, the first being temporal sequence. A cause precedes its consequences in time. The second element is that of intervention, or change in a temporal antecedent, with a corresponding change in a following event. The term "cause" embraces an elusive concept that has been elaborated upon from antiquity, with Aristotle, Galileo, Hume, and J. S. Mill, among others, providing influential interpretations. Nagel (1965) has averred that there is no uniquely correct explication of the term.

The probabilistic approach to cause and effect provides an interpretation that emphasizes the concept of contributing cause. Suppose that y denotes a 0–1 response, indicating, for example, the presence or absence of disease, such as the occurrence of stroke, diabetes, or some form of cancer. Let x denote some other factor. One may say that x is a cause of y if the probability (relative frequency) that y occurs is increased as a consequence of the presence of x. If x is a continuous variable, such as the duration of use of exogenous estrogens or cumulative dose of exposure to ionizing radiation, then the probability that y occurs may vary with the levels of x. If y is a continuous response variable, such as vital capacity or creatinine clearance, a causal relation may imply that as x increases, the average value of y increases, or some other feature of its distribution changes, such as its variance. The relationship between x and y may be affected by the levels of other variables; it may be strengthened, weakened, or may entirely disappear, depending on their levels. The idea easily becomes tortuous (Cochran 1972).

At times an isolated case report can definitively establish causation. In particular, an adverse drug effect is considered to be established if the drug and the event are temporally related, the effect disappearing when the drug is stopped and reappearing when the drug is readministered (Temple, Jones, and Crout 1979).

Experimental Criteria for Causation of Disease

Experimental criteria for the causation of disease have changed with time. The Henle-Koch postulates, comprising the classical point of reference for medical studies, were based on nineteenth-century knowledge of bacterial disease. The criteria proposed that a parasite be regarded as a cause of a disease if: (1) it occurs in every case of the disease, and under circumstances that can account for the pathological changes and clinical course; (2) it occurs in no other disease as a fortuitous and nonpathogenic parasite; (3) after being isolated from the body, grown in pure culture and repeatedly passed, it induces the disease anew.

At the time these postulates were presented in 1890, Koch realized that the causes of anthrax, tuberculosis, erysipelas, tetanus, and most infectious diseases in animals fulfilled these criteria. He was also aware that a number of infectious agents failed to satisfy all of them. (The suspected causes of typhoid fever, diptheria, leprosy, relapsing fever, and Asiatic cholera had not fulfilled the third condition.) Particularly noteworthy is cholera. Koch, the first to isolate the *Vibrio*, had identified its relationship to an epidemic in India, but could not experimentally reproduce the disease in any animal (Evans 1976, 1978).

The discovery of viruses in the early twentieth century required broadening the concept of causation in medical investigations. Emphasizing that criteria change with technology, Evans (1978) noted that it was particularly ironic that Werner Henle, a grandson of Jakob Henle, established with two other investigators the causative role of the Epstein-Barr virus in the development of infectious mononucleosis without fulfilling a single one of the postulates advocated by his grandfather and by Robert Koch.

Observational Criteria for Causation

The experimental approach provides a direct method for establishing or refuting whether an association between two factors is causal. In the absence of experimentation, several lines of reasoning have been advocated for assessing causality. Hill (1965, 1971) and Lilienfeld and Lilienfeld (1980) provide excellent general discussions, and the reviews by Evans (1976, 1978) should be consulted for further background references.

TEMPORAL SEQUENCE

A causal association requires that factors thought to be causative must precede those events that are regarded as their effects. This requirement is basic to all explications of the causal concept. Occasionally a definite temporal sequence may be difficult to establish, particularly for chronic disease. For example, is hypertension a cause or a consequence of the disease process that leads to renal disease? This question is difficult to answer because one is dealing with a continuous, evolving process that involves several self-regulating systems with feedback loops.

CONSISTENCY

A second condition that supports a causal interpretation of an association is the repeated observation of the association under different conditions of study. In commenting on the requirement for consistency, Hill (1965) has observed that we have the "somewhat paradoxical position that the different results of a different inquiry certainly cannot be held to refute the original evidence; yet the same results from precisely the same form of inquiry will not invariably greatly strengthen the original evidence." As a resolution to the paradox, one might argue that diverse studies yielding the same association support the plausibility of a causal interpretation, in that any counter-hypothesis based on an argument of study bias or spurious association is less likely to apply to each of the varying conditions of study. On the other hand, similar studies that yield diverse results weaken a causal interpretation.

STRENGTH OF ASSOCIATION

The larger the value of the relative risk, the less likely the association is to be spurious (Cornfield et al. 1959, Bross 1966, Schlesselman 1978). In this connection Hill (1965) discusses Percival Pott's conclusion that tar and mineral oils were the cause of scrotal cancer in chimney sweeps. He attributes this correct conclusion to the enormous increase in scrotal cancer in chimney sweeps, quoting Doll (1964): "Even as late as the second decade of the twentieth century, the mortality of chimney sweeps from scrotal cancer was some 200 times that of workers who were not specially exposed to tar or mineral oils, and in the eighteenth century the relative difference is likely to have been much greater."

BIOLOGICAL GRADIENT

The existence of a biological gradient or dose-response curve makes a causal interpretation more plausible. Cause-and-effect relationships in physics and biochemistry commonly have a dose response, and the use of medical treatment for therapy or prophylaxis is based on this concept.

SPECIFICITY OF EFFECT

A fifth consideration, often cited with reservations about its application (Lilienfeld 1959, Hill 1965, Susser 1973) is specificity of effect. A cause is "specific" to an effect if the introduction of the putative causal factor is followed by the occurrence of the effect, and if removal of the factor is followed by the absence of the effect. Berkson's (1958) arguments against cigarette smoking as a cause of lung cancer were based partly on the absence of specificity.

The weakness of specificity is that the concept is generally too simplistic. Multiple causes and effects are more often the rule than the exception. Specificity of an association supports a causal interpretation, but lack of specificity does not negate it. Radiation, for example, is the cause of numerous conditions, including impairment of cell division and fertility, DNA damage, congenital malformations, leukemia, cataracts, hypothyroidism, neoplastic skin changes, and cancers of the thyroid, salivary glands, lung, bone, and female breast tissues (Wald 1979).

COLLATERAL EVIDENCE AND BIOLOGICAL PLAUSIBILITY

In practice, collateral evidence and biological plausibility are used extensively to support or refute a hypothesis of cause and effect. The review by Doll and Vessey (1970) of rare adverse effects associated with oral contraceptives gives a good application of this approach, and the text by Lilienfeld and Lilienfeld (1980) should be consulted for a general discussion.

For example, the association between oral contraceptive use and the development of venous thrombosis and pulmonary embolism was initially established by three British case-control studies (Royal College of General Practitioners 1967, Vessey and Doll 1968, 1969, Inman and Vessey, 1968). Doll and Vessey (1970) argued that in addition to the results of these three studies, there was a substantial body of evidence that indirectly supported an interpretation of cause and effect. (1) Studies in the United Kingdom and in the United States had shown a trend in the national death rates from venous thromboembolism in young women compatible with the increase in the use of oral contraceptives and the estimates of the risks associated with them. (2) Two studies had shown evidence suggesting that estrogens used to supress lactation were a factor in the causation of puerperal thromboembolism. (3) Estrogens had been implicated as a cause of venous and arterial thromboembolism when they were administered to elderly men with arterial disease or cancer of the prostate. (4) Laboratory studies had shown that oral contraceptives may cause an increase in the level of some clotting factors in the blood and also an alteration in platelet behavior. Another study had demonstrated that changes in venous distensibility and blood flow were produced by the use of oral contraceptives by women.

Proof of Causation

The reader should recall that the tradition of scientific explanation requires that a claim of proof of cause and effect must specify the mechanism by which the effect is produced. The path of reductionism, whereby disease processes are explained in biochemical terms, virtually requires an experimental study. Thus, most observational studies end with an opinion or judgment about causality, not a claim of proof (Cochran 1965).

1.5 HISTORY OF CASE-CONTROL STUDIES

The case-control method has two distinctive features. First, it proceeds from effect to cause, attempting to identify antecedents that led to the disease or condition of study. This technique of looking retrospectively arises naturally. It is used daily by clinicians when they take case histories as an aid to diagnosis, a medical practice common since the time of Hippocrates, and undoubtedly an approach to reasoning in general use since the emergence of civilization. Second, the case-control method uses a comparison group (controls) to support or refute an inference of a causal role for any particular factor. The explicit use of a control appears to be of recent origin and was particularly emphasized in the experimental method formalized in the eighteenth and nineteenth centuries (Sartwell 1974).

Modern case-control studies date from the Lane-Claypon (1926) paper on reproductive factors in relation to breast cancer. This report was significant because it proposed methods for selecting matched hospital controls to address specific study objectives (Mantel and Haenszel 1959, Cole 1979). An earlier report that also used the case-control approach was that by Broders (1920) concerning squamous-cell epithelioma of the lip. Comparing 537 cases with 500 controls taken from male patients without epithelioma, Broders found that the percentage of tobacco use was similar in cases and controls (80.5% vs. 78.6%). However, he pointed out a remarkable difference in the method of smoking. Among the cases, 78.5 percent smoked pipes, whereas among the controls, only 38 percent were pipe-smokers, which suggested that pipe smoking played a role in the development of cancer of the lip.

Within the field of sociology, the case-control method was formalized and used in the 1920s and 1930s (Lilienfeld and Lilienfeld 1979). Epidemiologic applications of the case-control method increased greatly after World War II. A case-control study of carcinoma of the penis, reported by Schreck and Lenowitz (1947), emphasized the importance of using a control group for comparison with a case series, and identified the absence of circumcision and poor sex hygiene as etiologic factors. The relation of hepatitis to prior transfusions was first shown by a case-contol study (Sartwell 1947). Three case-control studies reported in 1950 cited cigarette smoking as a likely cause of lung cancer (Schreck et al. 1950, Wynder and Graham 1950, Levin, Goldstein, and Gerhardt 1950). In addition to leukemia, other primary cancers that were studied in the 1950s by the case-control method included cancers of the bladder, breast, cervix, larynx, lung, and stomach.

A landmark in the analysis of case-control studies is the paper by Cornfield (1951), which demonstrated that the relative risk can be estimated from either a case-control or a cohort design. In 1954 Cornfield applied direct standardization to control for extraneous variables in the analysis of case-control data (Wynder et al. 1954). Mantel and Haenszel (1959) later showed how to efficiently estimate the relative risk from stratified data, and gave chi-square tests for association. Their paper continues to serve as an authoritative introduction to the strengths and deficiencies of the case-control method.

Rare adverse drug effects, notably those associated with the use of synthetic hormones and oral contraceptives, have been investigated by numerous case-control studies reported in the 1960s and 1970s. Recent applications of the case-control method have been quite diverse. A brief listing of some investigations may give the reader an impression of the scope of the method: maternal smoking and congenital malformations (Kelsey et al. 1978), low-dose radiation and leukemia (Linos et al. 1980), oral contraceptive use and hepatocellular adenoma (Rooks et al. 1979), behavioral factors and urinary tract infection (Adatto et al. 1979), herpes simplex virus and Bell palsy (Adour, Bell, and Hilsinger 1975), induced abortion and spontaneous abortion (Kline et al. 1978), the HLA-system and asbestosis (Merchant et al. 1975), allergins and sudden infant death (Turner, Baldo, and Hilton 1975), physical activity and coronary death (Hennekens et al. 1977), toxic shock syndrome and use of tampons (Davis et al. 1980), artificial sweeteners and bladder cancer (Hoover and Strasser 1980) and protective measures for avoiding injuries in tornadoes (Glass et al. 1980).

2 Basic Concepts in the Assessment of Risk

2.0 INTRODUCTION

This chapter sets forth several approaches to evaluating the effect of exposure on the risk of disease and points out the manner in which an assessment can be made on the basis of a case-control study. The case-control approach is compared with follow-up studies in terms of their sampling schemes. The problem of interpreting an apparent effect of exposure, in view of potential bias from extraneous variables, is addressed in a discussion of confounding. Individual and joint effects of a set of variables are explained along with the concept of interaction.

An exposure may increase, decrease, or have no effect on the risk of disease, and a case-control study is equally well suited to assessing any one of these possibilities. Although our exposition is often couched in terms of assessing an increase in risk, this is strictly for convenience of expression. The reader should continually recall that a decrease in risk may be equivalently addressed (e.g. Weiss et al. 1980). The term "risk" is used in the sense of its common English usage, referring to the chance or probability of an event.

2.1 DISEASE OCCURRENCE

Incidence

An assessment of the risk of disease is best made in terms of the number of new cases that occur during a specified period of time—the *incidence*. To adjust for the size of the population at risk and the duration of time at risk, two distinct measures of disease occurrence may be calculated, both commonly (and confusingly) referred to as the *incidence rate*. The first, sometimes termed the *incidence rate*, the *cumulative incidence rate* (Miettinen 1976a, Morgenstern, Kleinbaum, Kupper 1980), or the *attack rate* (Lilienfeld and Lilienfeld 1980), is the proportion of persons in a population subgroup, initially free of disease, who develop the disease within a specified time interval. The cumulative incidence rate is calculated as the ratio of the number of new cases occurring over the time period to the number *initially* at risk. Thus, consider a group of individuals free of disease at the start of an observational period. An estimate of the cumulative incidence rate, denoted by $\hat{p}$, is the number of new cases occurring within the interval, d, divided by the number initially at risk, n. That is,

$$\hat{p} = d/n. \qquad (2.1)$$

This ratio may be interpreted as an estimate of the (average) conditional probability that disease develops within the interval. (The probability is "conditional" on the absence of disease at the start of the interval. Furthermore, since each individual may be considered to have a distinct risk of disease during the interval, $\hat{p}$ may be interpreted as an estimate of the average risk of disease for individuals in the group.)

Table 2.1 shows for each of three age groups the number of men who developed coronary heart disease during 12 years of follow-up in Framingham, Massachusetts (Truett, Cornfield, Kannel 1967). The fourth column shows that the cumulative incidence rate was .051 (40/789) among the 789 men aged 30–39 who had no evidence of CHD at a baseline examination. Thus, the conditional probability of a coronary event occurring within 12 years is estimated to be .051. The corresponding values of the cumulative incidence rate among men aged 40–49 years and 50–62 years are .119 (88/742) and .198 (130/656) respectively. The trend of increasing values of $\hat{p}$ with increasing age indicates a strong dependence of twelve-year risk on age. (Note that although the age groups in Table 2.1 are not of uniform width, the time period of risk is held constant at 12 years.)

In situations where losses, deaths due to causes other than the one under study, or other sources of withdrawal occur, refinements of the estimate (2.1) should be made. If w denotes the number of "withdrawals" (losses, deaths, etc.) during the period of observation, then

$$\hat{p} = d/(n - \tfrac{1}{2}w)$$

Table 2.1. Incidence of Coronary Heart Disease Observed in 12 Years of Follow-Up in Men Living in Framingham, Mass., by Age at First Exam

	Number at risk	Number of CHD events	Cumulative incidence rate	Person-years of observation[1]	Person-time incidence rate[2]
Age (yrs)	n	d	$\hat{p}$	T	$\tilde{p}$
30–39	789	40	.051	9228	4.3
40–49	742	88	.119	8376	10.5
50–62	656	130	.198	7092	18.3

1. Estimated
2. Cases per 1000 persons per year

Source: Truett, Cornfield, and Kannel 1967.

provides a refined estimate of the cumulative incidence rate. The adjustment of the denominator from n to $(n - \frac{1}{2} w)$ is made because the w withdrawals are at risk for only part (assumed to be $\frac{1}{2}$) of the interval. Additions to the study population can be analogously treated. Armitage (1971) and Chiang (1968) further discuss the underlying assumptions and rationale of this adjustment.

The second measure of disease occurrence, variously termed the *incidence rate*, the *person-time incidence rate* (Greenland 1981), the *instantaneous incidence rate* (Morgenstern, Kleinbaum, Kupper 1980), the *force of morbidity* (Chiang 1968), the *incidence-density* (Miettinen 1976a), or the *hazard* (Gross & Clark 1975), is the number of new cases divided by the population-time (e.g., person-years of observation) over which they occur. To be more specific, suppose that one observes a subgroup of individuals over a specified time interval. Within the interval, the amount of disease-free time observed for an individual is the *person-time at risk* of that individual. The sum of the individual person-times at risk represents the total person-time at risk over the interval. The number of new cases observed within the interval, divided by the total person-time at risk observed over the interval, may be interpreted as an estimate of the (average) person-time incidence rate over the interval. Thus, letting t_i denote the person-time at risk for the ith individual, the total person-time at risk, denoted by T, may be written $T = \Sigma t_i$, where the summation is over all individuals at risk. The person-time incidence rate, denoted by $\tilde{p}$ (p-tilde), is then given by

$$\tilde{p} = d/T. \tag{2.2}$$

Referring again to Table 2.1, the fifth column gives an estimate of the total person-time observed within each of the age groups. Since values of T were not reported by Truett, Cornfield, and Kannel (1967), the following approximation was used. First, suppose that all persons were followed either for the entire twelve-year period or until they had a CHD event. Thus, for simplicity, we assume that no losses to follow-up occur from deaths due to causes other than CHD, from inability to trace individuals over a twelve-year period, etc. Second, assume that on average the CHD events occurred at the midpoint of the twelve-year interval. Given these two assumptions, the person-time observed for an individual who developed CHD is $\frac{1}{2} \times 12$ years, and the total person-time for the d individuals who developed CHD is $d \times \frac{1}{2} \times 12$ years. Correspondingly, the person-time observed for an individual who did not develop CHD is 12 years, and the total person-time observed among the $(n - d)$ individuals who did not develop CHD is $(n - d) \times 12$ years. Thus, the total person-time observed among all individuals within an age group may be estimated by the sum of these two components, $(n - \frac{1}{2} d) \times 12$ years. For example, among the 789 men aged 30–39 years, an estimated $(789 - \frac{1}{2} 40) \times 12 = 9228$ person-years of observation was accumulated. The person-time incidence rate is therefore estimated by $\tilde{p} = (40/9228)/yr = (4.3/1000)/yr$. In other words, among every 1000 men 30–39 years of age, an estimated 4.3 developed clinically manifest CHD per year.

The cumulative incidence rate, being a proportion, always takes a value between zero and unity. Since it refers to a specific interval of time, however, its magnitude will be proportional to the length of the interval. Whereas the cumulative incidence rate has no unit of measurement, the person-time incidence rate is measured in units of $1/\text{time}$. Furthermore, the numerical value of the person-time incidence rate depends in part on the units (years, months, weeks, etc.) used for measuring the time interval of observation.

Although the cumulative incidence rate and the person-time incidence rate are not equivalent, they can be related to each other by means of an approximation. If $\tilde{p}$ is the average person-time incidence rate over a specified interval of length Δt, then the cumulative incidence rate p over the interval is given (Chiang 1968, pp. 60–61) by $p = 1 - \exp(-\tilde{p} \cdot \Delta t)$. If the cumulative incidence rate is small ($p < 0.1$), a simple approximation may be used: $p \simeq \tilde{p} \cdot \Delta t$ (Chiang 1968, Miettinen 1976a). In the remainder of this book, we shall use the term incidence rate to refer to either measure, explicitly distinguishing the two only when necessary.

Referring to Table 2.1, the person-time incidence rate of CHD for men aged 50–62 years is $\tilde{p} = 18.3/1000/yr$. For the 12-year period of observation, $\Delta t = 12$. Hence, $\hat{p} \cdot \Delta t = .220$ and $1 - \exp(-.220) = .197 \simeq \hat{p}$, to three decimal places.

One final point. An individual's risk often depends not only on the length of the interval at risk, Δt, but also on several other aspects of time: (1) an individual's age, (2) the date (calendar time), and (3) the time elapsed since an etiologic event, such as the initiation of smoking, for example. Table 2.1 shows that the incidence rate of coronary heart disease increases with advancing age. An age-specific incidence rate, however, may rise or fall over time due to changes in environmental or behavioral factors.

Prevalence

The *prevalence* of a disease is the frequency (number of cases) at a given point in time. The *prevalence rate* is the ratio of the prevalence to the number of persons at risk at that point in time. The determination of the number of persons at risk is subject to a variety of operational definitions that depend on a study's design (Hill 1971, MacMahon and Pugh 1970). The basic distinction between prevalence and incidence is that incidence is intended to refer to new cases that develop during an interval of time, whereas prevalence refers to all cases of disease at a given moment, irrespective of the time of onset. It is intuitively clear that prevalence depends on the duration as well as the incidence. For a stable disease process, in which neither the incidence rate (I) nor the mean duration (m) depends on time, the prevalence rate (P) may be written (e.g., Freeman and Hutchison 1980)

$$P = mI. \tag{2.3}$$

Equation (2.3) provides a basis for recommending that incident cases be used in studies of disease causation. The reason is that in a comparison of two groups, a higher prevalence rate in one may result from any one of three different circumstances: (1) a longer duration, but similar or lower incidence rate; (2) a higher incidence rate, with similar or shorter duration; (3) both a higher rate of incidence and a longer duration. If a factor were associated with an increase in the prevalence rate, then only in the second or third situation would it be regarded as possibly contributing to the cause of the disease. This point is discussed further in Chapter 5.

Table 2.2. Relationship of Disease and Exposure in a Target Population

A. *Frequency of Disease Among Exposed and Unexposed Individuals in a Target Population*

	Disease[1]		Total	Odds of disease
	Yes	No		
Exposure				
Yes	A	B	M_1	A/B
No	C	D	M_2	C/D
Total	N_1	N_2	N	
Odds of exposure	A/C	B/D		

B. *Hypothetical Data*

	Disease		Total	Odds of disease
	Yes	No		
Exposure				
Yes	8	992	1000	.0081
No	10	4990	5000	.0020
Total	18	5982	6000	
Odds of exposure	.80	.20		

1. Number of new cases during a specified period of time.

2.2 RELATIVE MEASURES OF DISEASE OCCURRENCE

Relative Risk

Imagine two groups of individuals, comparable in all respects relevant to the development of disease, apart from the presence or absence of exposure to some study factor at a specified point in time (t_0). Suppose that during a given interval of time, from t_0 to t_1, one observes the number of individuals who develop disease and who remain disease-free, as in Table 2.2. Among those exposed, the incidence rate (proportion of new cases) is

$$p_1 = A/M_1. \tag{2.4}$$

The incidence rate among the unexposed is

$$p_2 = C/M_2. \tag{2.5}$$

The ratio of the two incidence rates

$$R = p_1/p_2 \tag{2.6}$$

is called the *relative risk* (or "risk ratio"). It represents how many times more (or less) likely disease occurs in the exposed group as compared with the unexposed. If R differs from unity, then the study factor is associated with the risk of disease. For $R > 1$, a "positive" association is said to exist; for $R < 1$, there is a "negative" association.

Odds Ratio

The odds ratio is another measure of association that is closely related to the relative risk. If an event occurs with probability p, then the ratio p/q, where $q = 1 - p$, is called the *odds*. For example, if $p = 1/14$ represents the lifetime risk of breast cancer in U.S. women, then the odds of breast cancer are $1/13$. For rare diseases, the risk of disease p and the odds of disease p/q are virtually identical.

If p_1 denotes the incidence rate among exposed individuals, the odds of disease are p_1/q_1. Similarly, if p_2 denotes the incidence rate among the unexposed, the corresponding odds of disease are p_2/q_2. The ratio of the odds of disease in exposed individuals relative to the unexposed is called the *odds ratio* or *relative odds*. Using the Greek letter ψ(psi), the odds ratio may be written

$$\psi = p_1 q_2 / q_1 p_2 = AD/BC. \tag{2.7}$$

The distinction between relative risk and odds ratio is now standard, although the terms were often used interchangably in the early epidemiologic and statistical literature. The odds ratio is now commonly denoted by ψ, a convention that we shall follow.

The odds ratio is particularly important for two reasons. First, for rare diseases, it closely approximates the relative risk. Second, the odds ratio can be determined from either a cohort or a case-control study. In general, the relative risk can be exactly determined only from a cohort study, although it can be estimated from a case-control study by use of the odds-ratio approximation (Section 2.3).

As an example in which the odds ratio closely approximates the relative risk, consider a death rate of 7 per 100,000 per year, which prevailed among nonsmoking doctors in 1965 (Hill 1965). The risk of death for doctors smoking twenty-five or more cigarettes daily was 227 per 100,000 per year. The relative risk of death in smokers as compared with non-smokers was $R = 227/7 = 32.43$. The relative odds of death in smokers as compared with nonsmokers were $\psi = (227 \times 99993)/(7 \times 99773) = 32.50$. The percentage error in using ψ as an approximation for R is

0.2%. Using either measure, one estimates that the risk of death for heavy smokers is thirty-two times higher than the risk for nonsmokers.

The odds ratio ψ has been defined in terms of the *odds of disease* in exposed individuals relative to the odds of disease in the unexposed. An equivalent definition can be given in terms of the *odds of exposure.*

Among diseased individuals, the odds of exposure are A/C (Table 2.2). The odds of exposure are B/D among disease-free subjects. The ratio of the odds of exposure in diseased individuals as compared with the nondiseased is thus given by

$$\psi = (A/C) \div (B/D) = AD/BC. \qquad (2.8)$$

Thus the "exposure-odds ratio" defined by equation (2.8) is equivalent to the "disease-odds ratio" defined by equation (2.7). This important relationship is often useful in the consideration of the design and analysis of case-control studies.

2.3 COHORT AND CASE-CONTROL SAMPLING SCHEMES

The primary distinction between the cohort and the case-control designs is the method by which individuals are selected for study (White and Bailar 1956). The simplest paradigm that reveals this difference is one in which the study exposure and disease are dichotomous, each being considered either present or absent, as shown in Table 2.2.

The next two sections indicate similarities and differences between the cohort and the case-control methods in regard to the parameters that can be estimated from the two study designs. They show that a cohort study can estimate the *exposure-specific* incidence rates, p_1 and p_2, the *attributable risk* $p_1 - p_2$, the relative risk R and the odds ratio ψ. Typically, a case-control study can only estimate ψ. Since ψ is a good approximation to R for rare diseases, the case-control method can effectively estimate R in this circumstance. The reader who is uncomfortable with explanations that rely on algebraic manipulations may prefer to skip the next two sections on the first reading and proceed directly to the section entitled "Estimation of Relative Risk."

Cohort Sampling

Suppose that in a cohort study one takes random samples of exposed and unexposed individuals. If one samples a proportion f_1 of the total M_1

Table 2.3.   Cohort Study Based on Target Population of Table 2.2

A. *Expected Sample Outcome for a Cohort Study*[1]

	Disease		Odds of disease
	Yes	No	
Exposure			
Yes	n_{11} $(f_1 A)$	n_{12} $(f_1 B)$	n_{11}/n_{12} (A/B)
No	n_{21} $(f_2 C)$	n_{22} $(f_2 D)$	n_{21}/n_{22} (C/D)
Odds of exposure	n_{11}/n_{21} $(f_1 A/f_2 C)$	n_{12}/n_{22} $(f_1 B/f_2 D)$	

B. *Hypothetical Data*[2]

	Disease		Total	Odds of disease
	Yes	No		
Exposure				
Yes	2	248	250	.0081
No	1	499	500	.0020
Odds of Exposure ,	2.0	.50		

1. Random samples of $f_1 \times 100$ percent of the M_1 exposed and $f_2 \times 100$ percent of the M_2 unexposed individuals are taken from the target population in Table 2.2.
2. $f_1 = .25$ and $f_2 = .1$ applied to Table 2.2B.

exposed individuals in the target population and f_2 of the total M_2 unexposed, then on the average or in large samples one would have a sample outcome as in Table 2.3. It should be understood that the sampling fractions f_1 and f_2 are typically unknown. This is because one usually has uncertain knowledge of the total numbers of exposed and unexposed individuals in the target population, thereby precluding knowledge of the proportions of those totals that one is sampling. The quantities f_1 and f_2 are never used explicitly in computing estimates of the relative risk or odds ratio from the sample data. They are discussed here only to point out the differences between the cohort and the case-control sampling schemes and to indicate why only certain parameters can be estimated from the sample data.

Samples are "random" in the sense that, among exposed or unexposed individuals, a person who will develop disease has the same chance of being studied as does a person who will remain disease-free. That is, each of the M_1 exposed individuals in the target population has probability f_1 of being in the study, and each of the M_2 unexposed individuals has probability f_2 of being studied.

The incidence rates $\hat{p}_1 = n_{11}/(n_{11} + n_{12}) = A/M_1$ and $\hat{p}_2 = n_{21}/(n_{21} + n_{22}) = C/M_2$ estimated from the sample in Table 2.3 agree with the values in the target population in Table 2.2. The estimated relative risk and odds ratio from Table 2.3 similarly agree with the population values. (For simplicity our discussion ignores sampling variability.)

Sampling on the basis of exposure, as illustrated in Table 2.3, alters the estimated odds of exposure. In the target population, the odds of exposure are A/C in diseased individuals and B/D in nondiseased individuals. By contrast, the corresponding sample estimates from Table 2.3 are $n_{11}/n_{21} = (f_1/f_2)(A/C)$ and $n_{12}/n_{22} = (f_1/f_2)(B/D)$ respectively. As is evident in the numerical example, the sampling ratio f_1/f_2 distorts the exposure odds, unless $f_1 = f_2$.

Sampling on the basis of exposure does not affect the odds of disease. The sample values of the disease odds in Table 2.3 agree with the population values, $n_{11}/n_{12} = A/B$ for exposed individuals and $n_{21}/n_{22} = C/D$ for unexposed individuals.

Rather than taking samples of exposed and unexposed individuals, a cohort study often begins by taking a sample of all individuals, irrespective of exposure. Subjects are then followed over time to observe the occurrence of disease, and individuals are later stratified into various exposure groups. A table similar to Table 2.3 could be presented that would demonstrate that the incidence rates, relative risk, and odds ratio corresponding to this sampling scheme would also agree with the values in the target population. Furthermore, since sampling would not depend on either the exposure status or disease status of an individual, the odds of disease and the odds of exposure in the sample would agree (apart from sampling variability) with their values in the target population.

Case-Control Sampling

Suppose that in a case-control study one takes a random sample of incident cases of the study disease and a random sample of controls (individuals who are free of the study disease). With sampling fractions of f_3 (cases) and f_4 (controls), one expects on the average or in large samples an outcome as in Table 2.4. The sampling fractions are often unknown, but nonetheless are implicit in the sample design, insofar as one selects n_1 cases out of a total N_1 and n_2 controls out of a total N_2. The terms f_3 and f_4 are introduced here to indicate why only certain parameters can be estimated from a case-control study.

The proportion of incident cases among exposed individuals *in the sample* is $p_1' = a/(a + b) = f_3A/(f_3A + f_4B)$, which generally is not equal to the incidence rate in the target population, $p_1 = A/(A + B)$. Similarly, the sample proportion of incident cases among unexposed ind-

Table 2.4. Case-Control Study Based on Target Population of Table 2.2

A. *Expected Sample Outcome for a Case-Control Study*[1]

	Disease		
	Yes	No	Odds of disease
Exposure			
Yes	$a\ (f_3A)$	$b\ (f_4B)$	$a/b\ (f_3A/f_4B)$
No	$c\ (f_3C)$	$d\ (f_4D)$	$c/d\ (f_3C/f_4D)$
Odds of exposure	$a/c\ (A/C)$	$b/d\ (B/D)$	

B. *Hypothetical Data*[2]

	Disease		
	Yes	No	Odds of disease
Exposure			
Yes	8	3^3	2.67
No	10	15^3	.67
Total	18	18	
Odds of exposure	.80	.20	

1. Random samples of $f_3 \times 100$ percent of the N_1 diseased and $f_4 \times 100$ percent of the N_2 nondiseased individuals are taken from the target population in Table 2.2.
2. $f_3 = 1.0$ and $f_4 = .003$ applied to Table 2.2B.
3. Rounded to nearest integer.

viduals, $p_2' = c/(c + d) = f_3C/(f_3C + f_4D)$, generally is not equal to p_2. It is also clear that the ratio p_1'/p_2' does not correctly estimate the relative risk p_1/p_2.

Unless the ratio of the sampling fractions f_3/f_4 is known, is unity ($f_3 = f_4$), or can be estimated from ancillary sources, the incidence rates p_1 and p_2 in the target population cannot be determined from a case-control study. Equal sampling fractions ($f_3 = f_4$) are unrealistic for rare diseases, since this would imply that hundreds or thousands of controls would be taken for each case. Since cases generally are few compared with potential controls, the value of f_3 is often close to unity, whereas the value of f_4 is close to zero. Thus the ratio f_3/f_4 is usually a very large number.

Random sampling in a case-control study implies that among cases and controls, an exposed individual has the same chance as an unexposed individual of being in the study (see Table 2.4). Thus, the sample estimates of the odds of exposure for the cases and for the controls agree with the population values under this sampling scheme.

For convenience of expression, we shall refer to the odds of "disease" (in quotes) in a case-control study, realizing that, strictly speaking, one can only determine the odds of being a "case." A "case" represents an individual who not only has the study disease, but is also *selected* for study. The sampling ratio f_3/f_4 alters the odds of disease in the case-control sample as compared with the population. Whereas the odds of disease in the population are respectively A/B and C/D among exposed and unexposed individuals, in the sample the corresponding odds of "disease" are $(f_3/f_4)(A/B)$ and $(f_3/f_4)(C/D)$. The sampling ratio f_3/f_4 cancels on division in the calculation of the odds ratio, so that the sample estimate of ψ agrees with the population value apart from sampling variability.

Estimation of Relative Risk

The sample outcome for a case-control study consisting of n_1 cases and n_2 controls will be represented in general by Table 2.5. Among the n_1 cases are a exposed and c unexposed individuals. The corresponding odds of exposure are a/c in the cases. Similarly, among the n_2 controls are b exposed and d unexposed individuals, with corresponding odds of exposure of b/d. The sample estimate of the odds ratio in the target population is given by

$$\hat{\psi} = ad/bc. \tag{2.9}$$

Note that the relative odds of disease in exposed individuals as compared with unexposed individuals ($a/b \div c/d$) equals the relative odds of exposure in diseased individuals as compared with nondiseased individuals ($a/c \div b/d$).

For rare diseases, ψ estimates the relative risk. From the discussion in the preceding section, one observes that a/m_1 and c/m_2 *do not* estimate the population incidence rates among exposed and unexposed individuals, because of distortion introduced by the implicit sampling ratio f_3/f_4. (The analysis for matched case-control studies differs from that given here, and the reader is referred to Chapter 7 for details.)

As an example, consider data in Table 2.6 based on a case-control study of artificial sweeteners and human bladder cancer (Hoover and Strasser 1980). All incident cases in ten geographic areas were ascertained during a one-year period beginning December, 1977. A random sample of controls, stratified by age and sex, and frequency matched at a 2:1 ratio of controls to cases, was selected from the general population of the ten areas. From the data in Table 2.6, one estimates that individuals who have used artificial sweeteners have virtually the same risk of

Table 2.5. Sample Outcome Based on n_1 Cases and n_2 Controls

	Cases	Controls	Total
Exposure			
Yes	a	b	m_1
No	c	d	m_2
Total	n_1	n_2	n

Table 2.6. History of Use of Artificial Sweeteners (AS)

	Cases	Controls
AS:		
Ever	1293	2455
Never	1707	3321
Total	3000	5776

Source: Hoover and Strasser 1980.

bladder cancer as individuals who have never used them, $\hat{\psi} = (1293 \times 3321)/(1707 \times 2455) = 1.02$. (Chapter 7 gives methods for calculating tests of significance and confidence intervals.)

Discussion

In general, one cannot determine from a case-control study the incidence rates of disease associated with the presence or absence of the study exposure. One can, however, estimate the ratio of the incidence rates (relative risk) in terms of its approximation, the odds ratio. The paradigm of simple random sampling of cases and controls from a target population can be readily extended to more complex sampling procedures, such as those involving stratified, cluster, or multistage sampling (Cochran 1977).

Our discussion of cohort and case-control studies presents a dichotomy of exposure and disease that is an unrealistic simplification in practice. With respect to exposure, it ignores factors such as duration or intensity, age at onset, and the presence of other variables that may modify the effect of exposure, such as conditions that predispose one to the development of disease. Furthermore, the paradigm in Table 2.2 ignores changes in an individual's exposure status and the time interval between exposure and the development of disease. It also does not distinguish factors that have been introduced by planned intervention (e.g., use of reserpine for treatment of hypertension), self-selection (e.g., choice of contraceptive method), or accident (e.g., ingestion of polybrominated biphenyls from contaminated food). With regard to disease, severity and age at onset are ignored, as is the complicating factor of concurrent diseases being manifested in the same individual. These issues, which impinge on the design, analysis, and interpretation of a case-control study, will be discussed in later sections.

There is another problem with the distinction between cohort and case-control studies based on the sampling paradigms in Tables 2.3 and 2.4. These tables suggest that both types of study can be completed contemporaneously, which is not generally true. The element of time is obscured in the simplification made by the 2 × 2 table. With a current cohort study, one must allow a lapse of time for cases of the study disease to occur among exposed and unexposed individuals. A historical cohort study, on the other hand, can be completed as quickly as a case-control study using incident cases, if not more so. With a historical cohort study, however, one must rely on available records of past exposure. These are often incomplete with regard to all relevant aspects of exposure and with respect to important covariables that may modify the effect of exposure or otherwise alter the interpretation of the study. Finally, random sampling does not guarantee comparability; it only assures unbiased selection of subjects for study and agreement, on the average or in large samples, between sample estimates and population values. Even with unbiased selection, however, a comparison may be biased because of intrinsic differences in the two comparison groups.

2.4 RISK OF DISEASE ATTRIBUTABLE TO EXPOSURE

Attributable Risk

A relative risk of $R = 2$ indicates that the incidence rate of disease is two times higher in the exposed group as compared with the unexposed. Equivalently, this represents a 100 percent increase in risk. A relative risk of $R = 0.25$ indicates a 75 percent reduction in the incidence rate in exposed individuals as compared with the unexposed.

Taken at face value, a relative risk of $R = 2$, for example, is not completely informative. Ratios (p_1/p_2) of .02/.01 and .00002/.00001 both result in the same relative risk $(R = 2)$, but have quite different implications in terms of an individual's risk due to exposure. In the first instance, the incidence rate has increased from 1 to 2 per 100 persons at risk, whereas in the second instance, the rate has increased from 1 to 2 per 100,000 at risk. In relative terms the increases are equivalent. However, if benefits as well as risks result from an exposure, individuals may regard an increase in the incidence rate to be personally inconsequential in the second instance, but an unacceptable increase in the first. This example points out the usefulness of a second risk parameter, the *attributable risk*, which shall be denoted by the Greek letter δ (delta).

The attributable risk (also called the "risk difference") is defined as the difference between the incidence rates, exposed minus unexposed (MacMahon and Pugh 1970, Mausner and Bahn 1974):

$$\delta = p_1 - p_2. \tag{2.10}$$

The term "attributable risk" has not had consistent usage (see Markush 1977).

Whereas the relative risk indicates the *percentage* change in risk compared with "baseline" (unexposed), the attributable risk indicates the magnitude of the *absolute* change. To clarify in what sense the parameter δ represents the risk of disease "attributable" to exposure, consider two individuals, both of whom are at equal risk of disease apart from the presence or absence of exposure to some factor. Suppose that the risk of disease is p_1 in the exposed individual and p_2 in the unexposed individual. Had the exposure not been present in the first person, his risk would have been equal to p_2. Thus, the difference $p_1 - p_2$ represents the increase or decrease in risk due to exposure.

The preceding discussion shows that knowledge of the baseline incidence rate p_2 allows one to place a relative risk in better perspective. Consider, for example, the finding of a case-control study (Rooks et al. 1979) that the risk of hepatocellular adenoma is increased 26 times among long-term users (> 5 years) of low-potency oral contraceptives. In U.S. women 16 to 30 years of age who have never used oral contraceptives, or who have used them for 2 years or less, this liver tumor develops at an annual rate of about 1.0 per million. Among women 31 to 44 years of age, the rate is about 1.3 per million per year (Rooks et al. 1979). Assuming a twenty-six-fold increase in risk, long-term users of oral contraceptives who are 16 to 44 years of age are estimated to have an annual incidence of hepatocellular adenoma of approximately 26 to 34 cases per million women. The risk attributable to oral contraceptive use is therefore 25 to 33 cases per million women per year.

The attributable risk can be expressed in terms of the relative risk by noting that $Rp_2 = p_1$. Thus from (2.10)

$$\delta = (R - 1)p_2. \tag{2.11}$$

Taking the odds ratio ψ as an approximation to the relative risk, one has

$$\delta \simeq (\psi - 1)p_2. \tag{2.12}$$

Since a case-control study generally can estimate only ψ, one needs information from other sources in order to determine a baseline rate p_2 and thereby derive an estimate of δ. Rooks et al. (1979) estimated the baseline incidence of hepatocellular adenoma by combining data from the American College of Surgeons Survey of Liver Tumors, the National Survey of Family Growth, and U.S. Census Data. The use of census data, special surveys, and disease registries represents a common approach to estimating baseline incidence rates for various target populations. However, unless one has a population-based case-control study, one is often uncertain whether the population incidence rate applies to the target population from which the cases and controls arose.

Exposure-Specific Risks

The term p_2 refers to the incidence rate in the unexposed. Incidence rates for the entire target population are invariably a weighted average of the *exposure-specific* rates, p_1 and p_2. Thus, in order to estimate a baseline rate p_2 from the population rate, one must adjust for the proportion exposed. The adjustment is given by equation (2.16) below, which is derived in the following paragraph.

Referring to Table 2.2, let

$$p_e = M_1/N = (A + B)/N \tag{2.13}$$

denote the proportion of exposed individuals in the target population, and let

$$p = N_1/N = (A + C)/N \tag{2.14}$$

denote the population incidence rate of the study disease. Then one can easily show that p is a weighted average of the exposure-specific rates p_1 and p_2:

$$p = p_1 p_e + p_2 (1 - p_e).$$

Making the substitution $p_2 R = p_1$ and solving for p_2, one has

$$p_2 = p/[Rp_e + (1 - p_e)]. \tag{2.15}$$

This equation is the basis for the estimate of p_2 given by equation (2.16) below.

In order to estimate the exposure-specific incidence rates p_1 and p_2 using data from a case-control study, one first needs an estimate of the incidence rate in the target population, $\hat{p}$. The population incidence rate will most likely be derived from two sources. The numerator, representing the number of incident cases in a specified interval of time, will ordinarily be based on a disease registry or on hospital admissions in a defined geographic area. The denominator, representing the size of the population at risk, will often be based on a census or sample survey. Next, the relative risk of disease associated with exposure is estimated from a case-control study by the odds ratio $\hat{\psi}$, given by equation (2.9).

Finally, as shown in Section 2.5, an estimate of the proportion exposed in the target population may be based on the exposure-rate in the controls,

$$\hat{p}_e = b/(b + d).$$

Substitution of these estimates into equation (2.15) gives an estimate of the incidence rate in the unexposed,

$$\hat{p}_2 = \hat{p}/[\hat{\psi}\hat{p}_e + (1 - \hat{p}_e)]. \tag{2.16}$$

Substitution of $\hat{\psi}$ and $\hat{p}_2$ into equation (2.12) then gives an estimate of the attributable risk. Finally, using the odds ratio as an estimate of the relative risk, one may estimate the incidence rate in exposed individuals, p_1, by substituting $\hat{p}_2$ and $\hat{\psi}$ into equation (2.6), giving

$$\hat{p}_1 = \hat{\psi}\hat{p}_2. \tag{2.17}$$

As a consequence of Bayes' Theorem from elementary probability theory, exposure-specific incidence rates can be determined from a case-control study without making any rare disease assumption (Neutra and Drolette 1978). However, one does need an external estimate of the incidence rate of disease in the target population. To see this, let E_i denote the ith category of exposure, and let D and $\overline{D}$ denote respectively the presence or absence of disease. Using standard notation for conditional probability, Bayes' Theorem states that

$$P(D|E_i) = P(E_i|D)P(D)/[P(E_i|D)P(D) + P(E_i|\overline{D})P(\overline{D})]$$

(Feller 1968). Estimating $P(E_i|D)$ and $P(E_i|\overline{D})$ respectively by the proportions of cases and controls in the ith exposure category, and given an estimate of the overall probability of disease, $P(D)$, the exposure-specific probability of disease $P(D|E_i)$ is determined directly from the equation above. Neutra and Drolette (1978) and Greenland (1981) provide further details.

Etiologic Fraction

The *etiologic fraction*, which we shall denote by the Greek letter λ (lambda), is the proportion of all cases in the target population attributable to exposure (Miettinen 1974a). This concept places the relative risk in a national or public health perspective, since λ represents the expected reduction in disease load following removal of the study factor.

Referring to Table 2.2, one sees that if the exposure were removed from the target population, a total of Np_2 individuals would be expected to develop disease in a specified period of time. With the exposure present, however, the number of persons developing disease is N_1. Thus, one may regard the difference $N_1 - Np_2$ as the number of cases in the target population that are attributable to the exposure. Expressed as a proportion of all cases in the target population, the etiologic fraction λ may be written

$$\lambda = (N_1 - Np_2)/N_1. \tag{2.18}$$

Equation (2.18) can be written in the algebraically equivalent form

$$\lambda = p_e(R - 1)/[p_e(R - 1) + 1]. \tag{2.19}$$

Numerous names and formulae have been proposed for parameters that are equivalent to the etiologic fraction defined by equation (2.18) or (2.19) [Leviton 1973, Markush 1977]. The concept of etiologic fraction comes from Levin (1953), but the terminology has not been standard. Cole and MacMahon (1971) refer to the quantity $\lambda \times 100$ percent as the "population attributable risk percent," whereas Walter (1976) and Lilienfeld and Lilienfeld (1980) call λ the "attributable risk."

In deriving the number of cases in the population that are attributable to exposure, $N_1 - Np_2$, one effectively assumes that causal factors other than the exposure in question are equally distributed in the exposed and unexposed groups. That is, the incidence rate of disease among the unexposed, p_2, is assumed to apply equally to exposed indiviuals in the event that the exposure were removed.

Provided that the association between disease and exposure is causal, and not merely artifactual, one interprets the etiologic fraction as being the proportion of disease in the target population that would not have occurred had the factor been absent. Stated another way, removal of the factor is expected to produce a $\lambda \times 100$ percent reduction in the total number of cases.

Table 2.7 shows the etiologic fraction, $\lambda \times 100$ percent, as a function of the relative risk R and the proportion of exposed individuals in the target population p_e. For example, if 1 percent of a population were exposed to a factor that increased the risk of disease tenfold, $p_e = .01$ and $R = 10$, one estimates that 8 percent of the cases of disease would be eliminated by removal of the factor. (The actual number of cases eliminated would depend on the size of the population and the incidence rate of the disease.) As another example, if 25 percent of a population were exposed to some other factor that increased the risk of disease only twofold, $p_e = .25$ and $R = 2$, then 20 percent of the cases would be expected to be eliminated upon removal of the factor. If these two risk factors were independent causes of the same disease, then from a public health perspective, the detection of a relative risk of 2 for the second factor would

Table 2.7. Etiologic Fraction ($\lambda \times 100$ percent) as a Function of the Relative Risk (R) and the Proportion of the Population Exposed (p_e).

p_e	R			
	1.5	2	5	10
.01	.5	1	4	8
.05	2	5	17	31
.10	5	9	29	47
.25	11	20	50	69
.5	20	33	67	82
.9	31	47	78	89

be more important than the detection of a relative risk of 10 for the first factor. Thus, the detection of a comparatively small relative risk may be important, if the study exposure is common in the target population. This consideration is pertinent to planning the size of case-control studies (Chapter 6).

The exposure-specific incidence rates p_1 and p_2 can be expressed in terms of the etiologic fraction. First, one can show that $1 - \lambda = 1/[Rp_e + (1 - p_e)]$. Hence, from equation (2.15),

$$p_2 = p(1 - \lambda). \tag{2.20}$$

Finally, substitution of (2.20) for p_2 in equation (2.6) gives $p_1 = Rp(1 - \lambda)$.

2.5 EXPOSURE

The precise meaning of "exposure" presents a common problem confronting the interpretation of risks. Take as an example the concern in the late 1970s over a potential association between the use of saccharin and the development of bladder cancer. Most likely every adult at risk of bladder cancer in the U.S. in 1980 had consumed saccharin to some degree, since this sweetener was distributed widely in processed foods. Thus, in one sense, probably all persons had been "exposed." To refine the issue of exposure, one therefore must consider such aspects as intensity, duration, and total dose. In effect, one must define a minimal exposure that shall be taken as the reference level. Risks are then expressed in relation to the reference.

As an example of the intensity dimension of exposure, Table 2.8 shows a dose-response relationship between current cigarette smoking and the

Table 2.8. Relation of Myocardial Infarction to Smoking Habits in 55 Cases and 220 Controls

Cigarettes/day	Cases	Controls	"Disease" odds	Estimated relative risk
Never smoked	4	73	.055	1.0[1]
Exsmoker	2	27	.074	1.3
1–14	8	33	.242	4.4
15–24	15	59	.254	4.6
25–34	12	16	.750	13.6
≥ 35	14	12	1.167	21.2
Total	55	220		

1. Reference category

Source: Slone et al. 1978

risk of myocardial infarction in women under fifty years of age. Taken from a case-control study of risk factors related to myocardial infarction (Slone et al. 1978), this table indicates that the odds of "disease" (i.e., the odds of being a "case") increase as the intensity of smoking increases. Expressed relative to women who have never smoked, the risk of disease varies from 1.3 times higher among exsmokers to 21 times higher among women currently smoking 35 or more cigarettes per day. (The estimated relative risks in the last column of Table 2.8 are based on the ratios of the corresponding odds of "disease.")

To recapitulate a point made in the section entitled "Case-Control Sampling" (Section 2.3), we use the expression *odds of "disease"* (in quotes) to refer to the odds of disease determined from a case-control study. Strictly speaking, in a case-control study one can only determine the odds that an individual is a "case." A "case" represents an individual who not only has the study disease, but is also *selected* for study. When one selects cases and controls, one is usually sampling them implicitly with unknown sampling fractions f_3 and f_4 respectively. The sampling ratio (f_3/f_4) alters the odds of disease in the case-control sample as compared with the target population. Whereas the odds of disease among exposed and unexposed individuals in the population are A/B and C/D respectively (see Table 2.2), the corresponding odds of "disease" in the case-control sample are $(f_3/f_4)(A/B)$ and $(f_3/f_4)(C/D)$, as shown in Table 2.4. The sampling ratio (f_3/f_4) cancels on division in the calculation of odds ratios, so that the sample estimate of ψ should agree with the population value, apart from sampling variability.

As an example of the time dimension of exposure, Table 2.9 shows a dose-response relationship in which the risk of hepatocellular adenoma increases with increasing duration of oral contraceptive (OC) use (Rooks et al. 1979). Compared with women who have used OCs for 0–12 months, the risk of hepatocellular adenoma is four times higher among OC-users of 13–36 months duration and 49 times higher in OC-users of 85 months duration or more. [The presentation in Table 2.9, which for simplicity of exposition ignores the matching used in the study design, underestimates the correct relative risks determined by the matched analysis of Rooks et al. 1979.]

Some aspects of time that relate to an exposure are whether it was continuous or intermittent, and its occurrence in relation to an individual's age or significant life events such as menarche, pregnancy, or menopause. With a drug or environmental exposure, one may want to know the effect of discontinuation, or whether there is a period of time that must elapse before the effect becomes evident (a latent period). To investigate such issues, one may stratify (form subgroups) the *exposed* cases and *exposed* controls on the basis of time of initiation or discontinuation in order to assess whether the odds of "disease" show any time trends.

Another aspect of time concerns the interval over which the risk may be elevated or reduced. For example, in a case-control study of oral contraceptive use in relation to myocardial infarction, Shapiro et al. (1979) found that there was no evidence that "past use" of oral contraceptives was associated with an increased risk of myocardial infarction: 37 percent of the 234 cases and 43 percent of the 1742 controls had last used oral contraceptives more than one month before admission. Adjusted for a number of potential confounding factors, the relative risk was estimated to be 1.2, with a 95 percent confidence interval of (0.8, 1.7). However,

Table 2.9. Relation of Hepatocellular Adenoma to Duration of Oral Contraceptive Use in 79 Cases and 220 Controls

Months of OC use	Cases	Controls	"Disease" odds	Estimated relative risk
0–12	7	121	.058	1.0[1]
13–36	11	49	.224	3.9
37–60	20	23	.870	15.0
61–84	21	20	1.050	18.1
≥ 85	20	7	2.857	49.3
Total	79	220		

1. Reference category.

Source: Rooks et al. 1979.

considering "recent use" of oral contraceptives (last use within the month before admission), the risk of a myocardial infarction was estimated to be four times higher in users as compared with non-users. This suggests that oral contraceptive use has an acute rather than long-term effect on the risk of myocardial infarction. (This conclusion must be tempered by the fact that the cited study did not consider specific aspects of "past use," such as long-term use. See Slone et al. 1981).

Estimation of the Population Exposure Rate from the Control Series

Use of the exposure rate in the controls as an estimate of the population exposure rate depends on two assumptions. First, the control series must be representative of individuals who do not have the study disease in the target population. Second, the disease must be rare. The estimate of the population exposure rate given by equation (2.23) which follows is justified in the next paragraph, which some persons may want to ignore at a first reading.

Let D and $\overline{D}$ denote respectively the presence and absence of the study disease, and let E denote the presence of exposure. Using standard notation for conditional probability (Feller 1968), one can write

$$P(E) = P(E|D)P(D) + P(E|\overline{D})P(\overline{D}). \tag{2.21}$$

[Verification of equation (2.21) can be made by referring to Table 2.2, noting that $M_1/N = (A/N_1)(N_1/N) + (B/N_2)(N_2/N) = (A + B)/N$.] Thus, the *unconditional* probability of exposure in the target population, $P(E)$, may be written as a weighted average of the conditional probabilities of exposure among diseased and nondiseased individuals, $P(E|D)$ and $P(E|\overline{D})$ respectively. If the probability of disease is small, then $P(D) \simeq 0$ and $P(\overline{D}) \simeq 1$. As a consequence, equation (2.21) gives the resulting approximation

$$P(E) \simeq P(E|\overline{D}). \tag{2.22}$$

If the control series is a random sample of individuals in the target population who are free of the study disease, then the discussion of Table 2.4 in Section 2.3 indicates that

$$\hat{p}_e = b/(b + d) \tag{2.23}$$

estimates $P(E|\overline{D})$, the proportion of nondiseased individuals in the population who were exposed to the study factor. If the disease is rare, then $\hat{p}_e$ also estimates the population exposure rate, as shown in equation (2.22).

The etiologic fraction can be estimated from a case-control study by using the odds ratio $\hat{\psi}$ as an estimate of the relative risk, and by using the observed proportion of exposed controls, $\hat{p}_e = b/(b + d)$, as an estimate of p_e, the proportion of exposed individuals in the target population. Substitution of these estimates into equation (2.19) gives

$$\hat{\lambda} = \hat{p}_e(\hat{\psi} - 1)/[\hat{p}_e(\hat{\psi} - 1) + 1]. \qquad (2.24)$$

Chapter 7 provides more details regarding the estimation of the etiologic fraction from case-control studies.

2.6 INTERPRETATION OF RELATIVE RISK (DATA EXAMPLE)

Additional insight into the interpretation of relative risk can be derived by contemplating the data in Table 2.10, taken from a case-control study that identified all newly diagnosed cases of bladder cancer over an 18-month period, ending June 30, 1968, among residents of the Boston and Brockton Standard Metropolitan Statistical Areas in Eastern Massachusetts (Cole et al. 1971). A stratified probability sample of controls, selected at random within strata of age and sex, was drawn from the target population and classified on the basis of whether or not an individual had smoked at least 100 cigarettes during his or her lifetime. A

Table 2.10. Association Between Cigarette Smoking and Bladder Cancer in Men of Various Ages

	Number of study subjects				Case-control estimates		
					$\hat{\psi}$	$\hat{p}_e$	$\hat{\lambda}$
	Cases smokers[1]		Controls smokers				
Age (yrs)	yes	no	yes	no	Estimated relative risk	Population exposure	Etiologic fraction
50–54	24	1	22	4	4.36[2]	.85[3]	.74[4]
55–59	35	2	35	4	2.00	.90	.47
60–64	31	5	38	3	.49	.93	−.90
65–69	46	7	42	15	2.35	.74	.50
70–74	60	13	51	28	2.53	.65	.50
75–79	39	14	32	20	1.74	.62	.31

1. Smoker: yes, if > 100 cigarettes during lifetime; no, otherwise.
2. Age-specific odds ratio: 4.36 = (24/1)/(22/4).
3. Estimated proportion exposed in target population: 0.85 = 22/(22 + 4) from equation (2.23).
4. Estimated etiologic fraction: 0.74 = (.85)(4.36 − 1)/[(.85)(4.36 − 1) + 1] from equation (2.24).

Source: Miettinen (1976a), based on the case-control study reported by Cole et al. (1971).

subset of data restricted to men 50–79 years of age from the full study is reported in Table 2.10.

The relative risk of bladder cancer associated with smoking is estimated for each age group. For example, men who are 50–54 years old and have smoked 100 or more cigarettes during their lifetimes are estimated to have a risk of bladder cancer that is 4.4 times higher than the risk for nonsmokers of the same age. The estimated relative risk, based on the sample odds ratio, is calculated from equation (2.9) as $\hat{\psi} = (24 \times 4)/(1 \times 22) = 4.4$. The relative odds of exposure, 24/1 for the cases as compared with 22/4 for the controls, gives the same result.

There is a fundamental and important difference between the estimated relative risk column in Table 2.10 and the columns of estimated relative risk in Tables 2.8 and 2.9. Whereas the odds ratios in Tables 2.8 and 2.9 are expressed relative to the *same* reference group, the odds ratios in Table 2.10 are expressed relative to *differing* reference groups. Each age-specific relative odds in Table 2.10 estimates the risk of bladder cancer for smokers relative to nonsmokers of the same age. Since the baseline rates (rates in nonsmokers) vary with age, a direct comparison of these odds ratios is not very informative. For example, the estimated age-specific relative risks corresponding to 50–54 years and 75–79 years are 4.36 and 1.74 respectively. This does not imply that smoking is "more important" as a risk factor for bladder cancer in the younger men, nor does it imply that smoking by men 50–54 years of age results in a higher risk of bladder cancer as compared with the risk in smokers 75–79 years of age. Since the baseline rates differ, both the ratio of the estimated relative risks (4.36/1.74) and the difference in the estimated relative risks (4.36 − 1.74) tell us nothing about the risks of bladder cancer in older smokers compared with younger ones.

Table 2.11 shows that among smokers 50–54 years of age, the incidence rate of bladder cancer is estimated to be 34 cases per 100,000 per year; among smokers aged 75–79, the incidence rate is estimated to be 260 cases per 100,000 per year. The estimated risk in the older smokers is not only higher but also shows a greater absolute increase when compared with nonsmokers of the same age. Thus, relative risks can be deceptive. When contemplating one or more of them, one must keep in mind the reference group and the baseline risks.

For each age group in Table 2.10, the estimated proportion of male "smokers" in eastern Massachussetts has been calculated from the proportion of "smokers" in the control group using equation (2.23). Thus, 85 percent $[22/(22 + 4)]$ of men between the ages of 50 and 54 are

Table 2.11. Risk of Bladder Cancer Among Male Smokers and Nonsmokers of Various Ages

Age (yrs)	Number of new cases within 18 months	Size of target population ($\times$ 1000)	Population incidence rate per 100,000 per year $\hat{p}$	Estimated exposure-specific incidence rates $\hat{p}_1$	$\hat{p}_2$
50–54	35	77.4	30.1	34.0[1]	7.8[2]
55–59	52	68.4	50.7	53.4	26.7
60–64	52	61.5	56.4	52.6	107.3
65–69	86	47.4	121.0	142.2	60.5
70–74	106	38.0	184.2	233.8	92.4
75–79	76	23.2	218.4	260.1	149.5

1. Estimated incidence rate (per 100,000 men per year) among "smokers": 34.0 = 4.36 $\times$ 7.8 from equation (2.17).
2. Estimated incidence rate (per 100,000 men per year) among "nonsmokers": 7.8 = 30.1(1 − .74) from equation (2.20).

Source: Miettinen 1976a, based upon the case-control study reported by Cole et al. 1971.

estimated to have smoked 100 or more cigarettes during their lifetimes in this target population.

The last column of Table 2.10 reports age-specific estimates of the etiologic fraction. For example, if smoking were eliminated in this target population, an estimated 74 percent of the cases of bladder cancer in men 50–54 years of age may be prevented. The computations are based on equation (2.24). The estimated etiologic fraction of −.90 for men aged 60–64 indicates that if smoking were eliminated, there would be a 90 percent *increase* in the number of men with bladder cancer in this age group. Since this estimate is implausible on biological grounds, one should consider the possibility of error arising from sampling variability, from failure to control for important confounding variables, or from biased ascertainment of cases and controls. (Chapter 7 gives further details on estimating the etiologic fraction, including adjustment for bias from extraneous variables, calculation of standard errors, confidence intervals and tests of significance, and methods for combining estimates across strata.)

Table 2.11 shows for each age group the total number of new cases arising within the target population during the 18 month study period. (The data reported in Table 2.10 are based on a sample of these cases.) The yearly incidence rate, expressed per 100,000 men at risk, is derived from the first and second columns. Thus, 30.1 = [(35/77,400)/1.5] $\times$ 100,000. The divisor of 1.5 is used because 18 months corresponds to 1.5

years. The estimated exposure-specific incidence rates $\hat{p}_2$ and $\hat{p}_1$ are calculated from equations (2.20) and (2.17) using the corresponding estimates of p, ψ, and λ in Table 2.10. Thus $7.8 = 30.1(1 - .74)$ from equation (2.20), and $34.0 = 4.36 \times 7.8$ from equation (2.17). Note that the trend in $\hat{p}_2$ with increasing age is interrupted by the discrepant value of $\hat{p}_2 = 107.3$ for the age group 60–64 years. This results from the aberrant estimates of relative risk for this age group ($\hat{\psi} = .49$), and further reinforces the impression of error in the estimate at this age.

2.7 CUMULATIVE RISK OF DISEASE

If a case-control study is based on incident cases occurring over a specified interval of time, with controls for each case being chosen from among those who are disease-free at the time the case is diagnosed, then the odds ratio determined from a case-control study can be interpreted as the ratio of the instantaneous rates of disease in exposed versus unexposed groups of individuals (Sheehe 1962). This interpretation does not require any rare disease assumption (Miettinen 1976a).

Since the incidence rate of disease often depends on age in addition to other factors, one may want to know the cumulative risk of disease over an age span. This may be determined as follows. Suppose that: (1) individuals are grouped by age intervals $a_1, a_2, \ldots, a_t$; (2) that the corresponding widths (in years) of these intervals are $w_1, w_2, \ldots, w_t$; and (3) that the age-specific incidence rates (cases per person-year) are p_1, $p_2, \ldots, p_t$. If one assumes that the risk of disease can be approximated by an exponential distribution within each year (Chiang 1968, Chapter 12), then conditional on survival from other diseases, the probability of developing the study disease at some time during the age span from a_j through a_k may be estimated by

$$\mathcal{P} \simeq 1 - \exp\left[-\sum_{i=j}^{k} w_i p_i\right]. \qquad (2.25)$$

When $\mathcal{P}$ is small, it may be approximated even more simply by

$$\mathcal{P} \simeq \sum_{i=j}^{k} w_i p_i. \qquad (2.26)$$

Using equation (2.26) as an approximation to (2.25) may be regarded as using the value x as an approximation to $1 - e^{-x}$. For $\mathcal{P} < .01$, the error in the approximation is less than 0.5 percent. Morgenstern, Kleinbaum, and Kupper (1980) give further details concerning the derivation of equation (2.25).

If one has estimates of the exposure-specific incidence rates across age strata, equation (2.26) can be used to calculate the cumulative risk of disease over an age span for exposed and unexposed individuals. The preceding development can be applied to any dimension of time, including duration of exposure and time since discontinuation. Miettinen (1976a) provides details regarding tests of significance and confidence intervals for $\mathcal{P}$.

An example of the preceding considerations may be based on Table 2.11. Suppose that one wanted to estimate for a 50-year-old "smoker" the risk of bladder cancer developing at some time from 50 through 64 years of age. Using equation (2.26), one calculates $\hat{P} \simeq .0070$. Hence, for every 1000 men who have smoked 100 or more cigarettes by the time they are 50 years of age, 7 are expected to develop bladder cancer from 50 through 64 years. Corresponding estimates may be similarly calculated for nonsmokers.

From equation (2.26) one sees that $\mathcal{P}$ is essentially a weighted average of the age-specific incidence rates. One caveat regarding the interpretation of $\mathcal{P}$ concerns the assumption that the age-specific incidence rates p_i, which are based on a cross-sectional sample of the population, can be used to derive a longitudinal estimate of risk. Further problems can arise when one considers issues related to the exposure variable, such as duration, intensity, or reasons for discontinuation.

Consider a case-control study restricted to individuals within a specified age range. Suppose that one takes a random sample of cases and controls without regard to age, except that individuals must fall within the designated age span. Further suppose that one does not stratify the analysis on the basis of age. Let p_{1i} and p_{2i} denote respectively the age-specific risks of disease (assumed to be rare) among exposed and unexposed individuals. Then the corresponding risk of disease over the entire age range is given by $\mathcal{P}_1 = \Sigma w_i p_{1i}$ for exposed individuals and by $\mathcal{P}_2 = \Sigma w_i p_{2i}$ for unexposed individuals. One can show that the odds ratio calculated from the simple 2×2 table that ignores the age strata approximates $\mathcal{P}_1/\mathcal{P}_2$, which is based on a stratification of the age range in question.

2.8 ASSOCIATION AND TESTING FOR SIGNIFICANCE

The concept of *association* refers to a dependence, which may or may not be causal, between two or more variables. A statistical explication is made in terms of various measures of association, the correlation coefficient

Table 2.12. Prenatal Exposure to
Diethylstilbestrol (DES) Among Young
Women with Adenocarcinoma of the
Vagina and Among Controls

	Vaginal Cancer	Controls
DES:		
Yes	7	0
No	1	32
Total	8	32

Source: Herbst, Ulfelder, and Poskanzer 1971.

being a familiar example. The odds ratio and relative risk are two others.
In the context of the case-control study design shown in Table 2.5, an
association between exposure and disease is said to exist if the odds of
exposure, or equivalently the proportion exposed, differs significantly
between the cases and the controls. This implies that both the odds ratio
and the relative risk differ significantly from unity, both being either
increased or decreased. The standard chi-square test for a 2×2 table or
Fisher's exact test (Armitage 1971) may be used to test this condition.

Consider the data in Table 2.12 from a case-control study of vaginal
cancer in young women (Herbst, Ulfelder, and Poskanzer 1971). Eight
cases and 32 controls are classified according to whether or not they had
an *in utero* exposure to diethylstilbestrol (DES). The fact that 7 of the
8 cases and none of the 32 controls had such an exposure suggests an
association between DES and the development of vaginal cancer. As one
step in the analysis, one may consider calculating a test of significance. If
the observed outcome falls within reasonable limits of chance variation
under the null hypothesis of *no* association, there is little point in defend-
ing too strongly an interpretation of association based solely on the data
at hand.

Suppose that one had taken a case series from a target population in
a manner that assured that each case, irrespective of exposure, was
equally likely to appear in the sample. Assume that a similar selection
procedure had been used for controls (see Table 2.4). A test of association
between exposure and disease in the target population may then be made
by comparing the sample frequencies of exposure among cases and controls by means of the chi-square test for association (Chapter 7, Section
7.1).

The continuity-corrected value of chi-square with one degree of freedom (Chapter 7, Section 7.1) is calculated for the data in Table 2.12 to be $\chi^2 = 28.15$, yielding a p-value (two-sided) of $p \simeq 1 \times 10^{-7}$. Thus, under the assumption of no association, the chance of observing an outcome as extreme (or more so) than a $7/8$ vs. $0/32$ split would be less than one in 10,000,000.

A more appropriate analysis retains the case-control matching that was used in the study design. The Mantel-Haenszel test for association in matched samples (Chapter 7, Section 7.8) gives a chi-square value of $\chi^2 = 23.2$, with a corresponding p-value of $p \simeq 1.4 \times 10^{-6}$. For practical purposes, both matched and unmatched tests of significance give equivalent results, and they eliminate sampling variability as a reasonable explanation for the excess frequency of exposure to DES among the cases. One must admit, however, that the tests have excluded only one of many possible explanations.

A test of significance does not address the issue of whether an association is causal or whether it is due to some error resulting from a deficiency in the design, conduct, or interpretation of a study. Nevertheless, a test of significance is useful, if only to thwart the tendency to rash generalization based on "two men and a laboratory dog." Furthermore, a significance test provides a systematic approach to assessing uncertainty.

Just as a statistically significant result is open to a variety of interpretations, so too is a "nonsignificant" finding. An apparent association that is not significant by a formal statistical test may nonetheless derive from a causal dependence. The magnitude of the effect or the size of the sample may be insufficiently large to assure a high likelihood of meeting the test criterion, which itself, insofar as one uses $\alpha = .05$ or $\alpha = .01$, is rather arbitrary. A confidence interval provides one advantage over a test of significance, in that the limits of uncertainty are clearly stated. However, neither procedure addresses the issue of whether a lack of association has resulted from a study bias or from failure to adjust for extraneous variables. Either condition could obscure a true association.

In any observational study, a test of significance provides an imperfect assessment of whether "chance" alone might reasonably account for an apparent difference. With a comparative experiment that includes randomization in its protocol, the validity of the p-value as an assessment of the effect of chance is assured by the physical act of radomization (Fisher 1935). With observational data, the calculations are based on a model that is hypothetical. The same difficulty occurs with the calculation of confidence intervals (Kempthorne 1977). At best, a significance test or confidence interval can only eliminate sampling variability or chance as an explanation for an apparent association, leaving aside the more important issues concerning study bias and substantive interpretation.

2.9 RELATIVE RISK AS A MEASURE
OF THE STRENGTH OF ASSOCIATION

Despite pitfalls in the interpretation of relative risk, this parameter possesses several desirable properties that support its use in studies of disease causation. First, knowing the magnitude of the relative risk is helpful in assessing whether an apparent association is spurious. To clarify this point, suppose that a study exposure E apparently increases the risk of disease, so that the relative risk exceeds unity, $R > 1$. Next, assume that some other uncontrolled variable X, which does not interact with E, is postulated to account for *all* of the increased risk that is thought to be due to E. Then both of two conditions must be met (Cornfield et al. 1959).

(1) The factor X must be R-times more common among exposed individuals as compared with unexposed individuals:

$$P(X|E) > R \, P(X|\overline{E}).$$

(2) The uncontrolled variable X must be at least as strong a risk factor for the disease as the study exposure appears to be.

Conditions (1) and (2) provide some justification for the often-stated belief that a "large" value for a relative risk is unlikely to be completely explained by some uncontrolled variable (Schlesselman 1978).

In the present circumstance, "no interaction" between E and X is interpreted to mean that the relative risk of disease associated with exposure in the presence of X equals the relative risk of disease associated with exposure in the absence of X:

$$P(D|EX)/P(D|\overline{E}X) = P(D|E\overline{X})/P(D|\overline{E}\overline{X}).$$

As an example of the application of conditions (1) and (2) above, consider the finding from an early case-control study that oral contraceptive (OC) users aged 40–44 years had 2.8 times the risk of death from myocardial infarction (MI) as compared with non-users (Mann et al. 1975). Since cigarette smoking, which is a risk factor for heart disease, was not measured in this study, one might question whether the apparent increased risk could be explained by an excess of smoking among users of oral contraceptives. If smoking were to explain all of the apparent risk associated with oral contraceptive use, then in the absence of an interaction between smoking and OC use, two conditions must be met. First, smoking must be more than 2.8 times more common in OC-users as compared with non-users. Second, smoking itself must increase the risk of an MI more than 2.8 times. [Schlesselman (1978) has also discussed this example in terms of a potential interaction between smoking and oral contraceptive use (see Simon 1980, Schlesselman 1980).]

The relative risk parameter possesses the attribute that the presence of multiple real causes reduces the apparent relative risk for any one of them. That is, if the exposure under study is only one of many independent factors associated with the study disease, then the relative risk of disease in exposed individuals as compared with unexposed individuals will be closer to unity than if this is not the case (Cornfield et al. 1959, Cornfield and Haenszel 1960). The following paragraph gives the mathematical details of this statement.

Suppose that there are two risk factors for the study disease, the study exposure E and some other factor X. Let p_{11} denote the risk of disease in the presence of both E and X. Similarly, let p_{10} denote the risk in the presence of E and absence of X, p_{01}, the risk in the absence of E and the presence of X, and p_{00}, the risk in the absence of both E and X. Suppose that the proportion of the population exposed to X is p_x. By assumption, this is the same whether E is present or absent.

The risk of disease among individuals exposed to E is $r(E) = p_x p_{11} + (1 - p_x)p_{10}$ and the risk among the unexposed is $r(\overline{E}) = .p_x p_{01} + (1 - p_x)p_{00}$. If one further assumes that $p_{00} < p_{10}p_{01}/p_{11}$, then

$$r(E)/r(\overline{E}) < p_{10}/p_{00}$$

(Cornfield et al. 1959). The ratio p_{10}/p_{00} denotes the relative risk of disease associated with exposure to E among individuals in whom the risk factor X is absent.

The relative risk is sensitive to refinements in a classification of disease that distinguishes subtypes that are specifically affected by a causal factor. The relative risk of developing the undifferentiated disease is less than the relative risk of developing the type of the disease that is specifically affected by the study exposure (Cornfield et al. 1959).

The appropriateness of the relative risk parameter as a measure of the strength of an association has been extensively debated. Berkson (1958) argued that a relative measure is inappropriate and has advocated the attributable risk parameter $\delta = p_1 - p_2$. Cornfield et al. (1959) recommended the use of the relative risk, p_1/p_2, as the best measure of association for studies concerned with disease etiology. The preceding properties of the relative risk, which are not shared by the risk difference, were the basis of their advocacy. Fleiss (1981) reviews some other issues relating to this matter.

2.10 CONFOUNDING

The term *confounding* refers to the effect of an extraneous variable that wholly or partially accounts for the apparent effect of the study exposure, or that masks an underlying true association. Thus, an apparent association between an exposure and disease may actually be due to another variable. Alternatively, the apparent lack of an association could result from failure to control for the effect of some other factor. To take a simple example, suppose that one wanted to investigate by means of a case-control study the relationship between alcohol consumption and heart disease. In a comparison of cases and controls, one might find that the case group contained a greater proportion of smokers than the control group, since cigarette smoking is a risk factor for heart disease. At the same time, smoking is also known to be correlated with alcohol consumption. Thus, an apparent increased risk of heart disease found to be associated with alcohol consumption in fact might be due to cigarette smoking (Dales and Ury 1978). To assess this possibility, one may use the standard technique of stratifying cases and controls by smoking status, looking for an association between alcohol consumption and heart disease separately for smokers and for nonsmokers.

A *confounder* (confounding variable) is an extraneous variable that satisfies *both* of two conditions: (1) it is a risk factor for the study disease; and (2) it is associated with the study exposure but is not a consequence of exposure. In the preceding example, cigarette smoking is a confounding variable with respect to an association between alcohol consumption and heart disease.

A confounder's association with the study disease may be either cause-and-effect or a noncausal relation resulting from the confounder's association with causal factors other than the study exposure. Furthermore, a confounder's association with disease must occur in the absence of exposure (Miettinen 1974c). Figure 2.1 shows path diagrams (Wold 1956, Susser 1973) that illustrate situations in which a factor F is or is not a confounder for a disease-exposure association. In practice, any extraneous risk factor, which itself is not a consequence of exposure, may be regarded as a confounder if its control appreciably alters the estimate of an exposure's effect.

To explain confounding in terms of a data example, consider Table 2.13, which reports recent oral contraceptive (OC) use (last use within the month before admission) among 234 cases of myocardial infarction (MI) and 1742 controls (Shapiro et al. 1979). The acute risk of an MI

Figure 2.1.

(A) Situations in which F is a confounder for a disease–exposure association. ($\leftrightarrow$) non-causal association; ($\rightarrow$) causal association.

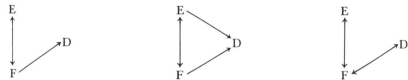

(B) Situations in which F is not a confounder for a disease–exposure association.

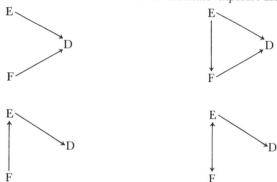

Table 2.13. Relation of Myocardial Infarction (MI) to Recent Oral Contraceptive (OC) Use

	MI	Controls	Estimated relative risk
OC			
Yes	29	135	$\hat{\psi} = 1.68$
No	205	1607	
Total	234	1742	

Source: Shapiro et al. 1979.

is estimated to be 1.7 times higher in OC-users as compared with non-users ($\hat{\psi} = 1.68$).

Suppose that one now stratifies cases and controls on the basis of current age (in years), as in Table 2.14. The age-specific relative risks exceed 1.7 in all but one instance, suggesting that the overall estimate $\hat{\psi} = 1.68$ is spuriously low. Table 2.15 confirms this impression and indicates the reason. Whereas controls are approximately uniformly distributed over the five age groups, roughly 20 percent occurring in each category, cases occur much more frequently in the older age groups. Furthermore, one

Table 2.14. Age-Specific Relation of Myocardial Infarction (MI) to Recent Oral Contraceptive (OC) Use

Age (yrs)	Recent OC use	MI	Controls	Estimated age-specific relative risk $(\hat{\psi})$
25–29	Yes	4	62	7.2
	No	2	224	
30–34	Yes	9	33	8.9
	No	12	390	
35–39	Yes	4	26	1.5
	No	33	330	
40–44	Yes	6	9	3.7
	No	65	362	
45–49	Yes	6	5	3.9
	No	93	301	
Total		234	1742	

Source: Shapiro et al. 1979.

Table 2.15. Distribution of Cases and Controls by Age, and Age-Specific Exposure Rates (%) from Table 2.14

Age (yrs)	Percent at each age MI	Controls	Age-specific percent of OC use MI	Control
25–29	2.6	16.4	67	22
30–34	9.0	24.3	43	8
35–39	15.8	20.4	11	7
40–44	30.3	21.3	8	2
45–49	42.3	17.6	6	2
Total	100.0	100.0		

sees that recent use of oral contraceptives is much less frequent among older women, both cases and controls. Thus, the analysis in Table 2.13 that ignores age is subject to a biased comparison, since there are proportionately more cases than controls in the older age groups. Because younger women are more likely to be recent users of oral contraceptives, the exposure rate in the controls is effectively overestimated relative to the case series.

Age, itself a risk factor for myocardial infraction, appears as a confounding variable in this example, because it is associated *in the sample* with both disease (case-control status) and exposure. The estimated relative risk, adjusted for age by the Mantel-Haenszel method (Chapter 7), is $\hat{\psi}_{mh} = 3.97$, suggesting a fourfold increased risk of an MI among recent OC users as compared with non-users.

A variable that is a confounder in the sample may be dealt with by adjustment procedures that rely on stratification or multivariate analysis (see Chapters 7 and 8), provided that one has data on the confounder in question. The need to control for a potential confounding variable by matching, stratification, or multivariate analysis depends on whether it has any residual association with exposure and disease after adjustment for other factors included in the analysis or sampling schemes. With correlated variables, adjustment for one may effectively dispose of the need to adjust for the other (Chapter 4).

In planning a case-control study, one should regard any known risk factor for the study disease as a potential confounder. The study design and analysis should be planned to either assess or eliminate the effects of such variables. The need to adjust for a potential confounder in the analysis depends on its association with disease (case-control status) and exposure in the sample. Variables that are not risk factors for the study disease may nonetheless be confounders as the result of unwitting selection bias introduced by the procedures used to obtain cases and controls. Thus, any variable that is related to exposure and that differentially affects the selection of cases or controls would be a confounder (Miettinen 1974c). [Yanagawa (1979) has discussed the concept of confounding in terms of a mathematical definition involving conditional odds ratios. Miettinen and Cook (1981) point out that the use of different measures of effect, such as the odds ratio, relative risk, and risk difference, can result in different assessments of confounding.]

Degree of Confounding

One should not think of confounding as an all-or-nothing property of any particular variable. It is a characteristic that occurs in varying degrees. An index of the degree of confounding is easily constructed. Let $\hat{\psi}_c$ denote the "crude" estimate of relative risk (odds ratio) based on an analysis that ignores a potential confounding variable, and let $\hat{\psi}_a$ denote the adjusted estimate, using, for example, the Mantel-Haenszel method (Chapter 7). One may consider the ratio $\hat{\psi}_c/\hat{\psi}_a$ as an index of the degree of confounding. For the data in Tables 2.13 and 2.14, $\hat{\psi}_c = 1.68$ and $\hat{\psi}_a = 3.97$. The ratio $1.68/3.97 = .42$ indicates that the crude odds ratio underestimates the adjusted value by 58 percent. Miettinen (1972) has proposed a similar method for assessing the extent of confounding (see Ejigou and McHugh 1977a, Miettinen 1977b).

Testing for Confounding

There is no generally agreed upon procedure for determining whether adjustment should be made for any given variable suspected of being a confounder. This is especially problematic when one has a comparatively large number of potential confounders. One common but questionable approach to screening such variables is to test for a significant difference between cases and controls. This approach to testing for confounding has been criticized on several grounds (Dales and Ury 1978, Greenland and Neutra 1980). First, even though a particular variable may show a statistically significant case-control difference, an adjustment may still be unnecessary because of a lack of association between that variable and the study exposure. Second, a nonsignificant difference may nonetheless be accompanied by a substantively important change between the adjusted and unadjusted estimates of the effect of exposure. Failure to achieve "significance," itself an arbitrary criterion with respect to the α-level, may simply be due to a comparatively small sample size. Third, the precise interpretation of a significance test based on observational data is moot. At best, the test can only address the issue of sampling variability, ignoring the far more important issue of study bias or errors of interpretation. Fourth, to conclude that a case-control difference could reasonably be due to "chance" is not pertinent to the question at issue, namely, "does $\hat{\psi}_c$ or $\hat{\psi}_a$ more correctly estimate the effect of exposure on disease?" Another complication arises if the effect of exposure is modified by the variable in question. If this occurs, then both a crude estimate and a summary adjusted estimate may be misleading.

In any analysis the choice of variables is largely a subjective matter. It should depend on one's hypothesized biological model for the disease process, and on one's assumptions regarding potential sources of bias that may distort the magnitude of the estimated association between exposure and disease. Beyond this, one can give little advice that will be incontrovertible. In practice, if adjustment for a variable makes no substantive difference in the analysis, then ignore it, even if the variable is "significantly" associated with both exposure and disease. Conversely, if adjustment for the variable yields a substantive difference, and if one's knowledge of subject matter indicates that the adjusted estimate is preferable, then adjust for the variable, even if the variable is not significantly associated with exposure or disease.

2.11 INTERACTION

One is often concerned with the way in which two or more potential risk factors act together. For example, consider two factors that are associated with the same disease. Suppose that some background level of disease is present in the absence of exposure to either factor, that persons exposed to both factors have the highest risk, and that persons exposed to only one factor have intermediate risk. The question arises whether persons exposed to both factors have a higher risk of disease than would be expected from a knowledge of their risks from exposure to each factor alone.

When the incidence rate of disease in the presence of two or more risk factors differs from the incidence rate expected to result from a combination of their individual effects, there is said to be *interaction* (MacMahon 1972). To the confusion of many, there is no single characterization of what to expect from a combination of risk factors. Expected behavior depends on the statistical model used to describe the biological process (Walter and Holford 1978). The statistical assessment of interaction, moreover, depends on the scale of measurement for the study variables and the measure used to assess a variable's "effect" (Mantel, Brown, and Byar 1977, Kupper and Hogan 1978). "Effect" may be measured in terms of a difference in risk, risk ratio, difference in log odds, etc. In practice, however, there are two alternative models, additive and multiplicative, that are often used to express the concept of interaction. They correspond to two different ways of measuring the effect of a risk factor. (The non-mathematically inclined reader may prefer to skip the next two sections at the first reading and proceed directly to the discussion that follows.)

Additive Model for Disease Risks

For simplicity, consider two dichotomous risk factors, x and y. Referring to Table 2.16, let p_{00} denote the incidence rate in the target population in the absence of both factors. Let p_{10} denote the rate when x, but not y, is present. Let p_{01} be the rate when y, but not x, is present, and let p_{11}

Table 2.16. Incidence Rates for Various
Combinations of Two Risk Factors, x
and y

	y	
x:	No (0)	Yes (1)
No (0)	p_{00}	p_{01}
Yes (1)	p_{10}	p_{11}

represent the rate when both x and y are present. Suppose that one uses a difference in incidence rates to measure the effect of one or more variables. Taking p_{00} as the reference, the difference $p_{10} - p_{00}$ represents the "individual" effect of x. That is, $p_{10} - p_{00}$ is the effect of x in the absence of y, but in the presence of other variables in the target population. Implicit in this definition is the assumption that, apart from the presence or absence of x, persons are otherwise at equal risk of disease, so that the difference in the rates measures the effect of x. As a practical matter, this assumption can never be completely verified in any observational study, and disputes over the interpretation of the apparent effect of a variable often center around the baseline comparability of the exposed and unexposed subjects. Putting aside this issue for the moment, and returning to the paradigm in Table 2.16, one may take the difference $p_{01} - p_{00}$ to be individual effect of y, and define $p_{11} - p_{00}$ as the *joint effect* of x and y.

If the joint effect of x and y equals the sum of their individual effects,

$$(p_{11} - p_{00}) = (p_{10} - p_{00}) + (p_{01} - p_{00}) \qquad (2.27)$$

then one may say that there is "no interaction." If the joint effect exceeds the sum of the individual effects, one may say that there is *synergism*, or that the two variables act synergistically. *Antagonism* may be said to occur if the joint effect is less than the sum of the individual effects (Blot and Day 1979). Synergism and antagonism are special cases of positive and negative interactions.

Table 2.17 gives a simple example of no interaction from the perspective of the additive model (2.27). Note that the additive model implies that the effect of x is homogeneous, in the sense that irrespective of the level y, the presence of x increases the risk by 6 units. A similar homogeneity of effect is also implied for y.

By dividing through by p_{00} in equation (2.27), a lack of interaction can be equivalently expressed in terms of *excess relative risk* (Cole and MacMahon 1971)

$$(p_{11}/p_{00} - 1) = (p_{10}/p_{00} - 1) + (p_{01}/p_{00} - 1). \quad (2.28)$$

Defining the relative risks $R_{xy} = p_{11}/p_{00}$, $R_x = p_{10}/p_{00}$ and $R_y = p_{01}/p_{00}$, one may express equation (2.28) as

$$(R_{xy} - 1) = (R_x - 1) + (R_y - 1). \quad (2.29)$$

Thus, an underlying additive model (2.27) for disease risks implies an additive relationship for the excess relative risks.

Multiplicative Model for Disease Risk

A second commonly used measure of effect is a multiplicative one, indicating by how much the baseline risk is multiplied in the presence of one or more factors. For example, suppose that the risk of disease in the absence of x and y is 3 per 1000, and that the presence of x increases the risk threefold, from 3 to 9 per 1000. Furthermore, suppose that the baseline risk of 3 per 1000 is increased fivefold by the presence of y, from 3 to 15 per 1000. If the effect of x is homogeneous, in the sense that its presence uniformly increases the risk threefold, irrespective of the level of y, then the risk of 15 per 1000 in the presence of y alone should be increased threefold by the presence of x, from 15 to 45 per 1000 (see Table 2.18).

Using a multiplicative measure, one may alegebraically express a homogeneous effect of x (no interaction with y) as follows:

$$p_{10}/p_{00} = p_{11}/p_{01}. \quad (2.30)$$

Table 2.17. Example of an Additive Risk Model

A. *Hypothetical Incidence Rates for Various Combinations of Two Risk Factors Based on an Additive Risk Model*

	Risk		Attributable risk	
	y		y	
x:	No	Yes	No	Yes
No	3.0	15.0	0.0[1]	12.0
Yes	9.0	21.0	6.0	18.0

B. *Measures of Effect Based on Attributable Risk*

Individual effect of x: $p_{10} - p_{00} = 6.0 = p_{11} - p_{01}$
Individual effect of y: $p_{01} - p_{00} = 12.0 = p_{11} - p_{10}$
Joint effect of x and y: $p_{11} - p_{00} = 18.0$ $(6.0 + 12.0)$

1. Reference group.

Table 2.18. Example of a Multiplicative Risk Model

A. *Hypothetical Incidence Rates for Various Combinations of Two Risk Factors Based on a Multiplicative Risk Model*

	Risk		Relative risk	
	y		y	
x:	No	Yes	No	Yes
No	3.0	15.0	1.0[1]	5.0
Yes	9.0	45.0	3.0	15.0

B. *Measures of Effect Based on Relative Risk*

Individual effect of x: $p_{10}/p_{00} = 3.0 = p_{11}/p_{01}$
Individual effect of y: $p_{01}/p_{00} = 5.0 = p_{11}/p_{10}$
Joint effect of x and y: $p_{11}/p_{00} = 15.0$ (3.0×5.0)

1. Reference group.

In words, the relative risk of disease associated with x in the absence of y is equal to the relative risk of disease associated with x in the presence of y. Referring to Table 2.18, $9/3 = 45/15$. Equation (2.30) implies that the effect of y is also homogeneous (no interaction with x). Rearranging terms, one has

$$p_{01}/p_{00} = p_{11}/p_{10}.$$

In words, the relative risk of disease associated with y in the absence of x is equal to the relative risk of disease associated with y in the presence of x. From Table 2.18, $15/3 = 45/9$. Either equation implies that no interaction between x and y involves a multiplicative relationship for relative risks. From (2.30), $p_{11} = (p_{10}/p_{00})p_{01}$. Dividing both sides by p_{00}, one has

$$p_{11}/p_{00} = (p_{10}/p_{00})(p_{01}/p_{00}). \tag{2.31}$$

Hence

$$R_{xy} = R_x R_y . \tag{2.32}$$

Using a logarithmic transformation, one has

$$\ln R_{xy} = \ln R_x + \ln R_y . \tag{2.33}$$

Thus, an underlying multiplicative model for disease risks

$$p_{01}p_{10} = p_{00}p_{11}$$

implies an additive relationship for the log relative risks.

Discussion

One sees from the preceding discussion that an assessment of interaction depends on the measure of effect. Since the statistical concept of interaction refers to departures from an additive relationship in a particular model, the presence or absence of interaction is a function of the chosen model or scale measurement (Mantel, Brown, and Byar 1977). For example, Table 2.18 indicates no interaction in terms of a multiplicative model. From the perspective of an additive model, however, one would argue that there is interaction between x and y.

As a public health concept, synergism refers to the situation in which the joint exposure to two or more factors results in a risk of disease that exceeds that expected from the sum of the risks from the separate factors. In this sense, synergism is a particular type of interaction, one based on departures from a model in which excess relative risks are additive [equation (2.28)]. We shall adhere to this distinction, even though it may result in speaking of synergism between factors that may not interact in a biological or mechanistic sense (Blot and Day 1979, Saracci 1980, Rothman, Greenland, and Walker 1980).

No exposure should be regarded in isolation from other factors that may affect the risk of disease. Furthermore, there is no a priori reason to expect that an exposure will elevate or decrease the risk by a constant amount or by a constant percentage irrespective of the baseline rates in the unexposed. This consideration is relevant when one encounters several case-control studies of a particular disease and exposure, each study being based on a different target population. The fact that the estimated relative risks may vary across the studies, assuming that they are consistently elevated or lowered, does not invalidate the existence of an association. What it does suggest is that the circumstances under which the risk is altered must be qualified. This emphasizes the need to state precisely the characteristics of the case and the control series that may relate to the development of disease.

A simple comparison of estimates of relative risk across several studies is often not appropriate. The size of a relative risk depends on the prevalence of other risk factors in the population and the magnitude of the risks associated with them. Although this point has been emphasized within the context of a particular model of risk (Peacock 1971), it applies generally and forms the basis for the recommendation that the characteristics of the population from which cases and controls derive be identified and temper the interpretation of a study (Dorn 1951). The comparison of relative risks across different studies should be based on estimates that have been adjusted for the same major confounding variables. The use of standardized rates rather than crude rates is a well-known and commonly employed technique of adjustment used to avoid biased comparisons of incidence and prevalence rates (Hill 1971, Fleiss 1981). The use of adjustment applies to a comparison of relative risks estimated from case-control studies. Techniques for estimating an adjusted relative risk, using stratification or logistic regression, are given in Chapters 7 and 8.

2.12 SUMMARY

Typically a case-control study can only estimate the relative risk in terms of its odds ratio approxiamtion, $\hat{\psi}$ from equation (2.9). However, if the control series can be regarded as a random sample from a defined population, then the exposure rate in the controls, $\hat{p}_e$ from equation (2.23), can be used as an estimate of the exposure rate among individuals in the population who are free of the study disease. Given estimates $\hat{\psi}$ and $\hat{p}_e$, one can then estimate the etiologic fraction λ by use of equation (2.24).

If, in addition to the estimates $\hat{\psi}$ and $\hat{p}_e$ based on a case-control study, one has an estimate, from an external source, of the disease incidence rate in the population of interest, $\hat{p}$, then one may estimate the exposure-specific incidence rates $\hat{p}_2$ and $\hat{p}_1$ by use of equations (2.16) and (2.17) respectively. The attributable risk can then be estimated as $\hat{\delta} = \hat{p}_1 - \hat{p}_2$.

3 Planning and Conducting a Study

Paul D. Stolley
James J. Schlesselman

3.0 INTRODUCTION

In this chapter, the reader will be taken step-by-step through the procedures necessary to plan and conduct a case-control study. These include: (1) stating the research question; (2) clearly defining the disease under study and the exposures of interest; (3) selecting the cases; (4) defining and selecting a control group; (5) developing and testing the research instruments; (6) conducting field operations; and (7) planning the analysis.

3.1 STATING THE RESEARCH QUESTION

Experienced researchers generally devote a considerable amount of time and energy to planning a study. A research question may be put forth first in a broad and ambitious fashion, unsuitable for a specific investigation. This initial formulation serves little purpose beyond pointing to a general problem of interest or a potential question. The original statement is inevitably narrowed and made more precise as a study is designed to evaluate aspects of one or more specific hypotheses. Issues such as the populations available for study, the possibilities of obtaining pertinent information on the exposures of interest, and other constraints such as time and cost, often lead to a modification of the original question, so that usually only a portion of the larger, more general question will be approached by any single investigation.

An example of this evolution is illustrated by the following reformulations of a research question, which successively reduce the scope of a study at the same time that they provide a feasible approach. Thus, "What are the causes of lung cancer?" may be restated with increasing specificity and precision as follows:

- Does exposure to products of combustion or particulates cause cancers of the respiratory system?

- Does smoking cigarettes or breathing asbestos fibers cause bronchogenic carcinoma?

- Is an increased risk of bronchogenic carcinoma associated with cigarette smoking and/or exposure to asbestos?

- Do persons who have developed bronchogenic carcinoma have a history of greater exposure to cigarette smoke and/or asbestos fibers than persons who are spared this disease?

A research question or group of questions should be a list of hypotheses that can be tested, at least within the limitations of the methods available to study the issue. A hypothesis is a predictive statement about relationships between independent and dependent variables. In the example above, cigarette smoking and exposure to asbestos fibers are the independent variables, whereas lung cancer is the hypothesized dependent variable. The predictive statement implicit in the research question is that "if one smokes cigarettes or breathes asbestos fibers, one increases one's risk of developing lung cancer." From the perspective of a case-control study, this statement may be rephrased as follows: "In comparison with individuals who remain free of lung cancer, individuals who develop this disease will have had a history of greater exposure to cigarette smoke and asbestos fibers."

The independent variable, cigarette smoking, can be categorized by type of cigarette (filter, non-filter), method of smoking (inhalation or not), duration of smoking in years, amount smoked (packs per day), and so forth. Exposure to asbestos might be expressed, for example, in terms of employment in occupations that handle asbestos, as in mining, manufacturing, or construction, the age at onset and duration of such employment, and the degree of contact with asbestos fibers. The separate and joint effects (interactions) of smoking and asbestos exposure may also be assessed.

In addition to collecting information on the primary exposures of interest, one should also gather data on potential confounding variables in order to rule out alternative explanations for the apparent presence or absence of an association. If the investigator does not list all of the hypotheses and subhypotheses at the beginning of a study, he or she runs the risk of not obtaining the requisite information. If the research question is not precisely defined, the approach to answering the question may also lack clarity, thereby jeopardizing the entire enterprise. A hypothesis must therefore be fully elaborated. Even within the confines of a study designed to address a narrowly specified hypothesis, one may want to gather some data on factors that may provide new leads regarding other potential causes of the study disease. Thus, an analytic study may well have an exploratory component.

3.2 DEFINITION OF CASES

Eligibility

The definition of a "case" is critical to the case-control study. It involves two distinct specifications: (1) establishment of objective criteria for the diagnosis of the study disease; and (2) a statement of eligibility criteria for the selection of individuals for study.

Eligibility criteria are established to restrict the study to persons who were potentially at risk of exposure. Such criteria *should be applied equally* to potential cases and controls. Thus, for example, in a study of a hypothesized association between recent (past-month) oral contraceptive use and myocardial infarction, all women who are postmenopausal, are surgically sterilized, or who have chronic diseases that contraindicate the use of oral contraceptives should not be eligible for study. Hence, a 35-year-old woman who was admitted to hospital with a diagnosis of definite MI would be ineligible if she had been sterilized one month or more before admission. Similarly excluded from study would be a 35-year-old woman admitted for treatment of a fractured arm (a potential control), if she were diabetic, this condition being a contraindication for use of the Pill. Such women (both cases and controls) would not have been at risk of recent exposure to oral contraceptives, and inclusion of ". . . them in a case-control study would represent effort wasted on studying persons whose experience was not pertinent to the investigation."

Criteria for exclusion depend on the definition of "exposure." Thus, if one were interested in past exposure to oral contraceptives, the exclusion of women who have been sterilized recently would be inappropriate if the operations occurred after the period of risk under consideration.

One must also be wary of excluding subjects on the basis of conditions that in fact may be consequences of the exposure under study.

Eligibility criteria can be applied either in the selection phase or in the analysis of a study, whichever is operationally more convenient. Exclusion of ineligible subjects in the selection (sampling) phase avoids the unnecessary collection of data on individuals who would later be ignored in the analysis. Although it is best to state clearly and in advance of the study the eligibility criteria to be used, one may nonetheless choose to apply them at the time of analysis, particularly in exploratory case-control studies in which several hypotheses may be under consideration, each implying a somewhat different set of exclusions.

Jick and Vessey (1978) have emphasized that cases included for study should have some reasonable possibility of having had their disease induced by the exposure under investigation. Failure to observe this restriction would dilute any association that might be present. For example, in a study of the relationship of oral contraceptive use to thromboembolism, cases of thromboembolism occurring during pregnancy or immediately postpartum should either be excluded or studied separately, since complications of pregnancy are the most likely causes. Similarly, postoperative thromboembolism should be considered separately from "idiopathic" disease, since surgery is a sufficient cause of the former condition and the effects of oral contraceptive use may differ for the two (Jick and Vessey 1978).

A criterion customarily employed in defining the case series is the requirement that they be newly diagnosed or incident cases of the disease. Since diagnostic fashions change periodically, one expects that recent diagnoses will be more uniform than those drawn from different time periods. Furthermore, recall of past events in personal histories should be more accurate in cases diagnosed close to the inception of an investigation, although if the latency period is long, recall of exposures in the distant past may still be inadequate. One can also be more certain that recalled exposures preceded the diagnosis, rather than followed it, in recently diagnosed cases. Other issues regarding the use of incident cases are discussed in Chapters 2 and 5.

Definition of Disease

Establishing objective criteria that lead to a reliable diagnosis of disease can be difficult at times. Consider, for example, rheumatoid arthritis. This exceedingly common disease can present with a myriad of signs, symptoms, and laboratory test results of varying sensitivity and specificity. In addition, the variation among different observers who interpret the physical signs can be very striking. Thus, the investigator is faced with the question of what evidence will be required for the diagnosis of rheumatoid arthritis. A partial list of the manifestations of this disease follows:

Symptoms

- Fatigue
- Morning stiffness
- Joint pain, warmth, and tenderness

Signs

- Fever
- Weight loss
- Joint swelling
- X-ray changes of osteoporosis and joint erosion

Laboratory Findings

- Positive test for rheumatoid factor
- Elevated erythrocyte sedimentation rate

What combination of signs, symptoms, and laboratory results will be chosen to define a "case" for an investigation? Will the definition be consistent with other studies previously reported? These are the questions the investigator must first ask.

Fortunately, for many diseases expert committees have established criteria for diagnosis that permit standardized definitions. These allow comparisons to be made among studies by different investigators. Table 3.1 shows an example of uniform criteria for the diagnosis of rheumatoid arthritis.

At times, a subclassification of the disease entity into "definite," "probable," and "possible" is needed, as shown in Table 3.2. This provides a breakdown by diagnostic certainty. If such a scheme actually distinguishes the certainty of diagnostic categories, the "definite" group should have fewer "false positives" among them, whereas the "possible" group would have more "false positives." The group of lowest diagnostic certainty, the "possible" group, is likely to be diluted with nondiseased individuals or individuals with a disease different from the one under

Table 3.1. American Rheumatism Association Criteria for the Diagnosis of Rheumatoid Arthritis

Criteria

Morning stiffness

Pain on motion or tenderness in at least one joint

Swelling (soft tissue thickening or fluid—not bony overgrowth alone) in at least one joint continuously for more than six weeks

Swelling of at least one other joint (any interval free of joint symptoms between the two joint involvements may not be more than three months)

Symmetric joint swelling with simultaneous involvement of the same joint on both sides of the body (bilateral involvement of proximal interphalangeal, metacarpophalangeal, or metatarsophalangeal joints is acceptable without absolute symmetry; distal interphalangeal joint involvement will not satisfy this criterion)

Subcutaneous nodules over bony prominences, on extensor surfaces, or in juxta-articular regions

Radiologic changes typical of rheumatoid arthritis (must include osteoporosis localized to, or greatest around, the involved joints, not just degenerative changes; degenerative changes, however, do not exclude the diagnosis of rheumatoid arthritis)

Positive test for rheumatoid factor (any test modification will suffice that does not give more than five percent positive results in nonrheumatoid control subjects)

Poor mucin precipitate from synovial fluid (shreds and cloudy solution)

Characteristic histologic changes in synovial membrane including three or more of the following: marked villous hypertrophy; proliferation of superficial synovial cells, often with palisading; marked infiltration of chronic inflammatory cells (lymphocytes or plasma cells predominating) with tendency to form "lymphoid nodules"; deposition of compact fibrin, either on the surface or interstitially; foci of cell necrosis

Characteristic histologic changes in nodules; granulomatous foci with central zones of cell necrosis, surrounded by proliferated fixed cells; and peripheral fibrosis and chronic inflammatory cell infiltration, predominantly perivascular

Diagnosis

Definite rheumatoid arthritis
    Diagnosis calls for at least five of the above criteria with a total duration of joint symptoms for a continuous period of at least six weeks

Probable rheumatoid arthritis
    Diagnosis requires at least three of the above criteria and a total duration of joint symptoms of at least four weeks

Possible rheumatoid arthritis
    Diagnosis requires two of the following criteria and total duration of joint symptoms of at least three weeks: morning stiffness, tenderness or pain on motion with history of recurrence or persistence for three weeks, history or observation of joint swelling, subcutaneous nodules, elevated sedimentation rate or C-reactive protein, iritis

Source: Ropes et al. 1959.

Table 3.2. Criteria for Classification of Pulmonary Embolism by Certainty of Diagnosis

Diagnostic Certainty	Evidence Required
Definite pulmonary embolism	A positive pulmonary angiogram and/or lung scan
Probable pulmonary embolism	ECG suggesting embolism and chest X-ray compatible with embolism and typical history
Possible pulmonary embolism	A typical history and chest X-ray, other studies not done

study. As a result, an effect of exposure would be diminished when estimated from a comparison of this group with the control series.

The classification of cases on the basis of diagnostic certainty provides one approach to dealing with misclassification, a problem that can occur for both the disease and the exposure variables. This can result in biased estimates of relative risk, and is discussed more fully in Chapter 5.

Sources of Cases

Cases can be identified through regional disease registries, records of large ambulatory-care practices, or admissions to one or more clinics or hospitals (Table 3.3) Each method of case finding has limitations and advantages. Ease of case finding may, for example, be balanced by biased referral or incomplete ascertainment. The potential biases and limitations of each method must be explored before committing the study to a particular case finding method.

In hospital-based case-control studies, cases and controls can often be selected from admission logs or lists of discharge diagnoses. If a disease registry is in existence, such as a tumor registry or registry of heart disease, cases can be selected from these specialized sources. On rare occasions, cases can be selected from communities where special surveys have been carried out and the health status of the resident individuals is known. In Olmsted County, Minnesota, all major medical care is obtained from a single source, the Mayo Clinic and its affiliated hospitals. Since medical information is centrally recorded, this system permits the identification of cases for case-control studies (Kurland, Elveback, and Nobrega 1970). Case-control studies have also been done within residential retirement communities served by a single health plan (e.g., Mack et al. 1976)

Table 3.3   Possible Sources of Cases for Case-Control Studies

Hospitals (all, or some, in a community)
Disease or tumor registries, such as the Surveillance, Epidemiology and End Results
    Network (SEER Network 1976)
Vital Statistics Bureau (all deaths in an area)
Ambulatory care practices (all cases seen in a large group practice)
Cases in a defined geographic area ascertained through record linkage, such as the
    Oxford Record Linkage System (Acheson 1967)

3.3 DEFINING A CONTROL GROUP

Definition

A control group is used to compare the history of exposure in the cases
with that in individuals who are free of the study disease. The control
series is intended to provide an estimate of the exposure rate that would
be expected to occur in the cases if there were no association between the
study disease and exposure (Chapter 1). Individuals selected as controls
should not only be free of the study disease, but should also be similar to
the cases in regard to past potential for exposure during the time period
of risk under consideration. Stated somewhat differently, controls should
be comparable to the cases in the sense that both groups would have been
at equal risk of exposure if there were no disease-exposure association
(Cole 1979). Unfortunately, these prescriptions fail to provide an
unequivocal criterion for the selection process. Furthermore, the achievement of comparability need not be restricted to the process of defining
and selecting the control series. It may be partially accomplished in the
analysis, either by exclusion of certain cases and controls through the use
of preestablished criteria, or by means of statistical adjustment for confounding variables (Chapter 7).

Sources

In general, controls may be selected either from hospitals or from the
community. If cases are chosen from a hospital or group of hospitals,
considerations of practicality and cost often confine the selection of controls to persons admitted to the same hospitals but with a disease or condition different from that under study. Such persons are called *hospital
controls*. The other source of a control group is the nonhospitalized community or geographic area from which the cases arose. Persons selected

from such a source are often called *community controls* or *population controls*. They are often chosen according to a probability sampling procedure based on census tracts or random digit dialing (Section 3.4).

In some circumstances, friends, neighbors, relatives, or associates of cases may serve as a convenient and appropriate source of controls. For example, in a study of the possible relationship of diethylstilbestrol to testicular cancer, controls might be selected by asking each friend who visited a case to nominate an individual who could be entered into the study as a control.

Jick and Vessey (1978) and Cole (1979) have stressed that past emphasis (Feinstein 1973) on the acquisition of a "representative" sample of cases and controls has been misplaced, since it has been urged not for reasons of generalizability, but rather for validity. In fact, a valid study may be carried out in a highly restricted group of individuals. Thus, a study of the relationship of benign liver tumors to the use of oral contraceptives could be confined to cases occurring in nurses (Jick and Vessey 1978). Since this occupational group may have distinctive contraceptive habits, one would likely also choose controls from among nurses. Although, strictly speaking, the findings would apply only to nurses, the detection of an effect of oral contraceptive use would probably be construed, on biological grounds, to apply more generally.

Eligibility Criteria

The requirement that controls be similar to the cases in regard to past potential for exposure during the time period of risk under consideration implies that certain individuals will be ineligible for study. For example, women who were more than one month pregnant or who are sterile would not be eligible as controls in a study of whether recent (past-month) use of oral contraceptives increased the risk of myocardial infarction. Similarly excluded would be postmenopausal women. Such exclusions *should* apply equally to the case series (Section 3.2).

The development of eligibility criteria tends to be more problematic in hospital-based studies, although some guidelines have been suggested. In principle, one wants to select a control series from hospital admissions that are likely to reflect the exposure rate to the study factor in the population from which the cases arose. The removal from the control series of individuals with conditions known to predispose to or against the study exposure is therefore often done.

Jick and Vessey (1978) have proposed that in hospital-based case-control studies, individuals who are identified by medical conditions or backgrounds that are known to be associated (positively or negatively) with the exposure under study should be excluded from the control series. For example, a study of the relationship of aspirin consumption to acute myocardial infarction *should* exclude from the control series patients admitted to hospital because of chronic arthritis (who would likely have excessive aspirin use) and those admitted because of chronic peptic ulcer disease (who would likely have decreased aspirin use). The reason for such exclusions is that an estimate of the exposure rate from a control group that includes individuals predisposed to or against the study exposure can be altered by simply adjusting the "patient mix" of the control series. Furthermore, the representation of such patients in the hospital setting as compared with their occurrence in the target population is unknown. As a consequence, one is quite uncertain whether the estimate of the exposure rate derived from hospital controls that include such persons, whether or not selected at random from within the hospital setting, would be similar to the exposure rate based on a sample of individuals from the target population who are free of the study disease.

An example of the problems encountered in deciding on exclusion criteria is provided by a hospital-based case-control study of the relationship of oral contraceptive use to thromboembolism (Stolley et al. 1975). Patients admitted for the treatment of biliary tract disease (cholecystitis) were initially eligible as controls. During the course of this investigation, however, another research group published a report that implicated oral contraceptive use with increasing the risk of cholecystitis (Boston Collaborative Drug Surveillance Program 1973). Stolley et al. (1975) were able to confirm this finding, and also demonstrate that retaining patients with biliary tract disease in their control series would have lowered the estimated risk of thromboembolism associated with use of oral contraceptives.

One tactic for minimizing bias due to overrepresentation of persons with diseases associated with the exposure variable is to take hospital controls from a variety of diagnostic groups that are believed to be unassociated with the study exposure (Mantel and Haenszel 1959, Jick and Vessey 1978). This protects against two sources of error: (1) claiming that exposure affects the risk of the study disease, when in fact the effect of exposure is really linked to the diagnosis from which the controls were drawn; and (2) failure to detect an effect of exposure because the study and the control diseases are both associated with it (Mantel and Haenszel 1959). When the control series comprises a variety of diagnostic groups, one may compare the rates of exposure across these subgroups. Adjusted for confounding factors, the exposure rates should be similar, if in fact the diagnostic categories are unassociated with exposure. Although this condition must be met to guarantee a lack of association, it is insufficient, because the exposure rate in all of the subgroups could be biased to the same degree.

The inconsistent findings with respect to an association between coffee drinking and myocardial infarction provides another example of the difficulties in the choice of hospital controls. Two hospital-based case-control studies estimated that the risk of myocardial infarction in heavy coffee drinkers was twice that in nondrinkers (Boston Collaborative Drug Surveillance Program 1972, Jick et al. 1973). Population-based studies, however, showed little or no association between coffee drinking and cardiovascular disease (Klatsky, Friedman, and Siegelaub 1973; Dawber, Kannel, and Gordon 1974; Hennekens et al. 1977). A subsequent hospital-based case-control study (Rosenberg et al. 1980) suggests a reason for the discrepancy in the findings. In this study, women 30–49 years of age with first infarctions were compared with controls whose admissions were for acute emergencies. The relative risk of a myocardial infarction in women drinking at least five cups of coffee daily, as compared with women drinking none, was 1.4, after adjustment for all identified potential confounding factors (95% confidence interval, 1.0–1.9). However, the frequency of coffee drinking among patients admitted for chronic conditions was lower than that among persons admitted for acute emergencies. Since patients of the former type may tend to avoid coffee, their inclusion in the control series of the previous hospital-based studies may have led to an overestimate of the relative risk.

There is still uncertainty concerning the extent to which persons with diseases known to be positively or negatively associated with the study exposure should be excluded from the control series. This is unquestionably one of the thorniest problems in hospital-based studies. Although general guidelines have been proposed, their specific application leaves considerable room for doubt. For example (Cole 1979), should one exclude persons with conditions believed to have very weak associations (positive or negative) with the study exposure? If so, what should be the cutoff point for making the decision? What about conditions for which an association is merely speculative? How does one establish exclusion criteria for exploratory studies that involve numerous possible causes, many of which are not highly credible? If exclusions are used, to what extent does one consider current conditions as opposed to the total medical history? If the latter were taken to be relevant, would one also exclude cases on this basis? The preceding questions inevitably arise at the stage of protocol development. The answers are often highly specific to the investigations being planned and invariably depend on one's understanding of the disease process and hypotheses concerning the pathways by which an exposure is presumed to affect the disease under study.

3.4 METHODS OF SELECTING CASES AND CONTROLS

Sampling Procedures

Having defined the eligibility criteria for cases and controls and having specified the sources from which they will be drawn, one must next specify a method for selecting the study subjects. (Discussion of the size of the investigation is deferred until Chapter 6.)

Ideally, one wants a method for the *unbiased ascertainment* of eligible cases and controls and a procedure for the selection of a sample from them in a manner that assures that each individual has an equal chance of appearing in the study. Unbiased ascertainment means that the identification of an eligible case or control does not depend on an individual's exposure status in regard to the study factor(s). In practice, most case-control studies use all eligible cases arising within a defined period of time. With cases derived from a disease registry that provides complete coverage for a geographic area, the only sampling involved is the implicit sampling on the dimension of time and, perhaps, severity of illness. With cases arising within a given hospital or medical practice, one is implicitly sampling from a subset of the total population of cases of interest.

Sampling considerations per se are often most pertinent to the selection of the control group, since with rare diseases the number of eligible controls available for study greatly exceeds the number of cases. Several strategies for the selection of subjects are available, and examples given later in this section will illustrate their application. Texts by Cochran (1977) and Kish (1965) may be consulted for details of sampling methodology; our discussion is taken from these sources.

One may regard a case-control study as an investigation of disease-exposure associations within some population. The term *population* refers to a collection of individuals defined by time, place, and characteristics such as race, sex, age, etc. We shall use the term *target population* to refer to a subset of the general population that is both at risk of the study exposure(s) and the development of the study disease.

A variety of sampling procedures can be used for the selection of cases and controls. In practice, several are often used at various stages in the sample design. Sampling is done from a *frame,* which conceptually is a list of potentially eligible cases and controls in the target population. An actual listing is often too difficult to establish, so that any procedure that is equivalent to such a list is also called a frame. A disease registry or hospital admission list often serves as a frame for the selection of cases. Controls may be selected from similar lists or by procedures that are conceptually equivalent. The frame may not provide complete coverage of the target population. As a result of incomplete ascertainment, the frame may be biased, often in unknown ways. This in turn can lead to a biased sample, even though probability sampling procedures are used.

Random sampling refers to a method of selecting individuals from a frame such that each possible sample has a fixed and determinate probability of selection. In practice, one often uses *epsem* (equal probability of selection method) sampling, in which each of the population elements has an equal probability of selection. In multistage sampling designs, epsem can result from either equal probability of selection throughout or from variable probabilities that compensate each other through the several stages of the selection process.

Systematic sampling refers to the sequential selection of individuals, conceptually separated on lists by an interval of selection. In brief, one selects every kth individual who is eligible for study. *Stratified sampling* involves the selection of individuals at random from defined subgroups (strata) of the target population. One may select a sample of different size from each stratum, so that the total sample size is made up of subgroups of possibly differing size. *Matched sampling* (matching) involves the pairing of one or more controls to each case on the basis of specified variables, the effects of which one wants to eliminate from the case-control comparison (Chapter 4).

The objective of any sampling procedure is the avoidance of biased selection. That is, each eligible case in the target population, irrespective of exposure, should ideally have an equal chance of appearing in the study. Similarly, each eligible control, whether exposed or not, should also have an equal chance of selection. (The selection probability for cases will ordinarily differ from that for controls; see Chapter 2.) Thus, a sampling procedure is intended to avoid overrepresentation or underrepresentation of exposed cases and exposed controls in the study at hand.

If one has a procedure for ascertaining all incident cases occurring within a geographic area in a defined period of time, then the use of controls selected at random from the general population is undoubtedly the option of choice. With a properly designed and implemented sampling procedure, an unbiased selection of controls can be assured. Furthermore, the absolute risks of disease associated with the presence or absence of exposure can often be determined, because the size of the populations at risk is frequently known from census information. Thus, one would have a sound basis for estimating not only the relative risk, but also the attributable risk, the exposure-specific risks, and the etiologic fraction (Chapter 2).

If cases are ascertained through admissions to a single hospital or network of hospitals, an imputed greater validity of a population-based control series, as compared with hospital controls, is often moot. In principle, a valid control series can be selected from hospital admissions. For some research questions, a hospital-based study is clearly the best approach. A study of the relationship of oral contraception to congenital malformations (Bracken et al. 1978), for which the sample design will be presented shortly, provides an example. One must admit, however, that in many situations the use of hospital controls leaves more room for doubt about the validity of the comparison, because it is a matter of judgment whether the procedures for the selection process are equivalent to a random selection from all potentially eligible controls in the target population (barring a design that employs both types of controls). Nevertheless, considerations of practicality and cost often lead one to the use of hospital controls.

Examples of Case-Control Selection

In practice, sampling procedures for the selection of cases and controls are implemented in diverse ways, and the reader can best gain some appreciation for this topic by reviewing several examples. The Prologue describes the sampling procedures for an exploratory case-control study (Herbst, Ulfelder, and Poskanzer 1971), done principally within a single hospital, which investigated various maternal and other factors potentially associated with vaginal cancer in young women. Other examples follow:

ARTIFICIAL SWEETENERS AND HUMAN BLADDER CANCER
(HOOVER AND STRASSER 1980)
Cases comprised all residents aged 21–84 who were newly diagnosed with a histologically confirmed carcinoma of the urinary bladder (or pap-

illoma not specified as benign) in designated counties in the metropolitan areas of Atlanta, Detroit, New Orleans, San Francisco, and Seattle, and in the states of Connecticut, Iowa, New Jersey, New Mexico, and Utah. Cases with previous lower-urinary-tract cancers were excluded. The cases were found through the Surveillance, Epidemiology and End Results Network (SEER Network 1976) and the New Jersey Cancer Registry.

Controls were an age- and sex-stratified random sample of the general populations of the ten geographic areas, frequency matched at a 2:1 ratio of controls to cases. Controls aged 65–84 were randomly sampled from the files of the Health Care Financing Administration, which enumerated an estimated 98 percent of individuals over age 65 in the United States. Controls aged 21–64 were selected in a three-stage process: telephone numbers were chosen at random from all residential telephones in the ten geographic areas; an interviewer called each number and recorded the age and sex of each household member aged 21–64; a stratified random sample was then selected from the household censuses.

ORAL CONTRACEPTION AND CONGENITAL MALFORMATIONS
(BRACKEN ET AL. 1978)
Cases of congenital malformations, confirmed by an examination by an internist or pediatrician associated with the study, were drawn principally from all newborns and stillborns delivered at five major Connecticut hospitals between November 18, 1974, and November 17, 1976. In addition, newborns and stillborns delivered at the same hospitals in the preceding six-month period were included, even though controls were not taken during that time. These sources provided 1189 cases. Two other sources provided 181 cases: (1) all newborns delivered elsewhere between May 18, 1974, and November 17, 1976, and referred to the five hospitals before one year of age, and (2) infants less than one year of age identified at two pediatric clinics.

Controls were obtained by sampling all unaffected newborns in the five study hospitals between November 18, 1974, and November 17, 1976. The number of controls required from each hospital was estimated as three times the anticipated case load. On each sampling day, controls were selected by systematic sampling of the patients who had delivered. The sampling days were rotated so that all days of the week were equally represented in each seven-week period. The total number of controls was 12.4 percent of all deliveries in the five hospitals, and the final control-to-case ratio was 2.3:1.

SMOKING AND CANCER OF THE LOWER URINARY TRACT
(COLE ET AL. 1971)

An attempt was made to identify all persons with a neoplasm of the lower urinary tract, newly diagnosed during the 18 months ending June 30, 1968, among 2,800,000 residents of the Boston and Brockton Standard Metropolitan Statistical Areas (SMSA) in eastern Massachusetts. All the 96 hospitals within and 15 of the larger hospitals peripheral to the study areas cooperated. To ensure maximum case finding, a search was made through the pathology log in each hospital for each day of the study period. In all, 722 cases were identified, but only 668 patients were deemed "eligible" for interview. They were 20 to 89 years of age and had cancer consisting of transitional or squamous-cell elements alone or combined. Of these, 657 cases were reviewed and confirmed as such. Eleven patients for whom histologic specimens were unavailable were included on the basis of hospital pathology reports.

For reasons of economy, it was decided to interview only about 500 each of the eligible cases and controls. These were selected at random from persons 20 to 89 years of age, since the rosters from which controls were selected did not include younger persons, and it was thought that older persons might give unreliable histories.

Each of 87 cities within the study area published an annually updated "residents list." These lists were expected to include all residents 20 years of age and over, whether citizens or not. Together, the lists constituted the roster from which controls were selected. Of the 458 cases of bladder cancer identified during 1967, 96 percent were located in the lists, suggesting that the lists were quite complete, at least for persons in the bladder-cancer age range, and that patients and controls were comparable in this respect.

For each calendar year of the study, every person included in the residents list of that year had a probability of being selected as a control equal to that of every other person of the same sex and age, irrespective of residence. This was done by a compilation of two sampling frames of names drawn at random from the residents lists of 1967 and 1968. The number of names included from each city was such that the total contributed to the sampling frame would be proportional to that city's contribution to the adult population of the study area.

Controls were drawn from the 1967 or the 1968 sampling frame for cases diagnosed in 1967 or 1968, respectively. For each of the 668 eligible cases, the sampling frame of the appropriate year was entered at random, and the first person listed of the same sex and year of birth as the patient was designated a control. Of 552 controls selected at random for interview from among these 668, 18 could not be located. Of the remaining 534, 500 (93.6 percent) were interviewed.

Random-Digit Dialing

The selection of controls from a population with extensive usage of telephones in households can be facilitated by the use of *random-digit dialing*. This is undoubtedly the most important innovation in survey sampling in the United States in the past decade. Random-digit dialing is based on the random selection of four-digit numbers within existing telephone exchanges. It avoids biases incurred in sampling from frames based on telephone directories, which do not contain unlisted numbers, and it is far more efficient than unrestricted random dialing, since approximately 80 percent of numbers are not assigned to households. Random digit dialing may be used for telephone interviewing or as a method for screening potential controls for eligibility. In the latter application, a sample of eligible controls for home interview is selected at a second stage of the sampling scheme, an approach used in the population-based case-control study reported by Hoover and Strasser (1980).

To implement the Waksberg (1978) method of random-digit dialing, one obtains from American Telegraph and Telephone a recent computer tape of all telephone area codes and existing prefix numbers within the target areas. To these one adds all possible choices for the next two digits, thereby obtaining a list of all possible first eight digits of the ten digits in telephone numbers. Treating the eight digit numbers as primary sampling units (PSU), one first selects a PSU at random (epsem), and then appends the two last digits, also selected at random. This number is dialed, and if a residence is reached, the PSU is retained in the sample. Additional last two digits are selected at random and dialed within the same eight-digit group. This continues until a fixed number, k, of residential telephones is reached. If the original number called was nonresidential, the PSU is rejected. The process is repeated until a predesignated number of PSUs, m, is chosen. The values of m and k are based on optimal design considerations (Waksberg 1978). The monograph by Groves and Kahn (1979) should be consulted for additional details.

3.5 DEVELOPING THE RESEARCH INSTRUMENT

Construction of a Questionnaire

The historical information sought in a case-control study can be obtained at times from existing documents such as hospital records, industrial work records, and health insurance records. More often, this information will supplement data obtained through direct communication with the study subjects, in person, by telephone, or by mail. Thus, the research instruments needed for case-control investigations usually include record abstract forms and standard interviews or questionnaires.

Although sociologists, as well as marketing research organizations and public opinion pollsters, have conducted extensive research on the personal interview as an information-gathering technique, medical scientists have only recently addressed this problem. A surprisingly modest amount of research has been devoted to establishing techniques for obtaining reliable and valid medical information, validating this information, and asking sensitive questions while encouraging high response rates. Fortunately, the emergence of medical sociology as a discipline has improved the situation. As a consequence, our knowledge of how to phrase questions, approach respondents to obtain accurate information, and establish unobtrusive measures and methods of checking the correctness of replies has grown. The book by Bennett and Ritchie (1975), which is devoted entirely to the medical questionnaire, is a brief, excellent, and valuable aid to the investigator; it served as the basis of this section.

A common error in developing a medical interview or questionnaire is to begin simply by writing questions. A more appropriate starting point is the construction of a list of pertinent variables, including the level and extent of information needed. One then writes questions that will obtain the required information as it is likely to be used in the analysis. For example, consider planning a study of the relationship of oral contraceptives to thrombophlebitis. Women would be questioned about their use of birth-control pills before the onset of the condition. The variable "use of oral contraceptives" can be categorized as follows:

1. Type(s) used (content and dosage):
   (a) sequential or combined
   (b) type of estrogen and dosage in micrograms.
   (c) type of progestogen and dosage in micrograms.

2. Number of months taken (duration of use).
3. Pattern of use (constant, interrupted, or discontinued).
4. Interval between initial use and development of disease.

Obviously, such a list dictates constructing a more detailed set of questions than merely "Did you ever use oral contraceptives?"

Investigators commonly employ two types of questions in interviews and questionnaires: *open-ended* and *closed* questions. The closed question allows a limited number of responses, leaving little room for the subject to volunteer additional information. The advantages of the closed format are greater precision, uniformity, and easier coding and tabulation of responses. Its disadvantage is limiting the variety and amount of data collected. For example, consider the following closed question:

When I climb three flights of stairs rapidly, I feel:

	Yes	No
Short of breath	——	——
Cramps in my calves	——	——
Pain in my chest	——	——
A rapid heartbeat	——	——

If the subject wishes to clarify or amplify his response (e.g., type of chest pain, location, severity, or radiation) he cannot do so. If climbing three flights produces an additional symptom, such as "light-headedness," it is lost to the investigator. If only one flight of stair-climbing produces symptoms, this detail is not obtained.

The open-ended question attempts to gather more information with minimal precategorization by the questioner. Using the same example as above, the open-ended approach might be:

"When you climb three or fewer flights of stairs rapidly, do you notice anything unusual happening to you?"

The questioner records the responses, which are then categorized and coded for analysis at the end of the study. While such a mode of questioning may provide more information, it may also present problems in coding responses. Instead of giving the forced response "short of breath," a patient with dyspnea may reply:

"I breathe hard"

"I gasp for breath"

"I am short-winded"

"I take deep breaths at the end"

"I wheeze"

"I am breathless"

Thus, the investigator must create a symptom dictionary that can be used to identify a patient's response as a synonym for dyspnea.

Open-ended questions require respondents to recall and explain things, whereas closed questions demand only recognition. Closed questions also discourage explanation and elaboration. Clearly, studies of attitudes and beliefs and attempts to describe or elaborate upon symptomology are restricted by the closed-question format. On the other hand, data collection for most large case-control studies is best accomplished by this approach. Open-ended questions are lengthy, require greater skill and probing by the interviewer, and are time-consuming to code.

Phrasing the question in a manner that can be understood by the respondent is an important consideration in questionnaire development. For example, if, in a general health questionnaire, one seeks to detect a recent decrease in libido, the question might be worded:

"Have you noticed a recent fall-off in your sexual urge or desires?"

For a different study population, the same information might be presented:

"Have you noticed a recent fall-off in your 'nature'?"

"Nature" is a colloquial term for libido among members of certain cultural groups. Using the term with college-educated persons, however, might totally mystify them.

The wording of a question should also strive for the least amount of ambiguity. An ambiguously worded question may ask:

"Do you have trouble with your muscles?"

But what muscles are referred to? The heart is a muscle as well as the biceps. Is the trouble a "charley-horse" of an athlete with well-developed muscles or atrophy and weakness in a polio victim? A common form of ambiguity results from questions in which the replies encouraged are not mutually exclusive, such as:

"Do you have trouble with your eyes, ears, or sense of smell?"

A positive reply may indicate difficulty with any one of the three sensory organs, or any combination of the three.

This last example points to the importance of properly sequencing questions. Doing so allows the questioner to cover all important variables and avoid wasting time on irrelevant items. To determine if a cough occurs in the morning, produces phlegm, contains blood in the phlegm, or leads to paroxysms of coughing resulting in fainting, one must start with "Do you cough frequently?" If the answer is negative, the sequence delineating the characteristics of the cough can be skipped, because a person who never coughs may find questions about the characteristics of a nonexistent condition very confusing.

The interviewer's attitudes as perceived by the subject and the phrasing of the questions are factors known to influence response. The respondent often wishes to please the questioner, and may give an answer that he believes will gratify the interviewer or gain approval. Sometimes the respondent wishes to conceal information, such as a psychiatric problem, venereal disease, or drug ingestion.

In a study investigating the relationship of excessive analgesic use with subsequent renal disease (interstitial nephritis), a review of previous work suggested that patients who used analgesics heavily had a tendency to conceal this behavior (Murray et al. 1980). To encourage full revelation of such habits, the questions broaching this matter were introduced as follows:

"When people have minor illnesses such as headache, backache, or joint pain, they often try to relieve their discomfort. We have all, at one time or another, been faced with an ailment that required relief. Here is a list of ways people try to relieve this kind of distress. . . ."

The whole tenor of this question is nonjudgmental. The approach encourages the respondent to view himself as part of a large group of persons whose acceptable behavior, in the face of certain afflictions, would include use of analgesics.

Another way of handling sensitive or embarrassing topics involves presenting cards that carry the possible responses. The subject points to the response relevant to his experience and need not articulate the sensitive response. This approach might be employed, for example, in a study of the relationship of cervical carcinoma to coital frequency and number of sexual partners.

Many studies have considered the relative merits and problems of collecting data through the self-administered questionnaire as compared with using a trained interviewer. The self-administered form often produces less information than one administered by an interviewer. It also eliminates the ability to probe for additional information or assess the emotional response to the questions. Advantages of the self-administered questionnaire versus the interview include:

1. Greater standardization in the presentation of material
2. Elimination of interviewer bias
3. Reduced cost through savings in time and effort in administering the questionnaire
4. Easier questioning of large numbers of persons
5. More leisurely, and possibly more careful, responding allowed.

In many studies, however, the disadvantages outweigh the advantages. They include:

1. General limitation to only simple, closed, and restricted choice questions
2. Requirement of a high rate of literacy and reading ability
3. Inability to probe for subtleties or qualification of response
4. Lack of assurance that the questionnaire is answered by the intended respondent, and alone
5. Lack of opportunity to observe emotional responses
6. Inability to clarify questions or responses.

Reliability and Validity

Concurrent with the development of the interview or questionnaire, the investigator should consider how a respondent's answer might be validated. Ideally, there should be some mechanism for checking the accuracy of the "soft" measurements that are obtained through such research instruments. The measurements are referred to as "soft" because, to a large extent, the data regarding exposure and other historical facts are made up of utterances based on fallible memories. These recollections may be made under conditions that pose, for the interviewed subjects, no special motivation to be precise, complete, and straightforward. Methods to validate responses vary from modest consistency checks built into the questionnaire to exhaustive searches for corroborating sources.

A *reliable* questionnaire is one that collects information that is replicable; checks on repeatability assure reliability. One approach to assessing reliability involves reinterviewing a sample of the respondents and comparing the responses given on the first and second interviews. The reinterviewing may be done using the same interviewers. This approach holds constant the effect of variability among interviewers, while measuring the consistency of the subject's recall. Alternatively, one may employ different interviewers on the first and second interviews of the same person. This approach not only measures consistency of recall but also variation in response to different interviewers. Another approach to assessing reliability involves repeating questions in a slightly different form at different points in the interview in order to check for consistency of response.

A *valid* questionnaire measures "that which it is purported to measure." Bennett and Ritchie (1975) subdivide validity into three components:

1. Relevance: Does the questionnaire obtain the information it was designed to seek?
2. Completeness: Was all desired relevant information obtained?
3. Accuracy: Can reliance be placed upon the responses to the questions?

One approach to assessing validity involves obtaining confirmatory information from several supplemental sources and comparing the rates of agreement. With this approach, a patient's recall of drug use is compared with the records of prescribing physicians, pharmacists, hospitals, or clinics. Interviews with close relatives may also corroborate some of the responses. This technique was employed in a study of the role of oral contraceptives in the development of thromboembolism (Stolley et al. 1978). Specifically, reports of oral contraceptive use were checked against the records of the prescribers with respect to the names of the drugs, the dates, and the duration of use. For women who reported a history of OC use within two years of hospitalization and who provided the names and addresses of physicians or clinics that prescribed hormones during the preceding two years, an attempt was made to contact the prescribers and request information on these prescriptions. It should be recognized that, strictly speaking, such a procedure measures the consistency between two sources rather than the accuracy of the user's statements, since the prescriber's records may be incomplete.

One aspect of research instrument validation concerns the possibility that the method of gathering information may differ between the cases and controls. A difference could result from interviewer bias (if the interviewer were aware of the hypothesis and probed more deeply when eliciting histories from the cases as compared with the controls), or from "wise" cases (who may deliberately overestimate or underestimate exposures to suspected causal factors if they are aware of the investigator's hypothesis). A validation strategy in this situation could compare the information obtained from cases whose diagnosis was confirmed with the information obtained from "false positives," cases whose first diagnosis was later altered. The consistency of interviewer probing of cases and controls could also be revealed from the interviews of the "false positives," since their responses should be similar to those of the control series. This tactic also provides a test for a respondent's bias in reporting a history according to whether he thinks that he does or does not have the disease in question.

An additional method for checking the veracity of data collected in an interview or from medical records uses research instruments with built-in test items that measure internal validity. Information can be obtained on the use of drugs directly relevant to the investigation, as well as on other drugs that are known to be irrelevant to the study disease or that are prescribed because of it. With this technique, a systematic bias can be examined, since cases and controls should be comparable in regard to histories of use of the irrelevant drugs and should show differences on those that are used for treatment. Finally, one may also ask questions that can have only one reasonable answer.

Whichever approach is adopted, the final reporting of study results should include a statement reflecting the attention given to the problem of validating the information, a practice that is commonly overlooked.

3.6 INFORMED CONSENT AND CONFIDENTIALITY

The medical questionnaire or interview must frequently probe the deeper levels of a person's private experiences. To reconstruct the milieu before the onset of disease, questions must often cover aspects of personal and family disease histories, including sensitive facts such as educational level attained, income bracket, age, and even, on occasion, sexual habits. Such intrusion inevitably raises issues concerning the right to privacy and to protection from exploitation of delicate material.

An investigator has a well-defined set of obligations to the individuals who become part of his or her study. These responsibilities are better delineated for experimental research and have been put forth in the Helsinki Declaration of the World Medical Assembly (Hill 1971), in the British Medical Research Council's Statement on Responsibility in Investigations on Human Subjects (Hill 1971), and by the Department of Health and Human Services (formerly Department of Health, Education and Welfare) of the United States of America (Code of Federal Regulations 45 CFR 46, 1978). Although case-control investigations do not involve administering or withholding therapies, they do obtain personal information and consequently involve ethical issues relating to "informed consent" and confidentiality.

The investigator must obtain an individual's consent before entering him or her into the study. Furthermore, in granting such consent, the individual should understand the general nature and purpose of the study, the possible risks and benefits, and his or her right to withdraw from the study at any time without prejudicing present or future treatment. The Clinical Center of the National Institutes of Health (USA) has published guidelines (NIH Clinical Center 1977) that define how and when informed consent should be obtained and how it should be documented.

Assuring informed consent is not always as straightforward as it sounds. Explaining complicated medical research problems can be difficult, requiring considerable planning and thought. Simple language, even slang or colloquialisms, are often necessary. Studies have shown that surprisingly large numbers of persons who give "informed consent," when tested a short time later, actually recalled very little of the document to which they affixed their signature (Robinson and Merav 1976). One should, however, distinguish between recall and understanding. The assessment of an individual's comprehension of material is far more problematic than measuring his ability to recall specific items on the consent form (Meisel and Roth 1980). Patients may well understand information at the time of giving consent but have difficulty recalling it later.

Before adopting a consent form, one should run a pilot test to remove ambiguities, complex language, and inconsistencies. Ideally, both a written document and an oral statement, with an opportunity to question the investigators, should be employed. An example of an informed consent statement is shown in Figure 3.1.

Numerous techniques can be used to help guarantee that the information collected from each individual is held in confidence. Almost immediately, the participant's name can be removed from documents and replaced by a code that is known only to the principal investigator or a key research associate. In the case of exceedingly sensitive information, elaborately "scrambled" or "hashed" codes can be used both for identification and for responses to questions. Original documents should be stored in locked file cabinets, with access to files and storage rooms made available to authorized staff only. Work areas for coding or review of data may be separated from other office functions. After the data are transferred to computer files, the original documents should be kept in a secure area or destroyed. Finally, all personnel should be instructed to refrain from discussing any personal aspects of the data collected. The best assurance of confidentiality undoubtedly lies in the quality and integrity of the research staff.

3.7 PILOT TESTING

After the study protocol and research instruments have been developed, they should be tested in a small-scale feasibility study ("pilot test") to allow for last-minute alterations in design. In the pilot testing phase, the investigator may uncover any number of problems. Following the protocol developed for case-finding and selection, he or she may have difficulty locating enough subjects with the disease of interest from the sources initially demarcated for study or encounter unexpected problems in verifying diagnoses. The pilot test may reveal that the procedure devised for control selection is inadequate; with case-control matching, for example, the criteria may prove too stringent to be productive. By administering the interview or questionnaire to a sample of study subjects, the investigator may find that too few relevant questions are asked or that some questions are improperly phrased. Items may be ambiguous or loaded with meanings that suggest unintended responses. The subjects may find the questionnaire too long and tiresome, or they may be upset by the manner in which embarrassing topics are handled.

Of course, a pilot test also strengthens the investigator's confidence in those procedures that run smoothly. Sometimes one unexpectedly discovers sources of supplemental data. For example, if valuable information

Figure 3.1

CONSENT FORM FOR INTERVIEW
(Cases)

I have been informed that (name of collaborating center), in collaboration with the United States Center for Disease Control, is
conducting a study of the health of women. The purpose of the study
is to look at why some women develop tumors and others do not. Women
with tumors and women without known tumors (who have been scientif-
ically selected) are being surveyed. I understand that I have been
asked to participate because I have recently been diagnosed as having a tumor.

I freely agree to take part in this study, understanding that it
involves: (1) Being interviewed for approximately 45 minutes concerning information about my medical history as well as other
information about my health, about my pregnancies, the medications
I use, and my monthly cycle; (2) Having my medical and laboratory
records reviewed.

I understand that my participation is entirely voluntary and that I
may refuse to answer any questions if I choose, or may withdraw my
consent to participate at any time without penalty or without in any
way affecting the health care I receive. I understand there are no
special risks involved in being a participant, and that, even
though I will not benefit individually, it is expected that other
women will benefit from the knowledge gained from the study.

I understand that the information collected about me will be
treated in a confidential manner and that I will not be personally
identified in the reporting of the results. Up to 20,000 women will
be interviewed and my answers will be combined with theirs to make
totals.

I understand that I may ask any questions I have about the study at
this time. If I have further questions about this study, I may contact (name, address, phone no. of appropriate person at the collaborating center).

_____   _____
Participant's signature & date   Interviewer's signature & date

1 copy for participant
1 copy for interviewer

Source: Ory 1979.

is found to be easily obtained from clinic records, a provision for abstracting this data may be added to the protocol. In any case, modifications in
design prior to launching the full-scale study may rescue an otherwise
problematic research effort and in the long run be cost-efficient.

Pilot testing is also useful for checking interviewer performance, standardizing techniques across different interviewers, and augmenting interviewer training and skills. The interviewer is the significant intermediary
between the investigator and the subjects, and any personal ineptitudes,
biases, or questionable integrity can defeat a study design that was otherwise carefully developed. The pilot phase can often reveal incipient
problems in this regard.

Some examples may best illustrate the importance of pilot testing. In
a questionnaire devoted in part to uncovering a patient's history of headaches, the following series of questions was developed:

—Have you ever had frequent headaches? (Yes)   (No)
  Age first noted
—Have you ever had very severe headaches? (Yes)   (No)
  Age first noted
—Have you had headaches once a week or more during the past
  month? (Yes)   (No)

After asking the third question, the interviewer was instructed as follows:

"If YES [on third question], ask Headache Series; otherwise, go to
page 9."

The intention underlying this sequence was to identify persons with
recurrent headaches, who consequently might be prone to use analgesic
drugs. The third question was included under the assumption that recall
is better for the most recent period, and that a person with a history of
recurrent headaches in the past would retain this pattern in the present.
Only when the questionnaire was pilot tested did the investigator realize
that the wording of this question led to a loss of information. Many
patients gave a positive response to having had frequent and severe headaches. However, the subsequent headache-related questions dealing with
drug use were often not asked, because for some subjects the past month
was atypical, headaches not occurring. The question was therefore modified to read:

Have you ever had headaches once a week or more for at least one month? (Yes) (No)

As another example, an investigator studying analgesic-associated nephropathy was interested in the history of drug use with respect to the time of disease onset. He needed to determine which of several dates to employ as the cutoff point for recording drug use and the proper source for this information. The following information was needed: (1) the patient's age when kidney disease was first noted; (2) the year the patient was first hospitalized for kidney disease (time of tests and diagnosis); and (3) the year the patient began renal dialysis.

The pilot test indicated which dates could be obtained reliably. Furthermore, the interview revealed that patients tended to recall better the date of first dialysis (the more recent event) than the date of the hospitalization when the diagnosis was made (the more distant event). The investigators also found that the medical records from the dialysis unit frequently replaced the "date-of-diagnosis" by the "date-of-first-dialysis" whenever information on "date-of-diagnosis" was unavailable.

3.8 PREPARING FOR AND CONDUCTING FIELD OPERATIONS

Before field operations can be initiated, the investigator must secure approval from the medical institutions responsible for the patients who will serve as cases or controls. The appropriate committees or individuals in the hospitals, clinics, or private medical practices should receive the study protocol, a copy of the questionnaire, the medical chart abstract form, the statement of "informed consent," and other relevant documents. The protocol and research instruments are then approved, rejected, or altered (in a mutually agreeable fashion) to conform to the institutions' research guidelines. Because the investigator usually encounters delays in obtaining institutional approval, it is wise to begin this process early.

If the study design calls for hospitalized patients, the protocol must be sent (together with a cover letter elaborating the nature, scope, and objectives of the study) to the approval boards of each hospital to be recruited for the study. The formal appeal to these boards usually consists of requesting permission to gain access to hospital records (such as daily admissions lists, discharge lists, and medical charts), and permission to approach the patients for interview. Sometimes separate approvals are required from the attending physicians of patients entering the study.

Once approval is received, additional solicitations for cooperation may be directed to the heads of the relevant hospital clinical departments (e.g., the head of the coronary care unit in a study of myocardial infarction), and to the head nurses of the hospital floors that may provide study subjects.

If the study plan involves cases from disease registries, approval of private physicians must usually be obtained before contacting the patient at home. If the study includes deceased cases, the investigator must obtain authorization from the State Health Department and the Vital Statistics Bureau to procure the death certificates of interest.

Quite often the investigator works from within a university setting. Most academic institutions require that research plans be submitted to a committee on human experimentation set up to review the ethics, motives, and conduct of medical research.

The preparation of the study materials for institutional review and the subsequent contact with committee chairmen to monitor the progress of the review requires a great deal of time, energy, and organization. A staff member should compile a formal record of all approvals and refusals to avoid confusion or possible litigation risks later. Occasionally, the investigator must adjust the sample composition, the size of the study, or the time frame for completing the field operations when hospitals initially counted upon to join decline to participate.

Once the process of approval is underway, the investigator should begin recruiting and training personnel who will interview subjects and abstract records. The text by the Survey Research Center (1976) provides a good source of information on interviewer training and technique. The interviewers most commonly sought are experienced nurses. Interviewer training involves an orientation to the study goals and familiarity with the questionnaire and all its subtleties. Usually the interviewers (or a supervisor) are given the responsibility for identifying, according to detailed sampling instructions, cases and hospital controls from the hospital admission or discharge lists. The interviewers should thus be trained in the principles of random selection and matching, as well as in interviewing techniques. The interviewers should also be impressed with the importance of the confidentiality and safety of the information entrusted to them by patients, physicians, and relatives.

Medical students or nurses are often recruited to abstract the medical charts. The abstractors are trained in the criteria used for the diagnosis of the disease in question and in the pertinent historical factors that must be compiled from the files. In multi-institution studies, assurance of standard procedures may require training key personnel, such as interviewers, abstractors, and supervisors, at a single site.

The compliance of the staff with established standards is best assured through regular monitoring during the conduct of the study. In view of the importance of their work, interviewers and abstractors should be carefully supervised and, at times, "refreshed" through special sessions.

The identification of cases and controls and the collection of data can become a complicated venture, particularly if a multicenter study is involved. As an example, one study of the relationship of endometrial cancer to estrogens was based on more than 500 cases occurring in six hospitals in Baltimore during a three-year period (Antunes et al. 1979). The logistics involved in organizing such a project were formidable. Each hospital required a unique system for both the identification of eligible cases and the random selection of eligible controls. Interviewers had to be sent to each hospital and to participants' homes in different parts of the city. Record abstractors had to visit each of the hospitals repeatedly in order to abstract patients' charts. The study necessitated interviewing the patients' physicians by telephone, and tissue specimens had to be collected from archives in the departments of pathology and transported to a central laboratory for independent review. As the initial field work got underway, preparations had to be made at the coordinating center for the receipt, checking, coding, and storage of documents arriving from the field. The development of computer programs for data editing and statistical analysis also had to be done prior to receipt of the data.

The importance of carefully planning each phase and operation of a study and attending to details at the outset cannot be overemphasized. Likewise, good management and organization are critical to a smoothly functioning enterprise, especially in studies involving large numbers of subjects or many separate centers. Planning, protocol development, and pilot testing can easily consume a year's effort in complex investigations.

3.9 PREPARATION FOR DATA ANALYSIS

Many investigators like to sketch the analyses of the major study questions by creating sets of skeleton or "dummy" tables. These are outlines of tables with the legends in place. This exercise forces the investigator to specify the important comparisons and categories required in the analysis, which in turn helps ensure that the needed data will actually be obtained. If crucial tables are not thought out and planned at the very beginning of an investigation, it is possible that important data will not be collected.

With the proliferation of "sophisticated" methods of data analysis, such as logistic regression or loglinear models (Chapter 8), the investigator is often tempted to immediately apply such techniques to the emerging data. We regard this approach as unsound, and instead recommend a more orderly application of analytic methods, beginning with simple descriptive statistical displays and summaries. Gaps, patterns, and inconsistencies in the data can be discovered and further analyses suggested by this examination. Next, relationships between variables can be explored by means of simple cross-tabulations, scatter plots, and measures of association, such as crude and adjusted estimates of relative risk (Chapter 7). Once again, patterns and inconsistencies are sought and, when found, lead to additional tabulations. Finally, multivariate methods may be applied to the data after a full exploration has been conducted using simpler techniques.

Concern is sometimes expressed that an early analysis of data may bias an investigator, since knowledge of preliminary results may affect the subsequent collection and interpretation of data. We find this to be a weak objection that is vastly outweighed by the advantages of interim analyses. Some of these advantages include the discovery of errors of omission of important data or other design errors. These can often be identified and corrected at an early stage, thereby salvaging that aspect of the study affected by such errors. An example of such an error involved coding "no use" of a drug as "continual use" due to a printing error. This mistake was detected in the preliminary analysis, which allowed an early correction to be made and avoided the loss of considerable staff time, which would have been needed to recode the data at the completion of the study. Sometimes leads are found in a preliminary analysis that suggest that insufficient detail is being acquired on important risk factors for the disease of interest. The questionnaire may then be revised at an early stage to collect the relevant information.

Much of the projected analysis can be planned and prepared for before the actual data are received. Often, the data will suggest further analysis, and rigid planning may commit the investigator to the use of inappropriate and uninformative analytic methods better avoided. While granting agencies demand a detailed plan of analysis before funding, considerable flexibility and multiple options should be preserved. There is undoubtedly no single "best" way to design a study of a particular question. However, "anticipatory" data analysis and planning tends to clarify the research design, prevents failure to collect crucial information, and promotes rigorous thinking about the relationships between variables.

3.10 CHECKLIST FOR PROTOCOL DEVELOPMENT

The following checklist is designed to assist the investigator in preparing a protocol for a case-control study. While some of the questions will not be appropriate to the particular investigation planned, most will be relevant, and perusal of this list should remind the researcher of points or issues that might otherwise be overlooked.

Checklist for Preparation of a Protocol for a Case-Control Study

I. Background

1. Have you comprehensively reviewed the literature concerning the problem? Have important previous findings been critically evaluated? Have you reviewed the results of animal and human experiments, clinical studies, vital statistics, and previous epidemiologic studies?
2. In what important areas is new knowledge needed? Will the proposed study answer previously unanswered questions or confirm work that requires additional corroboration?
3. What is the ultimate goal and significance of the research, and who will benefit from its findings?

II. Research Question

1. What is the immediate purpose of the investigation? Will the study be "exploratory" or "analytic"?
2. What are the major hypotheses? Are they stated clearly, concisely, and in such a way that they can be tested?
3. Are you trying to investigate too many questions in one research project?
4. Are both the disease and the exposure variables clearly defined? Is the exposure determined with respect to age at initiation of exposure, duration of time exposed, and time since discontinuation?
5. Do you plan to inquire about the reasons for initiation or discontinuation of exposures, such as drugs or medical devices?
6. Will a gradient of exposure be determined in the search for a dose-response relationship?
7. Do you consider investigating the joint effects of the risk factors under investigation?
8. Are all pertinent risk factors included in your investigation—environmental, genetic, and socioeconomic?

III. Research Design

1. Is the case-control strategy the method of choice? Is a cohort study or an experiment feasible or desirable? Justify the case-control approach.
2. Are the numbers of cases and controls required to answer the question possible to obtain? What is the smallest relative risk detectable by the study?
3. Does the study design incorporate blinding where feasible?

IV. Case Definition and Selection

1. Are the "cases" defined precisely? Are criteria for inclusion and exclusion comprehensive and clear?
2. Do the cases represent "incidence" or "prevalence" of the disease? Can the use of prevalent cases be justified?
3. Will cases be drawn from a population defined geographically and/or temporally?
4. What technique will be employed to ascertain cases and obtain a sample? Are the ascertainment and sampling techniques independent of the exposure status of the cases?

V. Control Definition and Selection

1. Will control subjects be hospitalized patients, residents of a community or geographic area, or both? How many controls per case will be selected? Can you justify the control:case ratio chosen?
2. Will control subjects, if selected from a hospital population, be drawn from a variety of admission diagnoses or from a few? What types of patients will be excluded, and why?
3. Do the exclusion criteria for the cases also apply to the controls, and vice versa?
4. Has a scheme for the random selection of controls been devised? Is the sampling technique independent of the exposure status of the controls?
5. Will individual or frequency matching of controls to cases be employed? On what variables, if any, will you match? Why? Could the purpose of matching be accomplished as well by analytic techniques such as post-stratification?

VI. Informed Consent and Confidentiality

1. Do all subjects have an opportunity to exercise their right to informed consent? Is the consent form likely to be intelligible to all subjects?
2. Has the consent form, as well as the entire study design, been approved by the appropriate review committee(s)?
3. How and where will completed data forms be stored to ensure confidentiality? Has a system been devised whereby each individual's identity will remain confidential throughout the analysis and reporting of study results?
4. Have steps been taken to secure the consent of participating hospitals and physicians whose patients will be approached to participate in the study?

VII. Resources Needed

1. What is the organizational structure for the study? How will it be managed? Are responsibilities clearly delineated?

2. Have you listed all the personnel and equipment needed for the study and explored their availability?

3. Have you budgeted realistically for the required resources?

4. Have you arranged for any needed collaboration? Are there written agreements with your collaborators? Have you obtained the required institutional approval for the investigation?

VIII. Study Conduct

1. Will the research instrument(s) be an interviewer-administered or self-administered questionnaire? Will the interview be conducted in person or by telephone? Will hospital records or other sources of information require abstracting? Do you need to develop special forms for recording data from slides, laboratory tests, or physical examinations?

2. Have you listed all the variables you wish to measure and checked to see if your instruments collect the required data with the detail necessary for the analysis? Will the data sources provide information of comparable detail for the cases and controls? Are you collecting information on possible confounding factors?

3. What are the logistic considerations in the efficient collection of data? Have items of questionable importance or those that are unnecessarily redundant been eliminated?

4. Have you pretested the research instruments? Can you employ any methods to improve recall, such as pictures, lists, etc? Can you evaluate the reliability and validity of the instruments?

5. Who will be responsible for collecting the data and maintaining quality control? Who will have responsibility for the daily supervision of staff?

6. Can variation within and among different observers influence the data? Can it be measured and controlled?

7. Have interviewer, abstractor, and coder manuals been written? Have all the variables been defined clearly?

8. Are the personnel collecting the data thoroughly familiar with the research instruments? Will special training sessions be conducted?

9. Does the research instrument lend itself to precoding?

10. Will computerized data files be established in such a way that information is easily retrievable through the use of standard data management and statistical packages?

IX. Data Analysis

1. How, in general terms, will the data be handled in the analysis? What are the exposure variables of primary interest, and how will they be defined for purposes of analysis? What provision has been made for the assessment of dose-response relationships, including intensity, duration, time of onset, and discontinuation of the exposure(s)?

2. In assessing a particular disease-exposure association, what other risk factors must be considered for adjustment to eliminate a biased comparison?
3. How will potential interactions among exposure variables and other risk factors be assessed?
4. Are matched or stratified analyses planned to correspond to a matched or stratified design?
5. Will the case series and the control series be subdivided to detect potentially different effects of exposure among hypothesized susceptible subgroups?
6. Can analyses be done to evaluate alternative hypotheses of how an exposure may alter the risk of disease?
7. What attempts will be made to investigate possible sources of bias and their influence on the results?
8. How will the effect of subjects refusing to participate be evaluated? Will data be collected in order to describe this group?
9. Will vital statistics or data from other sources be used for comparison with the study data? What precautions must be taken in doing so?

4 Matching

Definition of Matching

Matching refers to the *pairing* of one or more controls to each case on the basis of their "similarity" with respect to selected variables. Any characteristic or attribute of an individual, such as age, sex, race, blood group, hospital of admission, neighborhood, marital status, income, blood pressure, weight, occupation, parity, personal or family history of disease, and so on, may serve as a basis for pairing. To the extent that cases and controls are similar on the matching variables, their difference with respect to disease may be attributed to some other factor. Furthermore, if the cases and controls differ with respect to some exposure variable, suggesting an association with the study disease, then this association cannot be explained in terms of case-control differences on the matching variables.

We restrict the term matching to refer to the pairing of individuals in the sampling phase of an investigation, so that only those controls who "match" cases are selected for study. This procedure differs from *post-matching,* which refers to the selection of an unmatched sample of controls and the subsequent pairing of them to the cases at the time of analysis. This latter approach was used, for example, in a case-control study of artificial sweeteners and bladder cancer (Wynder and Stellman 1980). Althauser and Rubin (1970) and Smith et al. (1977) describe methods for implementing post-matching.

When matching multiple controls to each case, one usually attempts to have a constant case:control ratio, such as 1:2 or 1:3. Despite this objective, one often ends up with incomplete matching, so that some cases may have 3 controls, others 2 or 1, and some may remain unmatched. As a consequence, one often has a variable matching ratio.

Objectives of Matching

Although the primary objective of matching is the elimination of biased comparisons between cases and controls, this objective can only be accomplished in general if matching is accompanied by an analysis that corresponds to the matched design. Unless the analysis properly accounts for the matching used in the selection phase of a case-control study, the estimated relative risk of disease associated with exposure can be biased as a consequence of matching (Section 4.2). Thus, matching is only the first step of a two-step process that can be used to control for confounding: (1) matched design, followed by (2) matched analysis.

Even though the ultimate objective of matching may be the elimination of biased comparisons, the immediate consequence of matching is the achievement of "balance" in the numbers of cases and controls that occur at each level of the matching variables. For example, if one pairs on age, then equal numbers of cases and controls will occur within any specified age group. If one pairs on both age *and* race, then cases and controls will be balanced on age within each racial grouping. Furthermore, within any specified age group, cases and controls will also be balanced on race. As a result of balance, a subgroup-specific estimate of the relative risk based on the sample odds ratio will often be more precisely estimated than if balance had not been achieved.

To show that balance tends to increase precision, let p_1 and p_0 denote respectively the proportions of exposed cases and controls in a target population. If random samples of size n_1 (cases) and n_0 (controls) are taken, then the asymptotic variance of the sample odds ratio ($\hat{\psi} = ad/bc$) is

$$\text{var}(\hat{\psi}) \simeq \psi^2[(n_1 p_1 q_1)^{-1} + (n_0 p_0 q_0)^{-1}]$$

(Gart 1962). The null hypothesis $H_0:\psi = 1$ implies that $p_1 = p_0$. Thus, for $n_1 + n_0 = n$ (fixed), the asymptotic variance of $\hat{\psi}$ is minimized under H_0 when $n_1 = \frac{1}{2} n = n_0$. Although equal sample sizes are not optimal in terms of minimizing var($\hat{\psi}$) when $\psi \neq 1$, Thompson (1980) provides simulation results that confirm the general desirability of achieving balance. He also extends the above analysis to the Mantel-Haenszel procedure, which provides an estimate of a combined odds ratio that is adjusted for confounding (Chapter 7).

As an example of how matching can increase the precision of the estimated odds ratio, suppose that one were interested in studying a postulated association between recent oral contraceptive use and an increased risk of myocardial infarction in women 20–44 years of age. Since age is related to both disease and exposure, it is a confounding variable that might be controlled in several different ways. Consider the following two.

First, one might take unmatched random samples of n cases and n controls and stratify the analysis on the basis of age. This approach would use post-stratification to control for confounding. Second, one might take a random sample of n cases and match each to a control within $\pm$ 2 years in order to obtain n pairs. Suppose that one next formed subgroups of individuals by age strata (such as 20–24, 25–29, 30–34, 35–39 and 40–44 years) ignoring the pairing in the matched study. Then the analysis of either the matched or unmatched study may be done in terms of a combined estimate of the odds ratio based on the Mantel-Haenszel method (Chapter 7).

In the unmatched study, cases will predominate at the older ages, whereas controls will be approximately uniformly distributed over the entire age range. In fact, at the younger ages 20–24 and 25–29 years, there may be few cases, if any. If no cases occurred in the younger age groups, then information on the controls within these subgroups would be wasted, since the Mantel-Haenszel estimate effectively ignores such strata. Irrespective of whether this occurs, however, the post-stratified estimate will generally have a larger variance as a consequence of the imbalance in the numbers of cases and controls within the age strata. From the perspective of a stratified analysis, matching is essentially a form of stratified sampling that assures that no large imbalances occur.

Matching may be used in special circumstances to rule out some particular mechanism in a postulated causal pathway between exposure and disease. For example, if the effect of cigarette smoking on coronary disease is thought to be mediated by an elevation of serum cholesterol levels, then one might deliberately match on cholesterol to see if the association of smoking with coronary heart disease is eliminated or diminished (Miettinen 1968a).

Chapters 7 and 8 give methods for the analysis of matched case-control studies and discuss in further detail some of the issues raised in this chapter.

4.1 CRITERIA FOR MATCHING

Variables to be considered for matching are those that independently of exposure are risk factors for the study disease. A matching variable need not be a "cause" of the disease, but may derive its risk-factor status as a result of associations with other causal variables, excluding the study exposure (Miettinen 1974c).

In considering criteria for matching in case-control studies, it is helpful to think in terms of how one might control extraneous factors in an experimental setting. Figure 4.1 shows an aid to conceptualizing the problem in terms of path diagrams (Wold 1956, Susser 1973). The letters E, F, and D denote respectively exposure, potential matching factor, and disease. The symbols $\rightarrow$ and $\leftrightarrow$ represent causal and noncausal associa-

Figure 4.1.

Two situations in which matching on a factor F is proper.

Figure 4.2.

Two situations in which matching on a factor F is unnecessary.

tions. Figure 4.1A shows a situation in which there is an indirect association between exposure and disease that is due to the factor F. Failure to match or otherwise control for F would result in a spurious association between exposure and disease. For example, a finding of an association between drinking alcoholic beverages (E) and lung cancer (D) would likely be explained in terms of an association between alcohol intake and cigarette smoking (F.)

Figure 4.1B shows a situation in which E and F individually alter the risk of disease and are also associated. Failure to match or otherwise control for F in this instance would result in a biased assessment of the *individual* effect of E. For example, use of oral contraceptives and cigarette smoking are both risk factors for myocardial infarction (Shapiro et al. 1979). Furthermore, OC use and smoking are positively associated, so that failure to adjust for the effect of smoking (F) results in an overestimate of the effect of the OC use (E) on the risk of a myocardial infarction (Chapter 7).

Figure 4.2 diagrams two situations in which matching is unnecessary. In Figure 4.2A, the factor F is associated with disease independently of exposure (E.) In this instance, it is correct to *consider* matching on F because it is a risk factor for the study disease. However, since F bears no relationship to the study exposure, matching on F would be unnecessary, because it would be done on the basis of a factor that is not associated with the exposure variable on which the cases and the controls are being compared (Hardy and White 1971).

A case-control study of venous thromboembolism and blood group O provides an example of avoiding unnecessary matching (Jick et al. 1969). Although age and sex are characteristics that bear a strong relationship to disease, they are practically unrelated to the exposure, blood group O, so that matching or other control for these factors is unnecessary (Miettinen 1970a).

As another example, consider a case-control study of the ABO blood group in relation to cervical cancer. Since blood group is unrelated to sex, healthy male controls would be acceptable, provided they were matched to cases on the basis of race, which is related to both blood group and the risk of cervical cancer (Hardy and White 1971).

Figure 4.2B provides a second instance of unnecessary matching, in which a variable (F) is associated with exposure (E), but is not a risk factor for the study disease. As an example of this situation, consider a hospital-based case-control study of myocardial infarction (MI) and oral contraceptives. Since the prescribing habits of physicians vary considerably, one expects an association between exposure (oral contraceptives) and medical practice. The question arises whether controls should be matched to cases on the basis of the medical practice from which the cases came. Although medical practice itself is not expected to alter the risk of an MI, it may nonetheless be associated with this disease as a result of its association with other risk factors, such as race, education or socioeconomic status. If controls were matched to cases on the basis of such factors, however, the residual association between medical practice and MI would be expected to be approximately zero, so that further matching on medical practice would be unnecessary. Conversely, in some settings it may be operationally easier to match on medical practice, with further control for potential confounders being made in the analysis. In summary, the need to match or otherwise control a given factor depends on its *residual* association with disease and exposure after control for other variables.

4.2 OVERMATCHING

The term *overmatching* has been applied to matching that reduces either the validity or the statistical efficiency of a case-control comparison (Miettinen 1968a, MacMahon and Pugh 1970). One might further extend the use of this term to matching that unnecessarily increases the cost or complexity of a study. Each of these situations is sufficiently different to warrant careful distinction in the sense in which one uses the term overmatching.

Matching that is accompanied by an unmatched analysis can reduce the validity of a case-control comparison. For example, suppose that one matches on a variable (F) that is intermediate in the causal pathway between exposure and disease $(E \rightarrow F \rightarrow D)$. An analysis that ignored the pairing would result in an odds ratio biased toward unity. This would occur because matching on a consequence of exposure would spuriously equate the proportion of individuals in the case and the control series who were "exposed." However, even if one performed a matched analysis, the disease-exposure odds ratio would tend to underestimate the correct value. (One can contrive examples in which the matched analysis will overestimate the correct value, but this is unlikely to occur in practice.)

Overmatching can also reduce the efficiency of a case-control comparison. First, suppose one matches on a factor that is associated with exposure but not disease (Figure 4.2B). An analysis that retains the pairing will correctly estimate the odds ratio, assuming that the disease-exposure odds ratio is constant across pairs or across strata of the matching variables. However, the variance of the matched estimate will be increased in comparison with the variance of the odds ratio based on an unmatched sample of equivalent size. The reason for the loss of efficiency in this circumstance is that overmatching unnecessarily increases the frequency of exposure-concordant pairs, which are discarded in the paired analysis (Chapter 7). The additional cost and complexity of doing a matched study would further weigh against matching in this instance. Having matched unnecessarily in this situation, however, one should nonetheless retain the pairing in the analysis. Assuming that the matching factor bears the same relationship to exposure among the cases and the controls, an analysis that ignores the pairing is expected to yield an estimate of the odds ratio that is biased toward unity (Sartwell 1971, Seigel and Greenhouse 1973a, Armitage 1975). In general, if one matches on a factor that is causally or noncausally associated with the study exposure, an analysis that ignores the matching will typically result in a disease-exposure odds ratio that is biased toward unity.

As a second instance of unnecessary matching, suppose one matches on a factor that is associated with disease but not exposure. The disease-exposure odds ratio will be estimated correctly whether or not one retains the pairing in the analysis (Gart 1962, Seigel and Greenhouse 1973b).

However, a paired analysis will generally be statistically less efficient than an unpaired analysis of the same data (Youkeles 1963, Chase 1968, Armitage 1975).

Matching on highly related variables will also result in unnecessary matching (Cochran 1953, Billewicz 1964). For example, given three correlated variables, matching on the basis of the first two automatically matches to some extent on the third. The third variable improves homogeneity between cases and controls only to the extent that it is not already accounted for through its association with the first two. Thus, matching variables should be selected from those that have the strongest relationship to the study disease and are least correlated.

4.3 ALTERNATIVES TO MATCHING

Although matching is commonly used in case-control studies, there is usually no simple answer to the question of whether or not one should match. There are several alternatives to controlling for confounding, such as the use of post-stratification or regression adjustment for unmatched, stratified, or frequency-matched samples. The use of a matched design and analysis is just one of several means to the same end. To assess the extent of bias reduction or increase in precision expected from a matched design and analysis compared with other methods of achieving these objectives typically requires more information than is available when a study is begun. At the very least, one needs an estimate of the proportion of cases and controls in the target population that occur in each of the subgroups defined by the cross-classification of the matching factors. Assuming that the disease-exposure odds ratio is constant across these subgroups, one also needs an estimate of the exposure rate among the controls within each of them. The differential costs and complexities in implementing matching and its alternatives further complicate the assessment.

Stratified Sampling

Stratified sampling involves the formation of subgroups by partitioning the ranges of specified variables and sampling a predetermined number of cases and a predetermined number of controls within cells created by the multiple cross-classification. Controls are usually sampled so that every subgroup has the same ratio of cases to controls, such as 1:1, 1:2, etc. The actual numbers of cases and controls may vary across the strata (subgroups), even though the case:control ratio is constant.

For example, suppose that one wanted cases and controls to be balanced on age, sex, and race in a study of dietary factors and heart disease in individuals 45 to 64 years old. Taking age (45–49, 50–54, 55–59, 60–64), sex (male, female) and race (northern European, black, Hispanic, Asian) gives $4 \times 2 \times 4 = 32$ subgroups from which predetermined numbers of cases and controls would be selected in a stratified sample.

Frequency Matching

Frequency matching is a variation of stratified sampling that is more commonly used in practice than is stratified sampling. Rather than predetermining the numbers of cases and controls to be selected within each of the strata, frequency matching involves the selection of cases at random, with controls being taken from the corresponding subgroups in proportion to the number of cases. To continue with the example of the previous paragraph, if 30 percent of the cases were males of northern European extraction aged 60–64 years, then 30 percent of the controls would be taken to have similar characteristics. The final sample might contain 80 percent males, rather than the 50 percent that one might otherwise take if there were equal interest in heart disease in women.

With frequency matching, the expected size of the case series in each subgroup is proportional to its population size. With stratified sampling, however, one may deliberately oversample certain subgroups to allow for their better representation in the study. Estimates of overall risk can then be derived by appropriately weighting the stratum-specific estimates by the sampling fractions, as is done in sample surveys (Cochran 1977).

In practice, before a study begins, there is often little information available about the distribution of cases and controls over the strata determined by the cross-classification of multiple variables. As a consequence, stratified sampling is not commonly used in case-control studies. Frequency matching is more practical, although it does require that one continually update information on the distribution of accumulating cases and controls. This must be done in order to adapt the control-selection procedures to maintain a fixed case:control ratio across the subgroups. Of course, the validity of a study does not require that equal numbers of cases and controls, or a fixed ratio, occur in each of the strata. Such balancing may increase the precision (reduce the variance) of the estimated odds ratio, although the gain is often marginal in comparison with case and control groups that are only approximately balanced.

Matching, stratified sampling, and frequency matching are related techniques that are used in the sampling phase of a study to achieve balance in the numbers of cases and controls across levels of potential confounding variables. Under the proper circumstances, such balance can reduce the variance of the estimated disease-exposure odds ratio, thereby improving the statistical efficiency with which the relative risk is estimated. However, each of the above techniques must be accompanied by the proper analysis in order to achieve this result and, more importantly, to eliminate bias in the estimated odds ratio (Section 4.2).

Post-Stratification

The use of matching, stratified sampling, or frequency matching requires that one identify variables to control before starting the investigation. Two methods that avoid this requirement, being used only in the analysis phase of a study, are post-stratification and regression analysis.

Post-stratification involves the classification of unmatched samples of cases and controls on the basis of their values on one or more variables ascertained during the study. This approach is similar to stratified sampling or frequency matching, except that (1) the variables used for grouping need not be specified at the time of case-control selection; (2) the case-control ratio is not constrained to be constant across the strata; and (3) there is no assurance that each of the subgroups will contain both cases and controls, thereby permitting a comparison of exposure in each of the strata.

The rationale for post-stratification as a means of controlling bias is as follows. Within each of the subgroups defined by the cross-classification of the variables used for post-stratification, cases and controls are similar with respect to each of the stratification variables. Thus, any difference between them with regard to exposure can be due only to some other factor. For example, simultaneous stratification on age (45–49, 50–54, 55–59, 60–64), sex (male, female), and race (northern European, black, Hispanic, Asian) results in 32 subgroups, within each of which cases and controls are assured of being relatively homogeneous on each stratification variable. Thus, within each subgroup, a difference between cases and controls with respect to some exposure cannot be due to age, sex, or race. Some dissimilarity within subgroups may still remain and may partially account for (or obscure) a difference in exposure between cases and controls. For example, within an age grouping, cases may be slightly older than controls. The maximum difference is five years in the above stratification, but in practice the average difference would likely be less.

Finer stratification on any of the variables can be used, if necessary, and the variables on which stratification is based can be changed at any stage in the analysis, thereby providing great flexibility (see Section 4.6).

There are basically two limitations to post-stratification. First, there is a loss of information resulting from subgroups in which only cases or controls occur. In this situation, a subgroup comparison cannot be made, and an estimate of relative risk that combines odds ratios across strata omits these subgroups from the analysis (Chapter 7). Post-stratification thus relies on overlap in the distribution of cases and controls after the sampling phase. Second, the number of variables on which one can simulataneously stratify and the fineness of the classification are restricted by the number of cases and controls. For example, if each of 5 variables has 3 subgroups, then simultaneous stratification on all 5 variables would create $3^5 = 243$ strata. With a small study of 50 cases and 50 controls, many of the strata would contain either no subjects or possibly only one, thereby incurring a loss of information in a combined odds ratio estimate.

Regression Analysis

Another analysis technique involves fitting the logistic regression model (Chapter 8)

$$y = b_0 + b_1 E + b_2 X. \tag{4.1}$$

The variable E indicates the study exposure, X denotes a confounding variable that one wants to control, and $y = \ln p/q$ is the logarithm of the odds of "disease" (the log odds of a "case"). Among exposed individuals ($E = 1$), the log odds of "disease" is $y_1 = b_0 + b_1 + b_2 X$. Among unexposed individuals ($E = 0$), the log odds of "disease" is $y_0 = b_0 + b_2 X$. Thus, equation (4.1) assumes that the log odds of "disease" has the same dependence on X (b_2 is constant) among exposed and unexposed individuals. Furthermore, the difference in the log odds (exposed minus unexposed) for individuals with the same value of X is simply $y_1 - y_0 = b_1$. Thus, the effect of exposure on the log risk of disease, adjusted for the (linear) effect of X, is represented by b_1. In fact, $\exp(y_1 - y_0) = \exp(b_1)$ is the disease-exposure odds ratio, adjusted for the (loglinear) effect of X. Adjustment for multiple confounding variables and the assessment of interaction is handled as in multiple regression (see Chapter 8).

A hybrid of matching and regression is the use of regression analysis based on matched pairs (Prentice 1976, Holford, White, and Kelsey

1978, Breslow et al. 1978, Holford 1978). This approach generally removes more bias than the use of matching alone. Depending on the closeness of the matching, however, the improvement over a simple matched estimate can be negligible or dramatic. The regression analysis of matched data is particularly useful when one wants to adjust for variables that were not included in the matching scheme. This approach often yields an estimate that has less bias than an estimate based on a regression analysis that ignores the pairing (Cochran and Rubin 1973, Rubin 1973).

The use of regression models assumes more importance as the number of variables used for adjustment or the number of subgroups used for stratification becomes large with respect to the available sample of cases and controls. However, such conditions are precisely those in which the validity of the assumed model cannot be evaluated thoroughly. In this situation, analyses and interpretations based on a regression model should be considered provisional.

4.4 EFFECTIVENESS OF MATCHING AND ITS ALTERNATIVES

Removal of Bias

The use of a matched design and analysis, compared with the use of regression adjustment based on unmatched samples, has been evaluated for its effectiveness in eliminating biased comparisons (Cochran 1953, 1965). [The analyses of Cochran, which were based on the paradigm of a comparative experiment, can be related to case-control studies in terms of a weighted least squares analysis (Cox 1970) based on the logistic regression model (4.1).] Whereas fitting a correctly specified regression model to unmatched data removes all of the bias due to X in the estimate of $y_1 - y_0$, some residual bias may remain with an analysis based on post-stratification. Since exact matching on a continuous variable X such as age rarely occurs in practice, a paired design and analysis may also remove only part of the bias due to X (Billewicz 1965).

When variables to be used for matching are either categorical or discrete, the use of a matched design and analysis is no more effective in the removal of bias than the use of post-stratification with an unmatched, frequency-matched or stratified design (Cochran 1965).

The effectiveness of regression analysis for the removal of bias depends to some extent on whether the relationships between exposure, disease, and the variables used for adjustment have been correctly specified in the model equation. Rubin (1973) has given examples in which the use of an incorrectly specified regression model can introduce more bias into a comparison than was originally present. The situations in which a matched design and analysis is expected to be superior to regression analysis based on unmatched data are not easily summarized. One should refer to Cochran (1965), Cochran and Rubin (1973), and McKinlay (1975a) for an overview. A regression adjustment based on unmatched samples can often be just as effective in removing bias as a paired design with a pair-matched analysis.

Reduction of Variance

Section 4.2 considered the issues of efficiency and bias when overmatching occurs in a case-control study. Overmatching refers to matching on the basis of a variable that is not a confounder for the disease-exposure association under study. This section discusses the statistical efficiency of matched vs. unmatched designs in the presence of confounding.

Thompson (1980) has compared the asymptotic variances of the disease-exposure odds ratio based on stratified analyses of unmatched and frequency matched case-control designs. The potential matching variable was assumed to be a confounder. That is, it was associated with disease in the absence of exposure and was also correlated with the exposure. If the cost of matching is negligible, then the following major findings emerge.

1. In most circumstances, a matched design results in a modest improvement in efficiency, typically resulting in a 5 percent to 15 percent reduction in variance of the estimated disease-exposure odds ratio. In certain situations, matching may yield a 25 percent to 40 percent reduction in variance [see items (3) and (4) below].
2. If the disease-exposure association is large (relative risk $\geq$ 5), an unmatched design may be more efficient because an equal case:control ratio is not the optimal way to allocate a fixed number of subjects. However, the improved efficiency (reduction in variance) of the unmatched design is likely to be less than 5 percent.
3. The greatest improvements in efficiency due to matching occur when there is a strong association between the study disease and the confounder, the range in the risk of disease across levels of the confounder being twentyfold or greater. If the disease-confounder asso-

ciation is weak, the range in the risk of disease across levels of the confounder being sevenfold or smaller, then matching produces marginal gains of efficiency, often 10 percent or less.

4. A matched design is especially efficient relative to an unmatched design when only a small proportion (≤ 10 percent) of the target population is exposed to the study factor.

5. The strength of the association between the confounding variable and the study exposure is not an important determinant of the relative efficiency of matched and unmatched case-control designs, provided that a stratified analysis is used for both.

Although properly done matching can reduce the variance of an estimated disease-exposure odds ratio, the added cost and complexity of matching should be weighed against any expected gains in precision (reduction of variance). If the resources available for control selection are limited, and if the cost of a matched control exceeds the cost of an unmatched control by 10 percent or more, then the resulting loss in the number of controls that can be studied in a matched design may offset any expected gains in precision due to matching (Thompson 1980).

Arguing that a researcher must often choose between the use of unpaired samples that are subsequently stratified in the analysis and a reduced sample of matched pairs selected from the same source, McKinlay (1975b) made a Monte Carlo study (computer simulation) of stratified samples of fixed size with smaller samples of matched pairs. The comparison was most appropriate to post-matching, since unmatched individuals were discarded from the paired analysis. In this circumstance, the precision (reciprocal of the variance) of the pair-matched estimate of the odds ratio was found to be consistently less than the precision of estimates based on post-stratification. McKinlay (1975c) has also given a general condition that must occur for the use of matched sampling and analysis to be more effective in detecting an association than the application of a stratified analysis to unmatched samples.

4.5 EXPECTED NUMBER OF MATCHES

Given a set of variables for matching, such as age, sex, and race, one simple matching scheme, called *category matching*, stratifies each of the variables and randomly pairs cases and controls that fall into the same cell created by the multiple cross-classification. Thus, taking age (20–24,

25–29, 30–34, 35–40 years), sex (male, female), and race (white, black, other) gives $4 \times 2 \times 3 = 24$ matching categories. One question that arises with respect to category matching concerns the size of the control series that must be available in order to guarantee that the entire case series will be matched. Although there can never be a definitive answer to this question, the results of Cochran (1965) and McKinlay (1974) suggest that in typical situations one should expect to screen five times as many controls in order to completely match the case series. This general guide derives from the assumption that the number of matching categories does not exceed the number of cases, and that the case and the control series are not "unusually disparate" with respect to their distribution over the matching categories. In certain instances one might expect to screen considerably more than five controls per case. For example, if a case that fell into a matching category containing only 5 percent of the control population were selected for study, then without special techniques for selecting matches, one would expect that 20 controls on average would have to be screened in order to find a match.

On occasion, situations arise in which obtaining matches is virtually impossible. If one were matching on sex, age (± 2 years), weight (± 10 lbs), and height (± 2 in.), one would have difficulty finding a normotensive control for a woman with hypertension who was 26 years old, weighed 250 lbs and was 5 ft 1 in. tall. This example points out a paradox of matching, namely, that matching is least easily accomplished when it is most needed.

McKinlay (1974) has derived equations for the expected number of matches using category matching applied to random samples of cases and controls, and Walter (1980a) has given simple and accurate approximations. Their application requires that one estimate the frequencies with which cases and controls occur in each of the matching categories. Carpenter (1977) gives formulae for the expected numbers of matches and the probability of obtaining a match when one uses post-matching of continuous variables that are normally distributed, and Rubin (1979) reviews multivariate matching and regression adjustment procedures for observational studies.

4.6 HOW CLOSELY SHOULD ONE MATCH?

Two factors will affect the difficulty of matching: (1) the number of variables used, and (2) the closeness with which a control must match a case on each of the variables. Previous sections have addressed the issue of diminishing returns obtained by increasing the number of matching var-

Table 4.1. Percent Reduction in Bias in Estimated Log Odds Ratio Due to Frequency Matching or Post-Stratification with Equal-Sized Strata Based on a Single Variable[1]

	Number of strata						
	2	3	4	5	6	8	10
% Reduction	63	79	86	90	92	94	96

1. Based on results of Cox (1957) and Cochran (1968).

iables, and we now turn to the question "how fine should one stratify or how closely should one match?". A partial answer is provided by the results of Cochran (1968) and Cox (1957), shown in Table 4.1. Assuming a linear relationship between a response y (such as the log odds of "disease," $\ln p/q$) and a single variable X, Table 4.1 indicates the percent reduction in bias that can be expected to be removed by a stratified analysis based on frequency matching or post-stratification with equal-sized strata based on X. For example, to remove 80 percent of the initial bias due to a single variable X, 3 strata should be used, whereas 5 strata are needed to remove 90 percent of the bias. Of course, if the bias component is small to begin with, removing approximately 60 percent with 2 strata may be more than adequate. Table 4.1 suggests that matching need not be close, particularly if one uses a further regression adjustment based on matched pairs or matched sets to remove any residual bias.

The values in Table 4.1 were derived under the assumption that the variable X is normally distributed with a common standard deviation and different means for cases and controls. Calculations made for X following various chi-square, t, and beta distributions suggest that the figures in Table 4.1 can be used as a practical guide, including the situation where X is an ordered classification (such as none, slight, moderate, severe) based on grouping an underlying continuous variable (Cochran 1968).

Rather than using equal-sized strata, one might consider an "optimal" choice of subclass boundaries. Results of Ogawa (1951) and Cox (1957) show that for 2 through 10 subclasses, an optimal choice for the division points that determine the strata reduces the bias by at most 2 percent below the reduction achieved with equal-sized strata. The figures in Tables 4.1 assume that cases and controls are correctly classified into subgroups. If errors of classification occur, the percentages in Table 4.1 may be changed only negligibly, or may be reduced to less than half the values shown (Cochran 1968).

4.7 ADVANTAGES AND DISADVANTAGES OF MATCHING

Matching has several advantages. First, the process of pairing to achieve balance is conceptually easy to comprehend and communicate. Second, one is assured that cases and controls will be comparable with respect to each of the variables used for matching. Nothing is left to chance in this regard. Third, matching eliminates the assumption of a specific functional relationship that is needed to perform a regression adjustment. Although post-stratification is an effective alternative to regression analysis, its main disadvantage is that only a few variables can be used, since the number of cells in the multiple cross-classification increases as the product of the number of categories for each of the stratifying variables. Fourth, matching may provide the best means of investigating a very specific hypothesis or postulated mechanism of action, allowing one to conduct a comparatively small study. With a relatively large number of variables that need control, matching may provide the only guarantee of comparability. Matching is undoubtedly most useful in small studies, where greatly disparate case-control series may easily arise unless special precautions are taken to assure uniformity on confounding variables.

Use of a matched design implies some noteworthy disadvantages, however. First, matching cases and controls on the basis of a variable assures that subjects cannot be distinguished on that basis. One thereby eliminates the opportunity to assess the individual contribution of a matched factor to altering the risk of disease. As a consequence, one also removes the opportunity to fully investigate interactions between other study factors and the matching variable(s).

For example, suppose that one wanted to study oral contraceptive use in relation to myocardial infarction (MI). Cigarette smoking among U.S. women is a confounding variable, since it is related to the risk of an MI and is also associated with oral contraceptive use. Although one might want the investigation to focus on the "individual" effect of OC use on the risk of an MI, matching cases and controls on the basis of smoking history would preclude an assessment of the effect of smoking. Since one would have to retain the matching on smoking in order to avoid a biased estimate of the MI-OC odds ratio, one could make only two comparisons with respect to OC use, as diagramed in Figure 4.3A. These allow one to determine smoking-specific estimates of the relative risk of an MI in OC-users as compared with non-users. One could also compute a combined estimate using the Mantel-Haenszel procedure (Chapter 7).

If the odds ratios varied across the smoking categories, one would have evidence of an interaction between smoking and OC use on a multiplicative scale. One could not express the interaction in terms of a change in risk on an absolute scale, however, since an estimate of the effect of smoking would not be available. Furthermore, since cigarette smoking alters the risk of disease, the presence or absence of a constant odds ratio across

Figure 4.3.

Comparisons that can be made in matched and unmatched case-control studies of oral contraceptive (OC) use and smoking in relation to myocardial infarction.[1]

A. Matched on smoking   B. Unmatched[2]

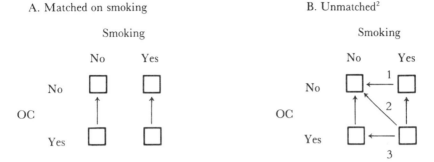

1. The symbol □ denotes the odds of "disease" within each subgroup.
2. The comparisons 1, 2, and 3 cannot be made in a case-control study matched on smoking (see text).

smoking strata in the matched study provides no information about whether smoking and oral contraceptives act synergistically. Information from an external source on the risk of disease associated with smoking, properly adjusted for other variables controlled in the study design or analysis, would be needed to address this issue.

Figure 4.3B shows the comparisons that one would want to make in order to fully assess the individual and joint effects of smoking and OC use on the risk of an MI. Taking nonsmoking women who have not used OCs as the reference group of primary interest, a case-control design that is matched on smoking precludes two important comparisons: (1) estimation of the relative risk (odds ratio) of an MI associated with smoking among women who to not use oral contraceptives, and (2) estimation of the relative risk of an MI associated with smoking among users of oral contraceptives. If one ignores the matching in a matched design, making the comparisons (1), (2), and (3) shown in Figure 4.3B, the estimate of relative risk will be biased toward unity.

Other arguments against the use of matching have considered the increased costs in time and labor required to form matches and the loss of information on unmatched individuals (Billewicz 1964, 1965, McKinlay 1974). Matching increases the complexity of the control selection process, since the eligibility criteria for controls change constantly as a function of the unmatched cases. For example, on one day a black married woman between the ages of 37 and 43 years may be sought as a control, whereas on another day one may be looking for a white bachelor between 54 and 60. Unless one uses post-matching, which invariably results in discarding unmatched cases and controls, a matched control can be selected only after a case has been enrolled in the study. Extensive matching can thus prolong the data collection phase while controls are sought to match "unusual" or late-entry cases. A certain fraction of the cases are often discarded as a result of failure to find a matching control within the time frame allowed for the study.

4.8 SUMMARY

Apart from variables such as age, race, and sex, which usually have a strong relationship to the study disease and exposure, additional variables that should be matched and the closeness with which pairs should be formed are often matters of doubt. Unnecessarily stringent matching increases the effort and reduces the available sample size with no corresponding gains in study precision or removal of bias.

The effort required for matching depends on the particulars of the study. For example, in a hospital-based case-control study, matching on sex, race, hospital, and date of admission will usually involve little, if any, increased effort. Incorporating age as an additional matching factor may only increase effort if one requires a stringent age match.

Since post-stratification and regression analysis can be used to control for confounding in the analysis of a case-control study, one is often uncertain of the necessity of using a matched design. Other means of avoiding large case-control imbalances on potential confounding variables involve selecting controls within a restricted range or the use of frequency matching or stratified sampling. The use of extensive matching criteria with population-based controls is unlikely to be either feasible or cost-effective.

Despite the intuitive appeal of matching, there is no unequivocal evidence in theory or practice that supports a general preference for this technique, and many writers have expressed reservations about the use of matching (Mantel and Haenszel 1959, Cochran 1965, Billewicz 1964, McKinlay 1977). Unless one has very good reason to match, one is undoubtedly better off avoiding the inclination.

Matching on a variable prevents an assessment of its effect on the risk of disease and also precludes a full assessment of potential interactions between the matching variables and the study exposure. Matching complicates both the case-control selection process and the data analysis. The analysis is complicated because matching is invariably done on the *presumption* that one or more variables are confounders. If in fact a matching variable were related only to the study disease, then an analysis that retained the pairing would suffer a loss of efficiency. If the matching variable were related only to the study exposure, then the pairing must be retained to avoid a biased estimate of the disease-exposure odds ratio. Since a matched analysis is based only on the exposure-discordant pairs (Chapter 7), one is often alarmed, though perhaps unjustifiably, at the number of pairs that are "discarded" because the case and control are either both exposed or both unexposed.

In the analysis of a matched study, it seems that one is forever trying to decide whether the pairing should be retained in any particular instance, especially when one is considering several different exposures. A matching factor may be a confounder with respect to one exposure variable, but not another. Furthermore, adjustment by stratification or regression analysis on unmatched factors may remove the confounding property of the matching variable(s), thereby removing the necessity to retain the pairing. One always seems haunted by the question whether one would have done better by simply taking a stratified sample of controls or a somewhat larger restricted random sample. Inevitably, economics and practicality intervene to thwart any initial tendencies to match on numerous factors. In general, frequency matching within rather broad categories of the matching variables will suffice for most studies.

5 Sources of Bias

James J. Schlesselman
Paul D. Stolley

5.0 INTRODUCTION

The validity of a case-control investigation depends partly upon the methods by which subjects are selected for study and classified by the four categories: (1) diseased; (2) nondiseased; (3) exposed; and (4) unexposed. Any number of errors in design can cause overrepresentation or underrepresentation of these categories. We shall use the term *bias* to refer to any systematic error in the design, conduct, or analysis of a study that results in a mistaken estimate of an exposure's effect on the risk of disease. Since there are endless ways in which a study can go awry (Sackett 1979), one can present only an outline of major sources of potential error that are relevant to most case-control investigations. To begin, we discuss sources of bias in the ascertainment and selection of cases and controls; we then proceed to a discussion of errors in the determination of exposure.

5.1 ASCERTAINMENT AND SELECTION BIAS

Case-control studies are vulnerable to misleading associations arising from the circumstances in which cases and controls are ascertained and selected for study. In particular, characteristics or exposures associated with differential surveillance, diagnosis, referral, or selection of individuals can lead to biased estimates of relative risk. These problems are not peculiar to case-control studies, since they can occur with follow-up studies as well.

Surveillance

If the disease or condition under study is asymptomatic, mild, or otherwise liable to escape routine medical attention, cases are more likely to be detected in persons under frequent medical surveillance. Reports of an apparent increased risk of endometrial cancer among women taking estrogens for menopausal symptoms were criticized partly on these grounds. It was argued presumptively that subclinical cancers were being diagnosed more frequently in exposed women as a result of closer surveillance and diagnostic thoroughness (Feinstein & Horowitz 1978). In fact, the increased risk cannot be explained on this basis (Shapiro et al. 1980; also see Hulka et al. 1980).

If more thorough follow-up examinations are done on individuals exposed to factors suspected of being toxic on the basis of theoretical considerations, animal experiments, or preliminary case reports, then exposed cases would have a greater likelihood of being diagnosed, compared with unexposed cases. For example, when the first reports linking phlebitis to oral contraceptive use were circulated, physicians might have been more cautious and thorough in the examination of women using oral contraceptives. Studies based solely on medical records are more likely to encounter this type of bias, since the recording of information tends to be selective rather than comprehensive in routine medical care.

As a consequence of differential surveillance, the estimated relative risk can be spuriously elevated, whether determined from a cohort or a case-control study (Schlesselman 1977). A direct assessment of this source of bias can be made by stratifying the analysis on some index of medical care, comparing cases and controls within subgroups having equal surveillance. Another tactic that can be used to control any bias that might arise from unusual publicity of a finding is to restrict the study to the time interval prior to publication of the finding.

In contrast to studying mild or asymptomatic conditions, suppose that one is investigating a disease that is progressive, eventually producing symptoms requiring medical attention. Then the number of new cases detected in a given period is little influenced by continuing surveillance. At the start of intensive screening of exposed individuals, there will be an initial increase in the number of cases due to their detection at earlier stages of the disease process. However, with continuing surveillance, the number of new cases found each year will be exactly the same as the number found annually before intensive screening (Hutchison and Rothman 1978).

Medical surveillance is often accompanied by therapeutic intervention, which itself may prove to be a source of bias due to initiation or discontinuation of therapies or other exposures. For example, women with benign breast disease are known to be at higher risk of developing breast cancer. Suppose that oral contraceptives have no effect on the risk of breast cancer, but that women taking oral contraceptives who develop benign breast disease discontinue usage on the advice of their physicians. One would then expect a resulting spurious protective dosage effect, with longer-term OC users being apparently at reduced risk of breast cancer. This emphasizes the importance of knowing why an agent was prescribed or discontinued. An agent found to be present or absent in association with a disease may have been started or stopped because of an early manifestation of that disease (Feinstein 1979).

In some situations, the intensity of medical follow-up will vary with the duration of exposure. Users of intrauterine devices (IUDs) will be closely watched immediately after an insertion, but subjected to no special examinations after the device has been used successfully for several months. In fact, some women may forget that an IUD has been inserted and consequently use two or more devices simultaneously. By contrast, individuals using drugs for which prescriptions need renewal by a physician will generally be followed more closely throughout the duration of use.

Diagnosis

The validity of diagnosis is another area in which bias may arise. For example, with conditions such as cervical dysplasia, it is conceivable that knowledge of exposure status may alter the histologic assessment. The simple precaution of using a standard review of slides by one or more pathologists who are unaware of a specimen's origin can eliminate this problem. Another tactic is to stratify cases on the basis of certainty of diagnosis or severity of disease since diagnostic bias will be increasingly unlikely as severity or certainty increases.

Initial reports of an association between oral contraceptive use and deep-vein thrombosis and pulmonary embolism were questioned partly on the ground that diagnoses may have been influenced by knowledge of a patient's contraceptive history. If this were true, one would expect that the association would be strongest in those patients for whom knowledge of their history could most influence the diagnosis, namely, in those patients for whom the physical basis of the diagnosis was least certain.

Table 5.1. Percentage of Cases Using Oral Contraceptives, by Type of Diagnosis and Certainty

Case diagnosis	Certainty of diagnosis		
	Possible	Probable	Certain
Idiopathic deep vein thrombosis only	3/9 (33%)	17/37 (46%)	1/1 (100%)
Idiopathic pulmonary embolism only	2/4 (50%)	5/10 (50%)	4/4 (100%)
Idiopathic deep vein thrombosis and pulmonary embolism	—	4/10 (40%)	10/17 (59%)
Postoperative deep vein thrombosis only	1/6 (17%)	3/8 (38%)	1/1 (100%)
Postoperative pulmonary embolism only	0/3 (0%)	5/8 (63%)	—
Postoperative deep vein thrombosis and pulmonary embolism	—	—	3/7 (43%)

Source: Vessey 1971.

To test this hypothesis, an independent review of cases was done without knowledge of patients' contraceptive practices. Not only was this hypothesis not confirmed, but the association was found to be strongest among those patients for whom the diagnosis was most firmly established, both in regard to idiopathic and postoperative disease (Vessey 1971). This is shown in Table 5.1, where the percentage of cases using oral contraceptives increases with increasing certainty of diagnosis.

As another example, biased clinical diagnoses were detected in the analysis of data from a case-control study of IUD usage and fetal loss. A fetal loss in a woman having a normal or slightly elevated temperature was more likely to be called septic on the basis of clinical diagnosis if the woman had an IUD in place since her last menstrual period (Schlesselman 1980). To assess the potential impact of this bias, the investigators conducted further analyses that restricted the definition of septic fetal loss to include only cases with documented temperatures of 103°F or greater. The results were essentially unchanged, indicating that the effect of this bias was negligible (Foreman et al. 1982).

The detection of misdiagnoses can be turned to one's advantage, since it allows one to check whether illness may bias the determination of exposure histories. In the absence of bias, one expects that the odds of exposure among false positive cases will equal the odds of exposure among the controls. For example, Doll and Hill (1952) showed that patients whose diagnosis of lung cancer was subsequently established to be erroneous had smoking histories characteristic of the control rather than of the lung cancer group. As another example, a collaborative case-control study of the sudden infant death syndrome (SIDS), being conducted by the National Institute of Child Health and Human Development, is using deaths among children originally thought to be cases of SIDS as one group of controls.

Referral

Differential referral patterns are another source of potential bias in hospital or clinic-based case-control studies. Table 5.2 shows that differential rates of hospitalization for exposed and unexposed cases and controls can distort the odds ratio determined in the hospital from that in the population. Whereas the population odds ratio is $\psi = AD/BC$, the odds ratio in hospital is

$$\psi' = b\psi \qquad (5.1)$$

where the bias term

$$b = (s_1 s_4)/(s_2 s_3) \qquad (5.2)$$

depends on the (usually unknown) differential referral rates s_1, s_2, s_3, and s_4 defined in Table 5.2.

Physician or self referral are two of many selective factors operating to produce the final case-control series in any hospital-based study. In general, if one regards the terms s_1 to s_4 as the sampling proportions for the four cells of the 2×2 table with population frequencies A, B, C, and D in Table 5.2, then a general condition for the absence of bias in the estimation of the odds ratio is that $b = 1$, implying that $s_1 s_4 = s_2 s_3$. For example, if among cases one is k times more likely to choose an exposed individual, and if among controls one is also k times more likely to choose an exposed individual, then $s_1 = k s_3$ and $s_2 = k s_4$, resulting in $b = 1$. Thus, in principle, a biased selection of cases can be compensated by a biased selection of controls. However, one usually strives to choose both cases and controls in a manner that assures that exposed and unexposed individuals have equal probabilities of selection, that is, $s_1 = s_3$ and $s_2 = s_4$ (see Chapter 2).

To put the consideration of compensating bias in more concrete terms, suppose that the study disease is sufficiently serious to require hospitalization for treatment. Then all persons with the disease will be admitted to some hospital. However, any particular hospital may have a peculiar referral practice, for example, taking referrals predominantly from upper-income individuals. If income is associated with the study exposure, then cases of the study disease at that hospital are more likely to be exposed to the study factor than are cases in the general population.

Table 5.2.   Population Frequency, Referral Rates, and
Hospital Frequency for Exposed and Unexposed Cases and
Controls

Exposure	Disease	Population frequency	Proportion referred	Hospital frequency
Yes	Case	A	s_1	$s_1 A$
	Control	B	s_2	$s_2 B$
No	Case	C	s_3	$s_3 C$
	Control	D	s_4	$s_4 D$

Population	$\psi = AD/BC$
Hospital	$\psi' = [(s_1 s_4)/(s_2 s_3)]\psi = b\psi$

However, other diseases or conditions based on referral to the same hospital are also more likely to be associated with the study exposure, because of their association in that hospital with individuals of upper income. Hence, an unbiased estimate of the odds ratio can be derived by taking hospital controls. If controls from the general population were selected, however, one would have to match or stratify on income in order to eliminate income as a source of selection bias operating on the cases, but not on the population-based controls. The rationale for matching cases and controls on the basis of source of referral or hospital of origin derives from the attempt to allow for such compensating bias.

The use of neighborhood or population controls will not compensate for biased referral of cases. Equation (5.2) shows that efforts directed to achieving equal selection probabilities for exposed and unexposed controls ($s_2 = s_4$) will be futile if the case selection probabilities are unequal ($s_1 \neq s_3$). For instance, if an exposed case is twice as likely as an unexposed case to be selected for study, the odds ratio will be overestimated by a factor of 2 in the presence of an unbiased selection of controls. This follows from equation (5.2), taking $s_1 = 2s_3$ and $s_2 = s_4$, yielding $b = 2$.

As a hypothetical example of differential referral, suppose that ectopic pregnancies believed to result from use of an intrauterine device are referred for detailed study to one particular hospital. A case-control study based on cases deriving from that hospital would overestimate the relative risk, irrespective of whether an unbiased series of controls from that hospital or the general population were used as the comparison group. However, since an ectopic pregnancy is a life-threatening condition, all cases are likely to be hospitalized. If the referral practices among hospitals in a given city or region differ, the overreferral of exposed cases to one hospital implies an underreferral of exposed cases to the others. As a result of differential referral, a factor may appear harmful when studied in one hospital and protective in another. Biased admissions can reduce an association as well as increase one. The solution to this problem for diseases or conditions that are invariably hospitalized is to establish a hospital network that captures all cases within a defined geographic area. Controls, whether hospitalized or not, should be taken from the same area. *Pooling* the data across hospitals, rather than stratifying on the basis of hospital, eliminates the bias from differential admission of cases.

Berkson (1946) pointed out that patients with two specific conditions requiring treatment are more likely to be hospitalized than persons with only one of these conditions. Thus a hospital-based case-control study could find an association between two diseases even if there were no association between them in the general population. The probability model upon which this conclusion was based specified that each condition be a force of hospitalization in its own right. Concern with the specific type of bias identified by Berkson is usually not germane to the typical hospital-based case-control study, since the characteristics of exposures being investigated for association with disease are not themselves conditions with a symptomatology that requires or leads to hospitalization (Kraus 1954, Walter 1980c).

A unique study of whether bias of the sort identified by Berkson might operate in practice has been reported by Roberts et al. (1978). Data on eight clinical conditions and six groups of medications, together with an indication of whether the respondent had been hospitalized at any time during the six months prior to interview, were recorded in interviews with 2,784 noninstitutionalized adults living in Ontario, Canada. There were 48 possible pairings of medication and clinical condition, resulting in 48 different relative risks. The estimates of relative risk based on the total survey population were compared with the estimates based on the hospitalized subset. Six of the total 48 comparisons showed a statistically "significant" ($p < 0.1$) difference between the hospital-based and the community-based estimates of the odds ratio. In three instances, the hospital-based estimate was significantly greater, and in three instances, the community-based estimate was significantly greater. Since no adjustment was made for potential confounding variables, one cannot be certain that the differences were due to differential referral as opposed to confounding. In any event, there was no consistent pattern of results, and the element of chance was not decidedly eliminated.

One sees from equation (5.2) that bias, corresponding to $b \neq 1$, results from *differential* referral rates of exposed and unexposed cases, or *differential* rates of referral for exposed and unexposed controls. As a group, exposed individuals may be more or less likely to be selected for study, but this does not in itself bias the estimated relative risk (odds ratio). For example, referring to Table 5.2, suppose that $s_1 = s_2 = s$ and $s_3 = s_4 = s'$. If exposed individuals are more likely to appear in the study sample, then $s > s'$. However, substitution of s and s' in equation (5.2) gives $b = 1$, indicating no study bias.

Selection

Differential surveillance, diagnosis, and referral all contribute to biased ascertainment of cases or controls. Equation (5.2) quantifies the magnitude of the bias expected to result from differential selection rates, which in turn may depend on case-control ascertainment. In practice, the selection probabilities $s_1, \ldots, s_4$ are never known precisely, if at all. The best one can do is to follow procedures in case-control ascertainment and selection that are likely to minimize bias.

Biased selection can occur in many ways. For example, in a case-control study of complications thought to be associated with usage of intrauterine devices (IUDs), some interviewers were found to be "keying" on cases who were exposed to the study factor. One nurse in particular was searching out all cases of ectopic pregnancy with an associated IUD usage (Schlesselman 1980). If all cases of ectopic pregnancy are ultimately selected, this causes no problem. If only a fraction of cases are selected, however, the sample is biased toward overexposure among the cases, thereby producing an overestimate of the relative risk. (This problem was identified and corrected at the initiation of the study.) To avoid such a problem, one must establish precisely and in advance the method by which cases and controls are identified and selected (Mantel and Haenszel 1959). One must also carefully train staff to do the field work properly and establish a system of quality control to maintain standards throughout the investigation (Chapter 3).

Nonresponse

Another source of selection bias derives from patient or control refusal or nonresponse to inquiries requesting participation in a study. The best-designed sampling scheme, assuring complete ascertainment of cases and a probability sample of controls, can be vitiated by high rates of refusal. One can attempt an assessment of the impact of nonresponse in the following way. Using assumed values for the exposure rates among the non-respondent cases and controls, one can add the refusals to the observed data to see the resulting distortion introduced under various assumptions of differential exposure. If the risk of the study disease were hypothesized to be increased as a result of exposure, then a "worst case" analysis could be performed that would assume that all the nonrespondent cases were unexposed and all the nonrespondent controls were exposed. (The reverse assumptions would apply for a worst case analysis for an exposure hypothesized to reduce the risk of the study disease.) If an observed odds ratio that differed from unity could be brought substantially closer to unity, reduced to unity, or even have its direction reversed, one could characterize the magnitude of the hypothetical odds ratio among the non-respondents that would be required to produce the effect. Whether such an occurrence would be "likely," however, would be a matter of judgment.

A refusal may be prompted by a temporary inconvenience in a person's schedule, by a particularly frustrating day with an unusual number of aggravations, or by some subliminal distaste for the tone or demeanor of the interviewer making the initial contact. Nonresponse arising from these circumstances can be reduced by tactful callbacks made at some other time of day by interviewers who have greater success in gaining cooperation. The characteristics of those persons who initially refused might provide some basis for assumptions regarding the intransigent refusals.

Different rates of nonresponse between cases and controls does not in itself introduce bias. For example, suppose that among eligible cases contacted for study, 10 percent refused to participate, while among eligible controls, 30 percent refused. If the exposure rates (proportions) were equal between refusing and participating cases, and the same were true of the controls (exposure rates need not be equal between cases and controls, however), then the odds ratio based only on the respondents would be equal to the odds ratio based on the entire set of eligible individuals.

Bias from nonresponse can occur irrespective of whether the response rates are identical or different in the case and the control groups. For example, suppose that both the case and the control groups selected for study represent 90 percent of the eligible subjects who were contacted, 10 percent refusing to participate in each group. If exposed cases were more or less likely to participate than exposed controls, then the odds ratio estimated from only the respondents would differ from the odds ratio based on the entire set of eligible individuals.

Length of Stay

For hospital-based studies, cases and controls should ideally be selected by a scheme that is equivalent to sampling from the admission logs (incident cases), rather than on the basis of a hospital register of current patients (prevalent cases). In the latter situation, patients who remain in the hospital for the longest period of time would have the greatest chance of selection. Cases of short duration, either because of early cure or early death, would tend to be underrepresented in this instance.

One reason for a greater length of stay may be the presence of other diseases as well as the one of interest. In a study of pulmonary embolism, patients who have this disease and also have other serious chronic illnesses such as diabetes, hypertension, or chronic obstructive pulmonary disease may require longer hospitalization. Concomitant disease may change both an individual's risk of the study disease and the likelihood of exposure to the study factor, thereby introducing confounding. If one selects patients on the basis of a hospital register of current patients, one can check for potential bias from length of stay by stratifying the analysis on the basis of the duration between admission and selection for study.

Survival

Neyman (1955) emphasized the importance of using incident cases by speculating, for the sake of argument, that case-control studies of an association between smoking and lung cancer based on prevalent cases could be misleading; a higher apparent risk of disease among smokers might be due to a lengthening of their survival, rather than an increase in disease incidence. Sartwell and Merrell (1952) have discussed further examples, one being the introduction of insulin, a factor protective from death due to diabetes, which was undoubtedly associated with a subsequent increase in the prevalence rate of diabetes. These concerns apply to any situation in which a disease accompanied by mortality is studied only in the survivors, a potential source of *survival bias*. Thus, in a study of survivors of myocardial infarction (MI), a case-control difference does not necessarily reveal factors that influence an individual's risk of sustaining an MI, but perhaps factors that increase a person's chance of surviving one (Taube 1968).

The preceding considerations are pertinent to the design of case-control studies. Unless one can justify the assumption that the study factors do not affect the duration of disease or survival, every effort should be made to limit recruitment to incident cases. If constraints on time or resources make the use of incident cases infeasible, one should choose prevalent cases occurring closest in time to the initiation of the study. This will tend to reduce any selective bias toward enrolling less severe forms of the disease.

A partial check on survival bias may be possible. One may stratify the cases by date of onset or date of diagnosis and compare the relative frequency of exposure across strata. If, among the cases, the relative frequency of exposure to a factor suspected of causing the disease increases with lengthening survival time, one has the potential for a biased inference.

Admission Diagnoses

With hospital-based case-control studies, the control group is taken from patients with diseases or admission diagnoses that differ from the study disease. The choice of such controls rests on the assumption that there is no association between the study exposure and the diseases that resulted in hospitalization of the control subjects (Cornfield and Haenszel 1960). If patients with diseases having an unsuspected positive association with the study exposure are overrepresented in the control group, then the apparent relative risk (odds ratio) will underestimate the correct value. This would be a consequence of the hospital control series overestimating the frequency of past exposure, as compared with past exposure among all individuals, hospitalized or not, in the target population. As an example of this, early case-control studies of smoking and lung cancer selected controls from patients with diseases other than lung cancer. It is now recognized that smoking is associated with a wide range of conditions that result in hospitalization. As a consequence, the effect of smoking on lung cancer was underestimated, although the positive association was correctly identified.

One must also take care that the study exposure is not protective against the diseases that are included among the controls. If this were true, the apparent risk of disease associated with exposure could be spuriously increased (Kraus 1954).

In practice, one attempts to avoid a biased control series in hospital-based studies by selecting controls from a wide variety of admission diagnoses, all of which are believed to be unrelated to the study exposure, in the sense that they are neither caused by nor prevented by it. Although a single type of admission diagnosis may fulfill this criterion, the prudent investigator will hedge his or her bet by taking controls with various diagnoses (Chapter 3).

5.2 BIAS IN THE ESTIMATION OF EXPOSURE

Recall

In case-control studies, medical records and interviews with patients and controls are the two main sources of information on past exposure. Erroneous estimation of exposure can occur for many reasons. Biased recall or faulty memory have been revealed by the comparison of subjects' responses to questions about exposure with documented records of exposure. For example, a woman who has a child with a congenital disorder and is trying to recall past exposures to pelvic X-ray may tend to overestimate her exposure as compared with a woman who has given birth to a normal child. Similarly, a woman questioned about frequency of coitus and number of different sexual partners may search her memory with more care and intensity if she has cervical cancer than would a healthy woman. The typical unstructured interview that forms the basis of medical and hospital records is particularly susceptible to biased recall.

The occurrence of a new case of disease within a family will stimulate its members to provide information to the diseased individual regarding a family history of illnesses and exposures believed to be associated with that disease (Sackett 1979). Thus, information on family history may vary on the basis of whether the respondent is a case or a nondiseased control. The use of controls with another disease can reduce this source of error, as well as compensate for the biased recall mentioned in the previous paragraph.

A subject responding to an interviewer's questions may give erroneous replies due to memory loss, confusion, or an effort to please the questioner. Several studies comparing women's responses to questions concerning use of oral contraceptives and prescribers' records suggest that recall of details of past use, such as different formulations, different brands, breaks in usage, and starting and stopping dates deteriorates with the passage of time (Stolley et al. 1978). One often finds in studies of drug use that many subjects tend to underestimate consumption and overestimate the cost of drugs. Studies of certain diseases have been hampered because the disease itself affects memory. Alzheimer's disease ("presenile dementia") is a disorder that causes severe impairment of memory, and although certain environmental exposures are under suspicion, questioning of the victims is likely to be a fruitless pursuit.

When planning a study, one should list potential sources of bias in the ascertainment of exposure in an effort to anticipate them and take steps to minimize their occurrence. If biased recall is anticipated, such as might occur in a study that involves obtaining information from mothers of children with a particular congenital anomaly, the control subjects could be chosen from among mothers with a different type of anomaly or adverse pregnancy outcome, in addition to using mothers of "normal" children as another control group. Independent verification of history of exposure can be sought, where possible, as a check on recall by the subjects.

Interviewer

The term *interviewer bias* has been loosely applied to several components of error arising in personal interviews. Biased recall can inadvertently be stimulated or encouraged by an interviewer who is privy to the hypothesis under consideration. Interviewers may tend to probe the diseased subjects more intensely for histories of exposure than they do the comparison or control subjects. Interviewers may even communicate their pleasure in receiving "positive" responses by their use of language, tone and inflection of speech, or even with unconscious use of "body language," such as smiles or frowns.

Interviewer bias can be reduced by training for even-handed probing. While some have advocated keeping interviewers ignorant of both the study hypothesis and the classification of the respondent as a case or a control, in actual field operations this is usually an unobtainable ideal. It requires more personnel and a greater expenditure of effort. Furthermore, it is hard to keep this kind of secrecy and maintain staff morale. There are also difficult logistic problems that interfere with accomplishing this masking of a subject's identity as either a case or a control. For example, an attempt to obscure subjects' case- or control-status in a study of the relationship of phlebitis to oral contraceptive use was defeated by the fact that phlebitis patients are often treated by leg elevation and ice pack, immediately identified by the interviewer. Use of a standardized interview form combined with intensive training are both feasible and effective ways to minimize biased patient recall and interviewer bias.

Prevarication

Subjects in a study may have ulterior motives for deliberately overestimating or underestimating exposure to a suspected causal agent. A worker who may receive disability pay or some other form of compensation might tend to exaggerate his exposure. Conversely, if exposure meant loss of his job, he might minimize it. Management of an industry where exposure to a harmful agent is suspected might feel a great impetus to underestimate exposures if asked to classify workers by history and extent of exposure. The estimate of the odds ratio will not be biased if the exposure rates for cases and controls are over- or under-estimated to the same degree (e.g. k-fold). Despite this, a proportionate over- or under-estimate will result in an incorrect assessment of the absolute risk of disease associated with exposure. The problem of incorrectly reporting exposure levels because of the influence of administrative rewards and penalties can sometimes be overcome by utilizing several independent raters.

Improper Analysis

If one matches cases and controls on a variable associated with the study exposure, an analysis that ignores the matching will yield a disease-exposure odds ratio that is biased toward unity (Chapter 4). Thus, in some circumstances, unmatched analyses of matched data can spuriously diminish the estimate of an exposure's effect.

5.3 MISCLASSIFICATION

The determination of an individual's exposure status or disease status may be subject to error. This can occur for diagnoses based on physical examination or laboratory findings, or for the estimation of past exposures based on recall in personal interviews or abstracted from written records. For example, the diagnosis of carcinoma in situ (CIS) from exfoliative cytology involves considerable error. Coppleson and Brown (1974) have estimated that the probability of correctly diagnosing CIS among patients who have the disease has varied from 0.55 to 0.80. As another example, Lilienfeld and Graham (1958) compared patients' statements regarding circumcision with physical examination findings.

Among 84 circumcised men, only 37 correctly reported their circumcision. Among 108 men who were not circumcised, 89 correctly reported the absence of circumcision.

Ordinarily, a disease is sufficiently well defined so that concern with bias deriving from its misclassification is more of an academic than a real problem. But this is not always so, and there have been issues in disease etiology where considerable controversy has resulted from speculation that extensive misclassification may have occurred. The apparent relationship of postmenopausal estrogen supplementation to the subsequent development of endometrial carcinoma has been questioned by critics who have suggested that many of the Stage 1 (low-grade) tumors might actually be misclassified endometrial hyperplasia of the atypical adenomatous type (Gordon and Greenberg 1976). Since this hyperplasia is known to be caused by estrogens, if such misclassification had actually occurred, then estrogens could be falsely indicted as a cause of cancer.

Although some controls may actually have the study disease, with rare diseases this is highly improbable. Thus, diagnostic tests are usually not carried out to guarantee the "purity" of the control group. This would represent a low-yield enterprise with unnecessarily incurred costs.

In case-control studies, the most likely source of classification error will occur in the determination of exposure. Interviewing technique and the phrasing of questions, the ages and educational backgrounds of the respondents, the time interval between the exposures of interest and the interview, and the degree of detail sought will all affect the validity of the responses. For example, although a well-educated woman may accurately recall aspects of recent (within 5 years) oral contraceptive use such as total duration, months since discontinuation, and the names of the most recent and least recent preparations she has taken, she is less likely to accurately remember breaks in use or the duration of use of specific preparations (Glass, Johnson, and Vessey 1974). As another example, one study found that 75 percent to 90 percent of a group of well-educated women recalled within one year their age at menarche, age at natural or surgical menopause, and age at first use of oral contraceptives. However, recollection of menstrual cycle length and variability was considered unreliable (Bean et al. 1979). Dietary histories are notorious for their error, and one would expect similar inaccuracy in the recollection of details of other complex exposures occurring in the far past.

Estimates of relative risk will be biased as a result of misclassification of subjects with respect to either disease or exposure status. Perhaps the most widely quoted consequence of classification errors is based on the results of Bross (1954), who demonstrated that random and independent errors tend to diminish the apparent degree of association between two variables (see Newell 1963). Such errors tend to equalize the observed counts a, b, c, and d in the 2×2 table representing exposure and disease (Table 2.5), thereby biasing the odds ratio toward unity. Thus, the existence of false positive or false negative diagnoses will result in a diminished estimate of relative risk, provided that errors of diagnosis occur equally for exposed and unexposed individuals. Similarly, errors in determining an individual's exposure status will also attenuate the estimated relative risk if they occur equally among cases and controls. If a true dose-response relationship exists that links exposure to disease, however, then random errors in the classification of exposure would not likely mask substantial risk increments (Marshall et al. 1981). In general, the odds ratio, relative risk, or risk difference may be spuriously increased or decreased if classification errors depend on either case-control status or exposure. Goldberg (1975) and Copeland et al. (1977) have reviewed this topic, and Greenland (1980) has extended the discussion to the effect of misclassifying subjects with respect to a potential confounding variable.

A simple adjustment for misclassification can be made if one assumes that cases and controls are correctly classified with respect to disease and that errors in determining exposure do not depend on case-control status. Unfortunately, the adjustment requires knowledge of two quantities that often can only be determined imprecisely: (1) the probability than an exposed individual is correctly classified as exposed, $p = P(+\,|\,E)$; and (2) the probability that an unexposed individual is correctly classified as unexposed, $p' = P(-\,|\,\overline{E})$. If errors in determining exposure depend on whether the individual is a case or a control, or if errors also occur in the diagnosis of disease, then the analysis is further complicated (Keys and Kihlberg 1963).

Suppose that one wants to estimate the attenuation in the odds ratio produced by errors in determining an individual's exposure status. For this purpose, assume that the probabilities p and p' defined in the preceding paragraph are the same for cases and controls. Further suppose that c of the n_1 cases and d of the n_2 controls are classified as unexposed. An adjustment for the average effects of misclassification with respect to exposure can then be made by calculating

$$A = (p'n_1 - c)/(p + p' - 1)$$
$$B = (p'n_2 - d)/(p + p' - 1)$$
$$C = n_1 - A$$
$$D = n_2 - B$$

from which an adjusted odds ratio is estimated by

$$\hat{\psi}_a = AD/BC. \tag{5.3}$$

In practice one may have to guess at values for p and p', perhaps calculating the adjusted estimate (5.3) over a reasonable range.

An adjustment for classification error does not eliminate the effects of other sources of bias. For example, if an exposed case were more likely to enter the sample than an unexposed case, the odds ratio would be upwardly biased. In this situation the presence of classification errors could fortuitously attenuate a biased odds ratio, and adjustment for misclassification could result in an estimate that was more discrepant with the correct value than the unadjusted odds ratio.

Concern with errors of diagnosis or reporting is best raised during the design phase of a study, since any mathematical adjustment of the odds ratio to correct for misclassification will be speculative. A pilot study can reveal many sources of error that can be eliminated during the full-scale investigation. For incident case-control studies, where cases are identified from hospital discharge diagnoses or pathology reports, one can make provisions for a standardized, independent review of records and material that formed the basis for the original diagnosis. On the other hand, information on past exposures reported in a personal interview may be difficult or impossible to validate.

5.4 OTHER SOURCES OF ERROR

A study may be faultlessly conducted but inadequately designed. For example, an investigation of insufficient size may contain no source of error other than an inbuilt predisposition to accept the null hypothesis of no effect (Chapter 6). On the other hand, an incorrect inference about an exposure's effect may derive from errors of interpretation or failure to properly account for the effect of extraneous variables. These sources of error are just as detrimental to an investigation as others resulting from deficient design or flawed execution of the study protocol.

A correct assessment of the effect of an exposure requires that at baseline (before exposure) both exposed and unexposed individuals be equally susceptible. If this does not occur, any factor that affects the risk of disease and that differs between exposed and unexposed individuals could cause a spurious positive or negative association between exposure and disease. This reasoning, applied to a case-control study, implies that cases and controls should have been similar with respect to factors that might have affected both the development of disease and the opportunity for past exposure. In particular, one must properly account for conditions in the cases and controls that predispose an individual to a disease and that consequently may preclude or modify usage of an exposure to a suspected causal agent. For example, although choice of a contraceptive method is partly based on personal preference, medical conditions such as hypertension, diabetes, or a family history of breast cancer will contraindicate use of oral contraceptives. Unless one accounts for this, a case-control study could either underestimate the effect of oral contraceptives on the risk of these diseases, or even find that pill use was apparently protective. This would be a consequence of users being inherently at lower risk. One way to adjust for this possibility is to restrict the analysis to individuals who had no predisposing conditions before exposure began or might have begun. In this regard, it is not *current* predisposing conditions but *past* ones that are important. In fact, one could unwittingly introduce a bias by excluding from analysis those individuals with conditions that arose subsequent to usage of oral contraceptives, if the risk of these conditions, themselves disease risk factors, were increased by OC usage. In this circumstance, exclusions could eliminate one of the pathways by which an exposure altered the risk of disease.

In some situations it may be difficult to disentangle the potential effect of predisposing conditions from the apparent effect of an exposure. This is likely to occur where a drug was prescribed as a treatment for a condition that itself may reflect an alteration in risk. For example, diethylstibestrol (DES) was commonly prescribed in the 1950s and 1960s to women with problem pregnancies in the belief that it would improve their reproductive outcomes. In 1980, the female offspring of DES-exposed mothers were themselves reported to be at increased risk of an unfavorable pregnancy outcome (Barnes et al. 1980). One might postulate a genetic basis that would explain this finding, hypothesizing, for example, that DES exposure had no effect on an offspring's reproductive capacity, but that its apparent effect was simply due to DES-exposed mothers being inherently at greater risk of bearing children who would have reproductive problems.

A related source of susceptibility bias derives from the possibility that an agent, later found to be present in association with the study disease, was actually prescribed because of an early manifestation of that disease. To check such a possibility, one must learn for each case and control why the agent was prescribed, avoided, or discontinued, and analyze data within strata of the manifestations leading to prescription, discontinuation, etc. For example, Gordon and Greenberg (1976) speculated that estrogens were prescribed for irregular bleeding that was the first symptom of undetected endometrial cancer. If this were true, then later diagnosis of the cancer would find an apparent association with estrogen usage. In a case-control study intended to address these and other criticisms, Antunes et al. (1979) reported on a series of 451 patients with endometrial cancer and 888 controls. None of the patients who received estrogens had them prescribed for the treatment of abnormal bleeding. Among both cases and controls, the most frequent indication for estrogen use was the relief of symptoms attributed to menopause, particularly "hot flashes" (vasovagal symptoms).

Certain symptoms of an underlying disease process may result in the discontinuation of a drug that was actually its cause. If the latent disease is subsequently identified long after discontinuation, and if use of the agent was not determined for the distant past, or if only *current* use of the agent is considered, cases of the disease would have a spuriously lowered frequency of prior exposure. Thus, a factor that was harmful might be found to be apparently protective. At the very least, the apparent risk would be biased downward. For example, hysterectomy removes a substantial number of women at risk of endometrial and uterine cancer. If use of oral contraceptives led to conditions that increased the frequency of hysterectomy, or if hysterectomies were otherwise performed preferentially on pill users compared with non-users, an association between oral contraceptive use and endometrial or uterine cancer may be missed. Hulka, Hogue, and Greenberg (1978) have discussed a variety of other issues related to this topic.

Arguments against a causal interpretation of the association between smoking and coronary disease were partly based on speculative differences in susceptibility between smokers and nonsmokers. Arguing in terms of a "constitutional hypothesis," critics of early observational studies suggested that underlying factors such as psychic stress could influence coronary disease and also affect one's tendency to self-select the alleged causal agent (smoking). Where feasible, the most direct approach to addressing the issue of suceptibility bias is to stratify the analysis (or match cases and controls) on the basis of the hypothesized confounder in order to assess the effect of exposure within strata of equal susceptibility. In practice this may be difficult, because the stratification or matching should be based on characteristics prior to the time that exposure occurred or might have occurred. Assessment of an individual's past susceptibility from personal interview or existing records may be infeasible or too unreliable to claim that comparisons are made within strata of equal risk.

5.5 SUMMARY

The case-control method is susceptible to many sources of bias, most of which are not peculiar to this form of investigation, occurring in cohort studies as well (Sartwell 1979). The establishment of the case and the control groups can be biased through improper ascertainment, diagnosis, or selection of study subjects. Error in correctly determining past exposures can derive from imperfect records, faulty recall, prevarication, or improper interviewing techniques. At the initiation of a study, one should list the likely sources of bias and plan the investigation and analyses as best one can to prevent errors that may invalidate one's findings. A review of the points of this chapter and use of the checklist at the end of Chapter 3 may assist in this endeavor.

6 Sample Size

6.0 INTRODUCTION

The number of subjects to be selected for study of a specific disease-exposure relationship is a fundamental consideration in planning a case-control investigation. A study should be sufficiently large to avoid two sources of error: (1) claiming that exposure is associated with disease when in fact it is not, and (2) claiming that exposure is not associated with disease, when in fact it is. When the frequency of exposure between cases and controls is compared by means of a statistical test, the probability of making the first error is called the *level of significance,* and is commonly denoted by "α." The probability of making the second error is represented by "β," and the quantity $1 - \beta$ is called the *power* of the study. Assuming that the relative risk in the target population differs from unity, the power ($1 - \beta$) is the probability of finding that the sample estimate of relative risk (odds ratio) differs significantly from unity.

Basically, an answer to the question of how many subjects should be selected for a case-control study depends on the specification of four values: (1) the relative frequency of exposure among controls in the target population, p_0, (2) a hypothesized relative risk associated with exposure that would have sufficient biologic or public health importance to warrant its detection, R, (3) the desired level of significance, α; (4) the desired study power, $1 - \beta$.

This chapter gives methods for the determination of sample size and power for unmatched and matched case-control studies. It also discusses sample size considerations relating to nonresponse, subgroup analyses, adjustment for confounding, multiple controls per case, differential case-control costs, and the use of sequential analysis.

6.1 SAMPLE SIZE AND POWER FOR UNMATCHED STUDIES

Sample Size

Suppose that one wants to assess whether a particular exposure, regarded simply as having been either present or absent, is associated with an alteration in the risk of a particular disease. For unmatched samples of cases and controls, the odds ratio in a simple 2×2 table can be tested by means of the standard chi-square test (Chapter 7). Let p_0 denote the estimated exposure rate (proportion exposed) among controls, and let R denote the relative risk corresponding to the smallest increase or decrease in risk of interest. Specifying desired values for α and β, such as $\alpha = .05$ and $\beta = .10$, and assuming that equal numbers of cases and controls will be selected, the required sample size for each group (n per group) is calculated as follows (Schlesselman 1974):

$$n = [z_\alpha \sqrt{2\bar{p}\bar{q}} + z_\beta \sqrt{p_1 q_1 + p_0 q_0}]^2/(p_1 - p_0)^2 \qquad (6.1)$$

where

$$p_1 = p_0 R/[1 + p_0(R - 1)] \qquad (6.2)$$

and

$$\bar{p} = \tfrac{1}{2}(p_1 + p_0) \qquad \bar{q} = 1 - \bar{p}$$

$$q_1 = 1 - p_1 \qquad q_0 = 1 - p_0$$

The quantities z_α and z_β are values from the standard normal distribution corresponding to α and β. For a one-sided test of the hypothesis that $R > 1$ (or $R < 1$), z_α is taken to be the value of the standard normal distribution that is exceeded with probability α. For a two-sided test, z_α is taken to be the value that is exceeded with probability $\alpha/2$. For either a one-sided or a two-sided test, z_β is taken to be the value that is exceeded with probability β. Table 6.1 gives selected values of z_α and z_β corresponding to commonly used values of α and β.

A formula that is simpler than (6.1), and for practical purposes equivalent, is given by

$$n = 2\bar{p}\bar{q}(z_\alpha + z_\beta)^2/(p_1 - p_0)^2. \qquad (6.3)$$

Corresponding to $\alpha = .05$ (two-sided) and $\beta = .10$, one has $z_\alpha = 1.96$ and $z_\beta = 1.28$, so that equation (6.3) reduces to a particularly simple formula: $n = 21\bar{p}\bar{q}/(p_1 - p_0)^2$.

Table 6.1. Unit Normal Deviates
z_α and z_β for Selected Values of α and β.

α or β	One-sided test z_α or z_β	Two-sided test[1] z_α
0.001	3.09	3.29
0.005	2.58	2.81
0.01	2.33	2.58
0.025	1.96	2.24
0.05	1.64	1.96
0.10	1.28	1.64
0.20	0.84	1.28
0.30	0.52	1.04

1. Values of z_β are the same for both one-sided
and two-sided tests of significance.

As an example of the application of equation (6.1), suppose that one is considering a case-control study of a potential association between congenital heart defects and maternal hormone exposure, particularly oral contraceptives, occurring around the time of conception. Further suppose that one estimates from data of Westoff and Bumpass (1973) that approximately 30 percent of women of childbearing age will have an exposure to oral contraceptives within three months of a conception. Taking this as an estimate of the expected rate of exposure among controls, that is, $p_0 = 0.30$, and specifying $\alpha = 0.05$ (two-sided) and $\beta = 0.10$, the sample sizes required to detect various hypothetical relative risks are shown in Table 6.2. The calculations corresponding to $R = 3$, for example, proceed as follows:

$$p_1 = 0.3(3)/[1 + 0.3(3 - 1)] = 0.5625$$

$$\bar{p} = \tfrac{1}{2}(0.3 + 0.5625) = 0.43125$$

$$n = [1.96\sqrt{0.4905} + 1.28\sqrt{0.2461 + 0.2100}]^2/(0.2625)^2 = 73,$$

where n has been rounded to the nearest integer. For comparison, equation (6.3) gives

$$n = 2(0.43125)(0.56875)(1.96 + 1.28)^2/(0.2625)^2 = 75.$$

The values of n given in Table 6.2 indicate the sensitivity of a calculation to the specified value of R. Depending on the minimum relative risk that one wants to detect, the sample size per group ranges from 18 to 188. The estimate of required sample size can also vary greatly with different choices for α, β, or p_0. Laird, Weinstein, and Stason (1979) give a detailed analysis of the sensitivity of sample size estimation in the context of a clinical trial of treatment for mild hypertension. The paper by the Multiple Risk Factor Intervention Trial Group (1977) is also instructive in this regard.

If one knows the rate at which cases accrue, determination of sample size will permit an estimate of the anticipated duration of study. One can therefore judge whether a single institution, group of institutions, or population base will be adequate to conduct a study within a reasonable period of time.

Although p_0 refers to the exposure rate among controls in the target population, when studying rare diseases, one may estimate its value from population information relating to the overall exposure rate, since cases would constitute a very small fraction of the total.

Use of Bayes' theorem (Feller 1968) allows one to express the preceding approximation algebraically and gives a slightly different perspective on the issue:

$$p_0 = P(E|\overline{D}) = P(E)[1 - P(D|E)]/[1 - P(D)] \simeq P(E).$$

Thus $p_0 \simeq P(E)$ whenever $P(D|E)$ is close to $P(D)$, which is true under the null hypothesis of no effect. If exposure increases the risk of disease, then $P(E) > p_0$, resulting in an overestimate of the exposure rate among controls based on population information. If the exposure is protective, then $P(E) < p_0$ (Schlesselman 1974).

Sample size formulae may be used to plan studies to detect either increased or decreased risks. For example, suppose that one hypothesized that long-term oral contraceptive use reduced the risk of benign breast disease, and that one wanted to detect at least a 30 percent reduction in

Table 6.2. Sample Size Requirement for a Case-Control Study of Congenital Heart Disease and Maternal Hormone Exposure

Relative risk	Case-control sample size[1] n (per group)
2	188
3	73
4	45
5	34
7	24
10	18

1. Equation (6.1) used with $p_o = .3$, $\alpha = .05$ (two-sided) and $\beta = .10$.

Source: Schlesselman 1974.

risk ($R = 0.7$). Then a case-control study would require $n = 1156$ women per group, assuming 20 percent were long-term oral contraceptive users, $p_0 = 0.2$, and specifying $1 - \beta = 0.9$ and $\alpha = 0.05$ (two-sided):

$$p_1 = 0.2(0.7)/[1 + 0.2(0.7 - 1)] = 0.1489$$

$$\bar{p} = \frac{1}{2}(0.2 + 0.1489) = 0.1744$$

$$n = [1.96 \sqrt{0.2880} + 1.28 \sqrt{0.1267 + 0.1600}]^2/(-0.0511)^2$$
$$= 1156$$

Appendix A gives tables of the sample size n (per group) based on formula (6.1) for selected values of R, p_0, α and β. This permits one to avoid computations in many instances and allows one to see at a glance how the sample size requirement changes for different parameter specifications. The exposure rate in controls, p_0, must be estimated from data sources or "expert opinion" in order to determine a sample size. Furthermore, specification of values for R, α, and β is a matter of judgment. For these reasons, one should regard a calculated sample size as a guide to planning and not an absolute requirement.

Study Power

In practice, the size of a study is often restricted by financial resources, the number of available cases, or a time limitation. For example, an important policy decision concerning an industrial, environmental, or drug exposure may require that a study be done quickly. In this situation the rate of accrual of cases will limit the size of the case series. Similarly, the number of cancers of a specific type in a tumor registry will restrict the size of a case series based on prevalent cases. If a study were proposed within a fixed administrative setting, cases arising within a given hospital, or from the facilities of a prepaid medical plan, the case series would be limited by the size and type of population covered. Although in principle one can always extend the duration of study or include more catchment units, such an option may not be considered practical. Finally, there are always financial constraints and limitations of staffing.

As a consequence of various constraints on the size of an investigation, a sample size analysis often begins with a fixed value for n, and then determines the resulting power ($1-\beta$) of detecting various values of R

(Walter 1977). Inversion of formulas (6.1) and (6.3) gives

$$\hat{z}_\beta = [\sqrt{n(p_1 - p_0)^2} - z_\alpha\sqrt{2\overline{p}\overline{q}}]/\sqrt{p_1 q_1 + p_0 q_0} \qquad (6.4)$$

and

$$\hat{z}_\beta = [n(p_1 - p_0)^2/2\overline{p}\overline{q}]^{1/2} - z_\alpha, \qquad (6.5)$$

respectively. The power is determined from tables of the normal distribution by finding the probability with which the calculated value of $\hat{z}_\beta$ is *not* exceeded:

$$\text{Power} = 1 - \beta = P(Z \le \hat{z}_\beta).$$

To continue with the example of congenital heart defects and maternal hormone exposure, suppose that one can only study case and control groups of size $n = 50$. Taking $p_0 = 0.30$ and $\alpha = 0.05$ (two-sided) as before, what is the power of a study with respect to detecting a twofold increased risk? Using equation (6.5) for simplicity, the calculations proceed as follows:

$$p_1 = 0.3(2)/[1 + 0.3(2 - 1)] = 0.4615$$

$$\overline{p} = \tfrac{1}{2}(0.3 + 0.4615) = 0.38075$$

$$\hat{z}_\beta = [50(0.4615 - 0.30)^2/0.47156]^{1/2} - 1.96 = -0.2970.$$

From tables of the normal probability function, given in Appendix B, one finds

$$\text{Power} = P(Z \le -0.2970) = 0.38.$$

Thus, if the relative risk in the target population is $R = 2$, a case-control study of $n = 50$ per group has only a 38 percent chance of finding that the sample estimate will be significantly ($\alpha = 0.05$) different from unity.

One should always consider the power of a study that finds no disease-exposure association. Failure to reject the null hypothesis ($R = 1$) may have resulted from an investigation that had insufficient power to detect an alteration in risk ($R > 1$ or $R < 1$) of biologic or public health importance. To evaluate the power of a completed study in which equal numbers of cases and controls have been used, one applies either equation (6.4) or (6.5), using the observed exposure rate among the controls for p_0 and the observed number of cases for n. Despite the intent to accrue equal numbers of cases and controls, a completed study may have groups of unequal size. In this situation one may apply equations (6.9) or (6.10) which are discussed in Section 6.2.

6.2 SAMPLE SIZE AND POWER WITH MULTIPLE CONTROLS PER CASE

Sample Size Determination with an Unequal Case-Control Ratio

A simple extension of equations (6.1) and (6.3) applies to the determination of sample size with multiple controls per case. With c controls per case, the sample size formula corresponding to (6.1) is

$$n = [z_\alpha \sqrt{(1 + 1/c)\, \overline{p}'\overline{q}'} + z_\beta \sqrt{p_1 q_1 + p_0 q_0/c}]^2/(p_1 - p_0)^2 \quad (6.6)$$

where

$$\overline{p}' = (p_1 + cp_0)/(1 + c), \quad\quad\quad (6.7)$$

$\overline{q}' = 1 - \overline{p}'$, and p_1 is calculated using equation (6.2).

The term n represents the number of cases to be taken, so that cn gives the number of controls. Note that when $c = 1$, indicating a 1:1 case:control ratio, formula (6.6) reduces to (6.1). The term c need not be an integer. Thus taking $c = 0.8$, implying more cases than controls, or $c = 1.5$ is perfectly acceptable. The sample size formula which corresponds to equation (6.3) is

$$n = (1 + 1/c)\, \overline{p}'\overline{q}'\, (z_\alpha + z_\beta)^2/(p_1 - p_0)^2. \quad (6.8)$$

Another useful formula that allows the determination of the sample size for a 1:c case:control ratio is given by equation (6.25) in Section 6.8.

Consider again the example of sample size determination for a case-control study of congenital heart defects, assuming that one desires to take 2 controls per case. Let $R = 4$ be the minimum value of relative risk that one would like the study to detect with $\alpha = 0.05$ (two-sided), $\beta = 0.10$ and $p_0 = 0.30$. Using equation (6.6) one has

$$p_1 = 0.3(4)/[1 + 0.3(4 - 1)] = 0.6316$$

$$\overline{p}' = [0.6316 + 2(0.3)]/3 = 0.4105$$

$$n = [1.96 \sqrt{0.3630} + 1.28 \sqrt{0.2327 + 0.1050}]^2/(0.3316)^2 = 34.$$

Thus one requires $n = 34$ cases and $2n = 68$ controls, resulting in a total study of 102 subjects. [For comparison, the use of equation (6.8) indicates $n = 35$ cases.] From Table 6.2 one sees that with a 1:1 ratio of cases to controls, a total of 90 subjects (cases plus controls) would be needed. If the number of available cases were restricted, or if a cost-differential existed, making controls relatively less expensive, a study with a 1:2 case:control ratio requiring 34 cases (68 controls) may be preferable to one with 45 cases (45 controls). This issue is discussed further in Section 6.4.

Study Power with an Unequal Case-Control Ratio

To evaluate the power of a study having unequal numbers of cases and controls, one inverts equation (6.6) or (6.8), solving for z_β:

$$\hat{z}_\beta = [\sqrt{n(p_1 - p_0)^2} - z_\alpha \sqrt{(1 + 1/c)\,\overline{p}'\overline{q}'}]/\sqrt{p_1 q_1 + p_0 q_0/c} \quad (6.9)$$

and

$$\hat{z}_\beta = [n(p_1 - p_0)^2/(1 + 1/c)\overline{p}'\overline{q}']^{1/2} - z_\alpha. \quad (6.10)$$

In the above formulae, the term n represents the number of cases, and the term c represents the number of controls per case. The power is determined from tables of the standard normal distribution (Appendix B) by finding the probability with which the calculated value of $\hat{z}_\beta$ is not exceeded: Power $= P(Z \le \hat{z}_\beta)$.

Equations (6.9) and (6.10) may be used either in planning an investigation or in evaluating the power of a completed study. An example of the latter application is provided by a case-control study of a postulated association between spontaneous abortion and prior induced abortion (Kline et al. 1978). A consecutive series of spontaneous abortions from three Manhattan hospitals was studied over a period of 2½ years, from April 1974 through August 1976. Controls matched to within two years of age of the cases were selected from pregnant women who registered for prenatal care before the 22nd week of gestation and delivered after 28 weeks. Extensive analysis of the data revealed no association between spontaneous abortion and prior induced abortion. [See Levin et al. (1980) for another case-control study of this issue.]

Table 6.3 shows previous induced abortions among multigravid cases

Table 6.3.   Prior Induced Abortion (PIA)
among Women Having a Spontaneous
Abortion (Cases) and Controls

	Spontaneous abortions	Controls
PIA:		
Yes	171	90
No	303	165
Total	474	255

Source: Kline et al. 1978.

and controls. (Primigravidae were excluded, since these women did not
have prior pregnancies.) The power of the study for detecting a relative
risk of $R = 1.5$ is calculated as follows:

$$c = 255/474 = 0.5380$$
$$p_0 = 90/255 = 0.3529$$
$$p_1 = (0.3529)(1.5)/[1 + 0.3529\,(1.5 - 1)] = 0.4500$$

$$\bar{p}' = [0.4500 + (0.5380)(0.3529)]/(1 + 0.5380) = 0.4160.$$

Using equation (6.10) for simplicity, we have for $\alpha = 0.05$ (two-sided)

$$\hat{z}_\beta = [474(0.45 - 0.3529)^2/2.8587(0.4160)(0.5840)]^{1/2} - 1.96 = 0.58.$$

From Appendix B, $P(Z \leq 0.58) = 0.72$. Thus the study had an estimated 72 per cent chance of detecting a 1.5 times increase in the risk of
spontaneous abortion.

6.3 SMALLEST DETECTABLE RELATIVE RISK

Our discussion of study power was premised on the existence of a constraint on the available sample size. Thus, given fixed values of n, α, and
p_0, equations (6.4), (6.5), (6.9), and (6.10) permit one to estimate the
power of an unmatched case-control study to detect any specified value
for R. A slight variation of this problem provides another useful perspective on the size of a study. Given fixed values of n, α, and p_0, what
is the smallest value of R that can be detected with a specified power?
The answer is given by equation (6.11) below.

Assume that the exposure rate among controls in the target population
is p_0, and that samples of size n per group are used. The smallest pop-

ulation relative risk greater than one (or the largest population relative risk less than one) that can be detected for specified values of n, p_0, α, and β is given by (Walter 1977)

$$\hat{R} = 1 + \sqrt{A}\{B\sqrt{A} \pm [AB^2 + 4C]^{1/2}\}/C \qquad (6.11)$$

where

$$A = (z_\alpha + z_\beta)^2$$
$$B = 1 + 2p_0$$
$$C = 2p_0[n(1 - p_0) - Ap_0].$$

Appendix C gives tables of $\hat{R}$ for selected values of n, p_0, α, and β. One may consider calculating $\hat{R}$ either in planning a study or at the completion of one. With c controls per case, substitute (cC) for C, $(1 + 2cp_0)$ for B, and $2(1 + c)$ for 4 in equation (6.11).

Kessler and Clark (1978) studied 365 males with bladder cancer and an equal number of controls, 35 percent of whom reported past use of nonnutritive sweeteners. Using a one-sided test at the $\alpha = 0.05$ level, the smallest relative risk greater than one that can be detected with 90 percent power is $\hat{R} = 1.55$:

$$A = (1.64 + 1.28)^2 = 8.5264$$
$$B = 1 + 2(0.35) = 1.7$$
$$C = 2(0.35)[365(0.65) - 8.5264(0.35)] = 163.9860$$
$$\hat{R} = 1 + 2.92[4.9640 \pm 26.0880]/163.9860$$
$$= 1.55 \text{ or } 0.62,$$

where 1.55 is obtained by addition and 0.62 by subtraction in (6.11). In other words, one is 90 percent sure that a relative risk of 1.55 or greater in the target population will be detected in a sample of $n = 365$ per group, using an $\alpha = 0.05$ one-sided test, and assuming an exposure rate of 35 percent among controls. The value $\hat{R} = 0.62$ is pertinent to the situation in which one is trying to detect a decrease in risk. It represents the largest relative risk less than unity that can be detected in samples of size $n = 365$, given the above specifications for α, β, and p_0.

Use of equation (6.11) will sometimes produce negative values of $\hat{R}$. These are associated with inadmissible parameter values in the equation for sample size from which (6.11) is derived. In those instances where $\hat{R}$ is negative and the plus sign is used in equation (6.11), replace the negative value by ∞ (infinity); where $\hat{R}$ is negative and the minus sign is used in equation (6.11), replace the negative value by 0 (zero) (Walter 1977). For example, if $n = 25$, $p_0 = 0.10$, $\alpha = .05$ (two-sided), and $\beta = 0.10$, then $\hat{R} = 1 + 3.24 [3.888 \pm 5.6812]/4.29$, giving values of $\hat{R}$ equal to -0.35 $(-)$ and

8.23 (+). Thus we take $\hat{R} = 0.0$ and $\hat{R} = 8.23$. This indicates that for the given specifications, no population relative risk less than unity is likely to be detectable. The study would have a 90 percent chance of detecting population relative risks greater than 8.23, however.

6.4 OPTIMAL ALLOCATION

Equal Case-Control Costs

Suppose that a case-control comparison will be made in terms of a single 2×2 table, that the costs of sampling individuals are the same for both groups, and that no prior information exists concerning the strength of the disease-exposure association. Then given a fixed *total sample size* of N, the selection of equal numbers $(N/2)$ of cases and controls minimizes the variance of the estimated odds ratio. In other circumstances, equal allocation is not optimal, but in practice, is often nearly so.

Suppose, on the other hand, that one wanted to confirm the results of a previous study, perhaps a pilot investigation, which suggested that the relative risk were equal to R. If the total sample size were fixed at N, and there were equal unit costs per case and control, the fraction of the total sample that should be devoted to the case group is (Walter 1977)

$$n/N = 1/[1 + \sqrt{p_1 q_1 / p_0 q_0}], \qquad (6.12)$$

where p_0 is the exposure rate in the controls and $p_1 = p_0 R / [1 + p_0 (R - 1)]$ is the exposure rate in the cases. Equation (6.12) is based on minimizing the asymptotic variance of the estimated log odds ratio. Values of expression (6.12) are shown in Table 6.4. The optimal percentage of cases does not differ greatly from 50 percent except for some extreme combinations of R and p_0. Table 6.4 may be used with relative risks less than unity by taking $1/R$ and $(1 - p_0)$ as the table entries. For example, if $R = 0.5$, and $p_0 = .10$, one would use the values $1/R = 2$ and $(1 - p_0) = .9$ in Table 6.4, which indicates that optimal allocation would place 57 percent of the total sample in the case group.

The objective of testing the null hypothesis of no association $(R = 1)$ is best attained by taking equal numbers of cases and controls. Although this allocation differs from that which is optimal for the estimation of relative risks that are expected to differ from unity, equal-sized samples will often be nearly optimal with respect to the precision of the estimated odds ratio (Walter 1977).

Table 6.4. Optimal Sampling
Percentages for the Case Group in a
Case-Control Study with Various Values
of R and p_0

p_0	\multicolumn{3}{c}{R}		
	2	5	10
0.05	43	35	31
0.10	44	39	38
0.25	47	47	51
0.50	51	57	63
0.75	55	64	71
0.90	57	67	74
0.95	58	68	75

Adapted from Walter 1977.

Unequal Cost: Maximum Power for Fixed Total Cost

The cost of a study will often be a factor limiting its size. Taking this constraint along with the possibility of differential costs for cases and controls, one is led to consider the following question. Given a fixed total cost, how many cases and controls should be selected in order to maximize the power of the study?

To answer the preceding question, suppose that c_1 is the unit cost per case, c_0 the unit cost per control, and T the total available budget. Then the sample sizes for the case group (n_1) and the control group (n_0) that maximize the study's power, subject to the fixed cost T, are given by (Winbush, Springer, and Liu 1978):

$$n_1 = T(c_1 - \sqrt{c_1 c_0})/[c_1(c_1 - c_0)] \qquad (6.13)$$

$$n_0 = T(\sqrt{c_1 c_0} - c_0)/[c_0(c_1 - c_0)]. \qquad (6.14)$$

The optimum ratio of controls to cases for arbitrary values of T is given by dividing n_0 by n_1:

$$n_0/n_1 = \sqrt{c_1/c_0}. \qquad (6.15)$$

The maximum power of the study, using case and control sample sizes of n_1 and n_0, is also easily determined. Let p_0 denote the exposure rate in the controls, and let R be the minimum relative risk of interest. Then for specified α, one first calculates

$$p_1 = p_0R/[1 + p_0(R - 1)],$$

$$q_1 = 1 - p_1$$

$$\bar{p} = (n_1p_1 + n_0p_0)/(n_1 + n_0)$$

$$\bar{q} = 1 - \bar{p}.$$

Next compute

$$\hat{z}_\beta = [\sqrt{n_1n_0(p_1 - p_0)^2}$$
$$- z_\alpha\sqrt{(n_1 + n_0)\bar{p}\bar{q}}]/\sqrt{n_0p_1q_1 + n_1p_0q_0}. \quad (6.16)$$

The maximum power is then determined from tables of the normal distribution by finding the probability that $\hat{z}_\beta$ is not exceeded: Power = $P(Z \le \hat{z}_\beta)$. Equation (6.16) is algebraically equivalent to (6.9).

As an application of the preceding formulae, suppose that the total budget available for a case-control study is \$250,000 and that the unit costs per case and per control are estimated to be $c_1 = \$170$ and $c_0 = \$140$. Then maximum study power will be achieved by taking 771 cases and 850 controls:

$$n_1 = 250000(170 - \sqrt{170 \times 140})/[170(170 - 140)] = 771$$

$$n_0 = 250000(\sqrt{170 \times 140} - 140)/[140(170 - 140)] = 850.$$

The total cost is \$250,070 = 771(\$170) + 850 (\$140). Due to rounding in n_1 and n_0, the total cost slightly exceeds the monetary constraint. The optimum ratio of controls to cases is 1.1 controls per case:

$$n_0/n_1 = 850/771 = 1.1.$$

This ratio can be determined directly from the unit costs, $\sqrt{170/140} = 1.1$.

A determination of the power of the study, given $n_1 = 771$ and $n_0 = 850$, requires specification of α, p_0, and R. Taking again the example of oral contraceptive use and congenital heart defects, discussed in Section 6.1, one has $p_0 = 0.3$. The power of the study for detecting a relative risk of $R = 2$ at the $\alpha = 0.05$ level (two-sided) is then calculated as follows:

$$p_1 = 0.3(2)/[1 + 0.3(2 - 1)] = 0.4615$$

$$\bar{p} = [771\ (0.4615) + 850\ (0.3)]/1621 = 0.3768$$

$$\hat{z}_\beta = 4.8 \qquad \text{Power} = P(Z \leq 4.8) = 1.00.$$

Thus, one is certain that a relative risk of $R = 2$ in the target population will be detected in the sample. Were this the sole objective of the study, one would conclude that it was overfunded. This leads to a related question, namely, what are the optimal numbers of cases and controls to be taken in order to minimize study cost for given power?

Minimum Cost for Fixed Power

As in the previous section, let c_1 and c_0 denote respectively the unit cost per case and per control. Suppose that one wants the study power to be $1 - \beta$. Then the minimum cost is achieved by selecting n_1 cases and n_0 controls where the values of n_1 and n_0 are determined through the following steps (Winbush, Springer, and Liu 1978): (1) given specified values for α, β, p_0, and R, first calculate the value n using equation (6.1) or (6.3); (2) next compute n_1 and n_0 as follows:

$$n_1 = n(1 + \sqrt{c_1/c_0})/(2\sqrt{c_1/c_0}) \qquad (6.17)$$

$$n_0 = n_1 \sqrt{c_1/c_0}. \qquad (6.18)$$

Note that with equal costs, $c_1 = c_0$, the optimal allocation is $n_1 = n_0 = n$. The minimum total study cost for the above design specification is $C = c_1 n_1 + c_0 n_0$.

Discussion

A problem with the preceding optimal allocation schemes arises in studies with several objectives. Case-control allocation that is optimal for one objective may not be optimal for another.

The sample size and power analysis based on the work of Winbush, Springer, and Liu (1978) closely approximates two other approaches to this problem (Meydrech and Kupper 1978, Pike and Casagrande 1979). Gail et al. (1976) have also given a general discussion of circumstances in which unequal sample size allocation may be preferred, considering cost and study power.

The application of equations (6.13) through (6.18) requires that one specify the expected costs per case and per control, c_1 and c_0 respectively. Thinking solely in monetary terms, the expense associated with contacting and interviewing a subject, and verifying information on disease (cases) and exposure (cases and controls), is only a fraction of the total study cost. Planning and coordinating a study, training interviewers, processing data, and writing reports of a study's findings represent some of the expenses that are incidental to those of case-control data collection, but that constitute a substantial proportion of the total study cost. Although there may be differential costs associated with selecting and gathering data on cases and controls, apportioning the incidental costs will attenuate this difference.

For hospital-based studies, one generally expects little difference in case-control costs. An exception might arise if one used matched controls. In this circumstance the unit cost of control selection might be much greater than that for the cases. Since pairing requires at least one control per case, the minimum cost in this instance would result from a $1:1$ ratio, rather than the use of multiple controls individually matched to each case.

Since incidental costs often represent a substantial fraction of the total study cost, one expects that planning a hospital-based study using equal allocation will be nearly optimal in regard to minimizing cost. For studies in which controls are population based, being selected from a stratified random sample of a target population, the cost of control selection may be substantially different from that for the cases. One would expect that cost considerations would be most relevant in these circumstances.

Brittain, Schlesselman, and Stadel (1981) have reviewed the actual costs incurred in some case-control studies. They estimated that when the cost of selecting and gathering data on a case is between ½ to 2 times the cost for a control, then the total study cost will be reduced by only 1 or 2 percent when optimal allocation is used instead of equal allocation.

Suppose that one partitions the total study cost T into a fixed cost F, which is independent of the case-control allocation, and a sampling cost S, which does depend on the allocation, where $T = F + S$. Then the percent reduction in S when using optimal as opposed to equal allocation is $D \times 100\%$, where $D = \frac{1}{2} - \sqrt{K}/(K + 1)$ and $K = c_1/c_0$. The percent reduction in *total* study cost with optimal as opposed to equal allocation will necessarily be less than $D \times 100\%$; it is given by $D_T \times 100\%$, where $D_T = D/(1 + F/S_e)$, and S_e is the sampling cost under equal allocation (Brittain, Schlesselman, and Stadel 1981).

6.5 ADJUSTMENT FOR CONFOUNDING

Occasionally one may want to determine the sample size required for a case-control study that will use stratified analyses to adjust for confounding. [The analysis of Whittemore (1981) may be adapted to estimate sample size in a case-control study when adjustment for confounding is made by means of logistic regression.] A combined estimate of relative risk, adjusted for confounding, is calculated as a weighted average of the stratum-specific odds ratios (Chapter 7). Thus, consider a study design in which cases and controls will be selected from k subgroups. These may be formed by the cross-classification of variables such as age, race, sex, or other factors. Suppose that within the jth subgroup, *equal numbers of cases and controls will be selected*, $n_{1j} = n_{0j} = n_j$, the subscript 1 denoting a case and the subscript 0 denoting a control. (This assumption implies that frequency matching or stratified sampling will be used.) Let the exposure rate among controls in the jth subgroup be p_{0j}, and further assume that the jth subgroup contains the proportion (fraction) f_j of the total observations. If one wants to detect a hypothetical relative risk R, assumed to be constant over the strata, then for specified α and β the total number of *cases* which must be selected is given from results of Gail (1973):

$$n = (z_\alpha + z_\beta)^2 / \Sigma f_j g_j \qquad (6.19)$$

where

$$g_j = (\ln R)^2 / [1/(p_{1j} q_{1j}) + 1/(p_{0j} q_{0j})]$$
$$p_{1j} = p_{0j} R / [1 + p_{0j} (R - 1)].$$

In brief, one must specify the following parameters in order to determine sample size in a stratified or frequency matched case-control study: (1) the relative risk (assumed constant) that one would like to detect, R; (2) the estimated exposure rates among controls in each of the k strata, $p_{01}, p_{02}, \ldots, p_{0k}$; (3) the estimated proportion of cases occuring in each of the k strata, $f_1, f_2, \ldots, f_k$; (4) the level of significance, α; and (5) the power $(1 - \beta)$.

As an example of the application of equation (6.19), suppose that one is considering the replication of a case-control study of myocardial infarction and oral contraceptive use, and that age is the major confounder for which an adjustment will be made. Based on the data reported in Table 2.15, the distribution of cases (f_j) and the exposure rate in controls (p_{0j}) are shown for each of the age strata in Table 6.5. In order to detect a

Table 6.5. Sample Size Calculation for a Stratified Case-Control Study of Myocardial Infarction and Oral Contraceptive Use[1]

Age (yrs)	f_j	p_{0j}	p_{1j}	g_j	$f_j g_j$
25–29	.03	.22	.46	.122	.0037
30–34	.09	.08	.21	.062	.0056
35–39	.16	.07	.18	.055	.0088
40–44	.30	.02	.06	.018	.0054
45–49	.42	.02	.06	.018	.0076
					.0311 (total)

$$n = (1.96 + 1.28)^2/.0311 = 328$$

1. Equation (6.19) used with $R = 3$, $\alpha = .05$ (two-sided), $\beta = .10$. Values of f_j and p_{2j} are based on Table 2.15.

threefold increased risk ($R = 3$) with $\alpha = .05$ (two-sided) and $\beta = .10$, the required total number of cases is $n = 328$.

Whenever all the n_j ($= f_j n$) exceed 15 and all p_{1j} and p_{0j} lie in the interval (0.1, 0.9), the sample size estimated from equation (6.19), although derived on the basis of unconditional tests of significance, should be appropriate for conditional tests, such as those suggested by Mantel and Haenszel (1959), Cox (1970, pp. 58–61), or Gart (1971). When some $p_{1j} > 0.9$ or $p_{0j} < 0.1$, equation (6.19) is expected to slightly overestimate the required sample size (Gail 1973).

6.6 SAMPLE SIZE AND POWER FOR PAIR-MATCHED STUDIES

Sample Size

For each pair in a matched case-control study, there are four possible exposure outcomes. Denoting an exposed individual by ($+$) and an unexposed individual by ($-$), one may write these as (case, control): ($++$), ($+-$), ($-+$), and ($--$). Thus, for example, ($+-$) indicates that the case was exposed and the control was not exposed. As shown in Chapter 7, McNemar's (1947) test of a disease-exposure association is based only on the exposure-discordant pairs ($+-$) and ($-+$). For specified α and β, the *number of discordant pairs* required to detect a relative risk R is given by

$$m = [z_\alpha/2 + z_\beta \sqrt{P(1 - P)}]^2/(P - \frac{1}{2})^2, \qquad (6.20)$$

where

$$P = \psi/(1 + \psi) \simeq R/(1 + R). \qquad (6.21)$$

The term ψ denotes the disease-exposure odds ratio and R denotes the relative risk. Letting p_e denote the probability of an exposure-discordant pair, the total number of pairs M required on average to yield m discordant pairs is $M = m/p_e$. Although strictly speaking p_e depends on the matching criteria, one may use as a crude approximation

$$p_e \simeq (p_0 q_1 + p_1 q_0), \qquad (6.22)$$

where p_0 is the estimated proportion of exposed controls in the target population and p_1 is the estimated proportion of exposed cases determined from equation (6.2). The quantities q_0 and q_1 are defined by $q_0 = 1 - p_0$ and $q_1 = 1 - p_1$, respectively. Thus

$$M \simeq m/(p_0 q_1 + p_1 q_0). \qquad (6.23)$$

Let m_{12} denote the number of $(+ -)$ pairs and m_{21} denote the number of $(- +)$ pairs, the total number of discordant pairs being $m = m_{12} + m_{21}$. Conditional on m, the observed proportion $\hat{P} = m_{12}/m$ has a binomial distribution. Expressed in terms of the odds ratio, the parameter P may be written (Cox 1970) as $P = \psi/(1 + \psi)$. Under the null hypothesis of no association ($\psi = 1$), $P = \frac{1}{2}$. Thus, using the binomial distribution, the conditional variance of $\hat{P}$ under the null hypothesis is $V_0 = 1/4m$, and the conditional variance under the alternative ($\psi \neq 1$) is $V_1 = P(1 - P)/m$. McNemar's test is based on the quantity $z = (\hat{P} - \frac{1}{2})/\sqrt{V_0}$ which has an approximate unit normal distribution when $\psi = 1$. Equation (6.20) thus follows directly from the normal approximation to testing a single binomial proportion.

Equation (6.22) assumes that the 0-1 outcomes (unexposed or exposed) for each case-control pair are independent and have constant probability:

$$\begin{aligned} p_e &= \text{prob} (+ -) + \text{prob} (- +) \\ &\simeq P(+ \mid \text{case})P(- \mid \text{control}) + P(- \mid \text{case})P(+ \mid \text{control}) \\ &= p_1 q_0 + q_1 p_0. \end{aligned}$$

Hills and Armitage (1979) give a related sample size estimate in the context of the two-period crossover clinical trial. The analysis of Cox (1958) and Gart (1969) is also relevant to the preceding development. Bennett (1967), Miettinen (1968b), and Bennett and Underwood (1970) give alternative analyses that can be applied to case-control studies, if one regards "exposure" as the outcome variable and uses the transformation given by equation (6.2). Walter (1980d) gives formulae for sample size and power in matched case-control studies with a variable number of controls per case.

As an application of the preceding sample size analysis, consider doing a matched case-control study of oral contraceptives and congenital heart disease, previously discussed in Section 6.1 as an unmatched study. Assume again that the proportion of exposed controls is $p_0 = 0.3$ and that $\alpha = .05$ (two-sided) and $\beta = 0.1$. In order to detect a twofold increased risk ($R = 2$) with these specifications, one needs 90 exposure-discordant pairs:

$$m = [1.96/2 + 1.28 \sqrt{(2/3)(1/3)}]^2/(2/3 - 1/2)^2 = 90.$$

As a crude approximation to the *total* number of pairs that are required, one calculates $p_e \simeq (.3)(.54) + (.46)(.7) = .484$ from (6.22), so that $M \simeq 186$ from equation (6.23). For an unmatched study with the above specifications, one estimates a sample size of $n = 188$ per group.

Power

Solving equation (6.20) for z_β allows one to calculate the power of a matched study based on m discordant pairs:

$$\hat{z}_\beta = [-z_\alpha/2 + \sqrt{m(P - \frac{1}{2})^2}]/\sqrt{P(1 - P)}. \qquad (6.24)$$

For specified values of m, R, and α, equation (6.24) can be used to calculate $\hat{z}_\beta$. The power is then determined from tables of the normal distribution by finding the probability that $\hat{z}_\beta$ is not exceeded, Power $= P(Z \le \hat{z}_\beta)$.

Equation (6.24) can be used directly to determine the power of a completed study, since in this situation the number of discordant pairs is known. To evaluate the power of a study that is being planned, the total number of pairs being fixed in advance at some value M, one may use equation (6.23) to estimate the expected number of discordant pairs as $\hat{m} \simeq (p_0 q_1 + p_1 q_0)M$. The value $\hat{m}$ may then be used in (6.24) to estimate the study power. In practice, the probability of an exposure-discordant pair will be better estimated from the initial data collection phase rather than (6.22), so that one may have to revise one's estimate of the required total numbers of pairs to be accumulated.

6.7 SEQUENTIAL CASE-CONTROL STUDIES

In situations such as postmarketing drug surveillance, a sequential approach to case-control studies may offer advantages over a fixed sample size design. Rather than wait until a predetermined number of cases and controls have accumulated for study, a sequential analysis proceeds as the data become available over time. Data collection continues until the null hypothesis of interest, such as $R = 1$, is either accepted or rejected with some pre-established values for α and β. On average, the sample size with a sequential test will be less than that required for a fixed sample size analysis. Bjerkedal and Bakketeig (1975) have described a system for monitoring birth defects in Norway based on a sequential case-control analysis of screening for potential teratogens, and O'Neill and Anello (1978) have given a general discussion of the application of sequential analysis to the design of pair-matched case-control studies.

Standard methods for sequential analysis apply to the situation in which case-control pairs are acquired one by one over time. In practice, a case-control study can often be more efficiently conducted if groups of cases and controls are selected in stages, with analysis occurring after every $2k$ observations (k per group) have accumulated. Pasternack and Shore (1979, 1980, 1981) have extended the work of Pocock (1977) to the application of group sequential methods for the planning and analysis of case-control studies. A *group sequential analysis* involves repeated tests of significance to decide whether to continue with data collection. After accumulation of every $2k$ observations, the standard one degree-of-freedom chi-square test (without continuity correction) for disease-exposure association, or the corresponding Mantel-Haenszel test (Chapter 7), is calculated. If the appropriate critical point of the χ^2 distribution is exceeded, data collection stops, there being a statistically significant case-control difference. If the value of the chi-square test is not significant, the next stage of data collection proceeds to accumulate an additional $2k$ observations. Data collection continues until one either obtains a significant case-control difference or until one reaches a predetermined maximum number of stages, S. If no significant difference has occurred by the end of the Sth stage, one concludes that there is no evidence of a statistically significant disease-exposure association. Either matched or unmatched designs may be used with the corresponding appropriate analysis.

Since the overall significance level is increased by repeated α-level tests,

Table 6.6. The Nominal Significance level α' and the Corresponding χ^2 Critical Point for Use in Group Sequential Testing for Various Numbers of Stages S and Overall Significance Level α.

	$\alpha = 0.05$		$\alpha = 0.01$	
S	α'	χ^2	α'	χ^2
2	0.0294	4.74	0.0056	7.68
3	0.0221	5.24	0.0041	8.25
4	0.0182	5.57	0.0033	8.64
5	0.0158	5.82	0.0028	8.92
6	0.0142	6.02	0.0025	9.14
7	0.0130	6.18	0.0023	9.32
8	0.0120	6.31	0.0021	9.47
9	0.0112	6.43	0.0019	9.60
10	0.0106	6.53	0.0018	9.72
11	0.0101	6.62	0.0017	9.82
12	0.0097	6.68	0.0016	9.90
15	0.0086	6.90	0.0015	10.13
20	0.0075	7.14	0.0013	10.39

Adapted from Pocock 1977, Table 1.

one makes an allowance by performing each test at a more stringent nominal level (α') in order to maintain an overall level of α. To do this, one must choose in advance the maximum number of tests to be made, S. For specified values of S, which also refers to the maximum number of stages, Table 6.6 shows the corresponding values of χ^2 which must be exceeded in order to maintain an overall $\alpha = .05$ or $\alpha = .01$ level test. For example, if a maximum of two tests are to be made, an actual $\alpha = .05$ (two-sided) overall significance level requires that each test be made at the nominal $\alpha = .0294$ level, with the corresponding value of χ^2 being 4.74.

For specified values of S, and selected values of α, β, p_0, and R, Appendix D gives the required number of persons per case and per control group (k) at each stage of a group sequential case-control study. For a predetermined value of S, the maximum sample size per group is kS, the maximum total sample size being $(2k)S$. In fact, the average sample size will be smaller than $(2k)S$, because of early stopping. Values of the average sample size for the group sequential design are also shown in Appendix D.

As an example of the use of Appendix D, suppose that one considers a group sequential case-control study that is to be sufficiently large to detect a hypothetical twofold increased risk ($R = 2$) with $\alpha = .05$ (two-sided) and $\beta = .10$. If the exposure rate among controls is estimated to be $p_0 = .10$, then for a 3-stage study ($S = 3$), one would take 146 cases and 146 controls at each stage ($k = 146$). The maximum number of subjects per case and control group that might be required is $n = 438$ (146 × 3). On average, however, only 274 subjects per group would be needed. With a nonsequential study ($S = 1$), 378 subjects per group would be needed. Thus, on average, a reduction in sample size of 27.5 percent would be expected.

The sample sizes for $S = 1$ in Appendix D correspond to those for a nonsequential fixed sample size analysis [equation (6.1)]. One sees from Appendix D that the greatest incremental reduction in average sample size is achieved by using a two-stage design ($S = 2$). The point of diminishing returns quickly sets in, so that use of designs with more than 4 or 5 stages is likely to have little further benefit. One may refer to Pocock (1977, Table 2) to determine sample sizes for the additional values of $1 - \beta$ equal to .5, .95 and .99. Other values of power or α-level require the application of numerical quadrature as described by Armitage, McPherson, and Rowe (1969). Pasternack and Shore (1979) have also presented tables of the smallest detectable relative risk (Section 6.3) that can be determined in group sequential case-control studies of various sizes.

The texts by Armitage (1971) and Wetherill (1975) provide introductions to the application and theory of sequential analysis. The suitability of sequential testing in case-control studies is likely to be restricted to special situations, and two caveats are particularly worth mentioning. First, the approach uses an analysis that is overly simplistic insofar as it emphasizes a test of significance. Second, choice of too large a value for R as the alternative of interest may lead to very early rejection of the null hypothesis. One might thus discontinue a study with some assurance that a difference exists but be unable to measure it with any precision (Armitage 1967). With this in mind, sequential estimation, as described in the text by Wetherill (1975), may be more appropriate to consider than sequential testing.

6.8 FURTHER CONSIDERATIONS IN ESTIMATING SAMPLE SIZE

Adjustment for Nonresponse

To anticipate the effect of nonresponse on the available sample size, one should make an adjustment to reflect the number of cases and controls that must be available in order to obtain a final sample size of n per group. Since the size of the available case series is ordinarily the limiting factor in case-control studies, an adjustment for nonresponse most likely will be of interest for the cases. For example, suppose that one determined for an unmatched study that 150 cases and an equal number of controls were required. If one anticipated 15 percent nonresponse among the cases, then 177 cases ($= 150/0.85$) would have to be available. In general, if the rate of nonresponse is $r \times 100$ percent, then the number of subjects that must be available for study in order to obtain a final series of size n is given by $n_a = n/(1 - r)$.

Factors other than nonresponse, particularly criteria for exclusion, may be pertinent to making an adjusted estimate of sample size. In practice it may be difficult to anticipate the fraction of potential cases and controls that will be excluded by the application of any particular set of criteria. A pilot study or the early stages of an ongoing study can resolve the matter.

Subgroup Analysis

The sample size analysis given thus far assumes that a single case-control comparison will be made. In practice, multiple comparisons are usually performed on various subgroups. For example, to study the association of menopausal estrogens and endometrial cancer, one may want to consider stratifying the analysis on the basis of factors such as stage of the disease, extent of invasion into the myometrium, type of estrogen (conjugated, combination, diethylstilbestrol), schedule of administration (intermittent, cyclic, continuous, combination), form of administration (oral, injection, cream), duration of use, dosage, and time since initiation of use or discontinuation. Such analyses often support the objective of determining whether an overall association exists and is likely to be causal. For instance, suppose that if an overall increased risk were found, one would want to assess whether low-dose preparations carried a significantly lower risk of cancer than high-dose preparations. Then a sufficient number of subjects should be selected to assure adequate power to test for this association. First, one may stratify the entire case-control series on the basis of high vs. low estrogen exposure, as shown in Table 6.7. Taking users of low-dose preparations as the reference group, the relative risk of endometrial cancer among users of high-dose preparations is estimated by the odds ratio $\psi = a_1 b_2 / a_2 b_1$. Since the odds ratio relates

Table 6.7. Distribution of Cases and
Controls by Estrogen Use

Estrogen use	Cases	Controls
High	a_1	b_1
Low	a_2	b_2
None	c	d

only to cases and controls who are *users* of estrogen (high vs. low dose),
the sample size analysis must be made on the basis of this subgroup.

If one defines high-dose to be an estrogen content of > 1 mg and low-
dose to be an estrogen content of .25 to 1.0 mg, then among users of
estrogen, an estimate of the proportion of high-dose preparations is given
by $p_0 = 0.5$ (Antunes et al. 1979). In order to detect a threefold increase
in risk of disease for high vs. low dose preparations, 62 *users of estrogen
among the cases* and 62 *users of estrogen among the controls* would be
required ($\alpha = .05$ one-sided; $\beta = .10$):

$$p_1 = (0.5)(3)/[1 + 0.5(3 - 1)] = 0.7500$$

$$\overline{p} = \tfrac{1}{2}(0.5 + 0.75) = 0.6250$$

$$n = [1.64 \sqrt{0.4688} + 1.28 \sqrt{0.43751}]^2/(0.25)^2 = 62.$$

If the proportion of ever-use of menopausal estrogens among the controls were 5 percent, whereas usage was 20 percent among the cases, then
one would need an estimated 1,240 (62/.05) available controls and 310
(62/.20) available cases in order to obtain a final sample size of 62 cases
and 62 controls who had used estrogen. One thus needs four times as
many available controls in order to expect equal numbers of cases and
controls within the subgroup of prior estrogen use. (There is no necessity
for an equal number of cases and controls in the subgroup, just a sufficient number to guarantee adequate power.) This example points to one
rationale for selecting multiple controls per case.

An interesting point (admittedly hypothetical) is that if the preceding
study were designed solely to investigate the effect of high vs. low dosage,
then cases and controls would be selected (without regard to dose) from
among the diseased and the non-diseased *estrogen users*. That is, the
absence of prior estrogen use could be used as an exclusion factor for
potential subjects. This would contrast with a study designed primarily

to establish whether estrogen use increases the risk of disease. In the latter situation, cases and controls would be selected without regard to prior estrogen use, and every effort would be made to assure that irrespective of whether an individual had used estrogens, an eligible case (or control) would have an equal chance of being selected for study.

Multiple Controls per Case

The sample size tables in Appendix A can be used to determine the number of cases and controls in a study with a case:control ratio different from unity. Suppose that for specified values of α, β, p_0, and R, the sample size per group based on a $1:1$ ratio is equal to n. Then if one were to use c controls per case, the corresponding sample size for the *case-group* would be given by

$$n' \simeq (c + 1)n/2c, \tag{6.25}$$

and the corresponding size of the control group would be cn'.

Equation (6.25) is an approximate formula that is derived from equations (6.3) and (6.8). Letting n and n' be the sample sizes corresponding to (6.3) and (6.8) respectively, one has

$$n/(2\bar{p}\bar{q}) = (z_\alpha + z_\beta)^2/(p_1 - p_0)^2 = n'/[(1 + 1/c)\bar{p}'\bar{q}'].$$

Using the approximation $\bar{p} \simeq \bar{p}'$, one derives equation (6.25). Equation (6.25) is often useful when one has performed a sample-size analysis assuming a $1:1$ case-control ratio, and the question arises regarding the corresponding sample size with a $1:c$ ratio. The relationship in (6.25) can also be applied directly to sample size analyses for matched studies.

Dependence of Sample Size on Parameter Specifications

The required sample size depends on one's specifications for α, β, p_0, and R. For example, fixing $\alpha = 0.05$ (two-sided) and $p_0 = 0.3$, Figure 6.1, based on equation (6.1), shows the sample size n (per group) as a function of the desired study power $(1 - \beta)$ and the hypothetical relative risk R. Changes in one's specifications for study power or the value of R can have dramatic effects on the required size of a study. Thus, if one fixes the study power at 90 percent, one needs $n = 568$ corresponding to $R = 1.5$. Taking $R = 2$ reduces one's sample size requirement to $n = 188$, and for $R = 3$ one needs only $n = 73$. Fixing the relative risk of

Figure 6.1. Case-control sample size as a function of study power and relative risk (α = .05, two-sided and p_0 = 0.3).

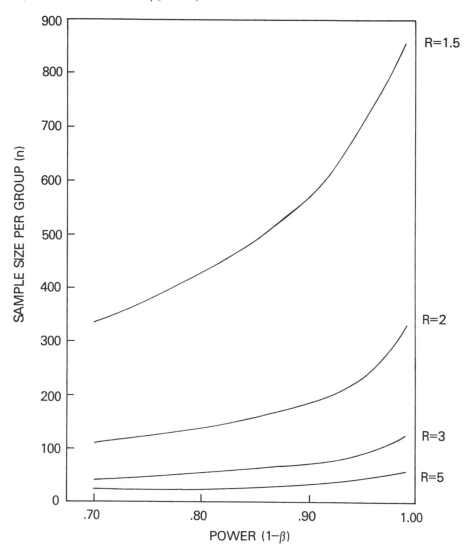

interest at $R = 2$, a study with 80 percent power requires $n = 140$, whereas $n = 105$ for 70 percent power and $n = 232$ for 95 percent power.

6.9 SUMMARY

An estimate of sample size for both matched and unmatched case-control studies depends on the specification of two key parameters: (1) the relative frequency of exposure among controls in the target population, p_0, and (2) a hypothesized relative risk associated with exposure that would have sufficient biologic or public health importance to warrant its detection, R. The exposure of interest may either increase ($R > 1$) or decrease ($R < 1$) the risk of the study disease. In practice, the size of a study is often constrained by financial resources, time, or the number of available cases. Thus, given a specified sample size, one will want to determine the smallest alteration in risk that can be reliably detected.

One should always calculate the power of a study that finds no disease-exposure association in order to determine whether the size of the investigation was sufficiently large. In some circumstances, such as postmarketing drug surveillance, one may want to establish a sequential case-control study in which the sample size is not fixed in advance, but accumulates until a decision can be made regarding the presence or absence of a disease-exposure association.

Cost considerations can be incorporated to estimate the optimal case:control ratio, but in many practical situations this added level of complexity is likely to produce only marginal gains of cost-efficiency. Because of imprecision or arbitrariness in one's parameter specifications, any estimated sample size should be considered as only a guide to planning a study and not an absolute requirement.

7 Basic Methods of Analysis

7.0 INTRODUCTION

Conducting the Analysis

The most effective way to proceed in the analysis of a case-control study is from the simple to the complex. For an unmatched study, the exposure of interest can first be dichotomized as present or absent among the cases and the controls, as shown in Table 7.1. One can then determine whether there is a crude disease-exposure association by estimating the odds ratio for a single 2×2 table. Next, one can investigate whether the presence or absence of a crude association continues to appear when adjustment is made for potential confounding variables, and whether the magnitude of the odds ratio is increased or diminished by adjustment. In practice, it is helpful to state a hypothetical causal pathway between the exposure and disease, including the effects of important extraneous variables. The analysis can then be guided by a sequence of hypotheses that attempt to refute or confirm an association. One's questions should become increasingly detailed, so that the circumstances in which an effect occurs can be precisely stated and the variables that alter its magnitude can be identified.

Where possible, one should look for evidence of a dose response by further characterizing exposure on the basis of factors such as dose, duration, and time of onset or discontinuation. The consistency of an effect can be examined within a study by stratifying cases and controls on the basis of variables such as age, race, sex, geographic area, and so forth, seeing whether the apparent effect of exposure is maintained across the strata. One may also want to look for an effect within subgroups of individuals who are thought to have particularly high susceptibility. This

Table 7.1. Frequency of Exposure in an
Unmatched Sample of n_1 Cases and n_2
Controls

	Cases	Controls	Total
Exposure:			
Yes	a	b	m_1
No	c	d	m_2
Total	n_1	n_2	n

leads one to the assessment of the effect of an exposure in the presence or absence of other risk factors for the study disease, so as to determine whether their joint effect exceeds that expected on the basis of their individual effects. Analyses may also focus on the identification of subgroups of individuals who have high susceptibility to the adverse or beneficial effects of the study exposure. Benefits or risks are not always spread evenly across members of a population. Although one may have a large study in terms of the total number of cases and controls, subgroup analyses often reveal an inadequate sample size, so that many comparisons of interest cannot be made precisely.

The observational criteria for assessing causality given in Chapter 1 should be kept in mind continually during the analysis of a study. Many variables in addition to the study exposure may show a positive or negative association with the study disease. With any association, one is always confronted with the problem of deciding whether the relationship is (1) causal; (2) noncausal, but due to an association with an underlying causal variable; or (3) an artifact of improper study design or analysis. The process of disentangling the causal effects of a set of variables and placing them in their proper sequence, relationship, and importance requires a thorough knowledge of the disease or condition under study and insight into potential sources of bias.

The statistical methods of this chapter, based on stratification or matching, may obviate the need for more complex analyses involving multivariate methods such as logistic regression or loglinear models (Chapter 8). At the very least, simpler methods of analysis should be used before more complex ones. They allow one to become familiar with the data and provide a basis for assessing the reasonableness of the assumptions underlying an analysis based on a multivariate model. Stratification on two or more variables, moreover, provides a basic form of multivariate analysis, through it is perhaps not quite as efficient as one based on a parametric model. On the other hand, a stratified analysis does not depend on the validity of mathematical assumptions regarding the particular form of the relationship between a set of variables and the risk of disease.

Limitations of Statistics

Before proceeding, one should keep in mind several points concerning the role of statistical methods. First, with respect to significance tests, the p-value should be considered only a guide to interpretation (Cox 1977). It is a summary measure of the consistency of the data with a null hypothesis H_0, usually taken to be one of no disease-exposure association ($H_0: \psi = 1$). Small p-values only indicate that "chance" is an unlikely explanation, leaving unanswered the question of whether an apparent association represents one of cause and effect. As an example, Hill (1953) cites an uncontrolled field experiment of vaccination against influenza and notes the impossibility of concluding that the vaccine was effective, despite a p-value of $p = .00567$. As another example, a 4.5-fold elevation ($p < .01$) in the reported occurrence of loss of libido among users of oral contraceptives, compared with never-users, was regarded as highly suspect (Royal College of General Practitioners 1974). Although OC users certainly complained of loss of libido more than non-users, they were considered to have many reasons and opportunities to do so that were unrelated to the pharmacological action of the Pill.

Statistical significance is quite different from scientific significance. Thus , it is important to estimate the magnitude of an effect, irrespective of whether a statistically significant departure from the null hypothesis is achieved. In this regard, a confidence interval is valuable, because it indicates whether the data are so limited that they are not only consistent with H_0, but also with departures from H_0 that are of scientific importance (Cox 1977). P-values are useful in conjunction with confidence intervals, however, because a confidence interval alone does not give precise information about how much H_0 is contradicted by the data (Spjøtvoll 1977).

The preceding considerations suggest that in an observational study one need not be too concerned with the problem of multiple comparisons leading to chance associations. A decision regarding some variable's effect should never be based solely on a p-value. Evidence of a dose response, biological plausibility, and consistency of the evidence within and across studies are important elements in the interpretation of an association.

Although statistical methods provide standard techniques for the numerical description of a study's findings, there is rarely a single way to proceed in an analysis. The results of one analysis often suggest further questions that lead to alternative analyses of the same issue. Analyses should be guided by an investigator's insight into potential biological mechanisms and an awareness of sources of study bias. The primary function of statistics is to provide clear and precise description. The calculation of a p-value to eliminate "chance" as an explanation for a finding is perhaps the least important role of a statistical analysis.

Even though statistical methods may facilitate the interpretation of a study, they do not generally give insight into a mechanism of action. This must be based on biological, biochemical, or other substantive grounds. Finally, any analysis is incomplete without a substantive interpretation of the results and a judgment regarding their plausibility.

7.1 UNMATCHED ANALYSIS OF A SINGLE 2 × 2 TABLE

Point Estimation of the Odds Ratio

The odds ratio ψ (psi) is a key parameter in the analysis of case-control studies, since it approximates the relative risk and is invariant across cohort and case-control designs (Cornfield 1951). A number of statistical procedures have been proposed for its point and interval estimation and for tests of significance (see Gart 1971). Taking the case-control design as our point of perspective, the sample data may be displayed as in Table 7.1 (p. 172). The number of exposed cases in the sample is designated by a; b denotes the number of exposed controls, and so forth. An estimate of ψ is given by the sample odds ratio,

$$\hat{\psi} = ad/bc. \tag{7.1}$$

The sample odds ratio $\hat{\psi}$ is a maximum likelihood estimate, assuming that the sample sizes for cases and controls are fixed at n_1 and n_2 respectively, and that simple random samples have been taken from theoretically infinite populations of cases and controls, or that random samples with replacement have been taken from finite populations. The sample odds ratio is also a maximum likelihood estimate under the assumption that a, b, c, and d follow a multinomial distribution with total sample size fixed at n.

To avoid asymmetry, Woolf (1955) proposed using the log odds ratio parameter as a measure of association,

$$\omega = \ln \psi. \tag{7.2}$$

If the relative odds of disease is ψ for exposed individuals compared with the unexposed, then a comparison of unexposed to exposed individuals results in an odds ratio of ψ^{-1}. By use of the transformation $\omega = \ln \psi$, the numerical value of ω will be retained with only a change in sign, $\ln \psi = -\ln \psi^{-1}$. Thus, on a log scale $\psi = x$ and $\psi = 1/x$ represent equal but opposite effects. No effect is indicated by $\omega = 0$, corresponding to $\psi = 1$. Estimates of ω can be converted to estimates of ψ by using the inverse transformation (antilogs) $e^{\omega} = \exp(\ln \psi) = \psi$.

Haldane (1955) and Anscombe (1956) have shown that an approximately unbiased (in the statistical sense of expectation) estimate of ω is derived from adding ½ to each of the cells of the 2×2 table and using

$$\hat{\omega}_h = \ln\{(a + \tfrac{1}{2})(d + \tfrac{1}{2})/(b + \tfrac{1}{2})(c + \tfrac{1}{2})\}. \qquad (7.3)$$

The antilog of $\hat{\omega}_h$, given by equation (7.4) below, can be used as an estimate of ψ which always has a finite value, there being no problem with infinite values arising from division by zero or from taking the logarithm of zero. Although the estimate

$$\begin{aligned}\hat{\psi}_h &= \exp(\hat{\omega}_h) \qquad\qquad (7.4)\\ &= (a + \tfrac{1}{2})(d + \tfrac{1}{2})/(b + \tfrac{1}{2})(c + \tfrac{1}{2})\end{aligned}$$

is often used, the practice of adding ½ can greatly distort one's estimate of ψ or ω in small samples. In general, we prefer to ignore the ½ correction factor (see Cox 1970, Mantel 1980). If one encounters a situation in which $\hat{\psi}$ is infinite as a result of division by zero, one may report a lower limit for ψ based on a confidence interval from the exact conditional distribution (7.17). One should not use the ½ correction factor in this calculation. (Section 7.8 gives an example with matched data.)

Table 7.2 shows a subset of data from a case-control study of menopausal estrogen use and endometrial carcinoma. A woman was regarded as having used oral conjugated estrogens if she had taken them at any time before diagnosis (cases) or entry into the study (controls). Although each case was matched to a hospital control on the basis of hospital, date of admission within six months, age within five years, and race, we shall ignore the matching in the analysis of this section. Since age (and possibly race) is associated with the study exposure, one expects that an unmatched analysis will underestimate the disease-exposure odds ratio (Chapter 4). A matched analysis is given in Section 7.7 for comparison.

Table 7.2. Use of Oral Conjugated
Estrogens (OCE) for Cases of
Endometrial Cancer and Controls

	Endometrial cancer	Controls	Total
OCE:			
Yes	55	19	74
No	128	164	292
Total	183	183	366

From equation (7.1), the estimated odds ratio is $\hat{\psi} = (55)(164)/(128)(19) = 3.71$. Use of equation (7.4) gives an alternative estimate of $\hat{\psi}_h = 3.63$. Both approaches suggest that the risk of endometrial cancer is almost four times higher in users of menopausal estrogens. We next present two methods for calculating approximate confidence intervals for the odds ratio. A third approach due to Miettinen (1974b, 1976a) is given in Section 7.5.

Approximate Confidence Intervals for the Odds Ratio

WOOLF'S METHOD
One approach to setting approximate confidence limits on ψ is based on a tranformation of approximate limits for $\ln \psi$ (Woolf 1955). An estimate of the variance of $\ln \hat{\psi}$ is given by

$$\text{var}(\ln \hat{\psi}) \simeq (1/a + 1/b + 1/c + 1/d). \tag{7.5}$$

Since $\ln \hat{\psi}$ in large samples has a normal distribution, an approximate $1 - \alpha$ confidence interval for $\ln \psi$ is

$$\ln \hat{\psi} \pm z_\alpha \sqrt{(1/a + 1/b + 1/c + 1/d)}, \tag{7.6}$$

where z_α is the point on the unit normal distribution that is exceeded with probability $\alpha/2$. (For $\alpha = .01$, $z_\alpha = 2.58$; for $\alpha = .05$, $z_\alpha = 1.96$, etc.) Approximate lower and upper confidence limits for ψ are found by taking antilogs of the lower and upper limits for $\ln \psi$:

$$\begin{aligned}
\hat{\psi}_L &= \hat{\psi} \exp[-z_\alpha \sqrt{\text{var}(\ln \hat{\psi})}] \\
\hat{\psi}_U &= \hat{\psi} \exp[+z_\alpha \sqrt{\text{var}(\ln \hat{\psi})}].
\end{aligned} \tag{7.7}$$

Woolf's method applied to the data in Table 7.2 gives an approximate 95 percent confidence interval for ln ψ of $1.31 \pm (1.96)\sqrt{0.0847} = (0.74, 1.88)$. Taking antilogs of the limits for ln ψ, or using equation (7.7) directly, gives approximate 95 percent confidence limits for ψ equal to (2.10, 6.55).

The estimated variance of the sample log odds ratio given by equation (7.5) shows that the precision of the estimate depends not only on the total number of cases $(a + c = n_1)$ and controls $(b + d = n_2)$, but also on the numbers that fall into the exposed and unexposed categories. The variance of ln $\hat{\psi}$ is approximately

$$\text{var}(\ln \hat{\psi}) \simeq 1/(n_1 p_1 q_1) + 1/(n_2 p_2 q_2), \tag{7.8}$$

where p_1 and p_2 are respectively the probabilities of exposure among cases and controls, and n_1 and n_2 are the corresponding sample sizes (e.g. Haldane 1955). Substitution of the sample estimates $\hat{p}_1 = a/(a + c)$ and $\hat{p}_2 = b/(b + d)$ into equation (7.8) yields the estimate in equation (7.5).

CORNFIELD'S METHOD

Cornfield (1956) has given a method for calculating approximate confidence limits for ψ which correspond to Fisher's exact test of significance of association in a 2×2 table, under which all the marginal totals in the table are considered to be fixed (e.g. Armitage 1971, pp. 135–138). Using the marginal totals n_1, n_2, m_1, and m_2 defined in Table 7.1, approximate lower and upper $1 - \alpha$ confidence limits for ψ are given by

$$\begin{aligned} \hat{\psi}_L &= a_L(n_2 - m_1 + a_L)/(m_1 - a_L)(n_1 - a_L) \\ \hat{\psi}_U &= a_U(n_2 - m_1 + a_U)/(m_1 - a_U)(n_1 - a_U). \end{aligned} \tag{7.9}$$

The values of a_L and a_U in equation (7.9) are obtained by using an iterative procedure. Let $a_0 = a$, the number of exposed cases in Table 7.1, and define for $i = 1, 2, \ldots$

$$\begin{aligned} a_i = a \pm 1/2 \pm z_\alpha [(a_{i-1})^{-1} + (m_1 - a_{i-1})^{-1} \\ + (n_1 - a_{i-1})^{-1} + (n_2 - m_1 + a_{i-1})^{-1}]^{-1/2}. \end{aligned} \tag{7.10}$$

The values of a_i converge to a_U by using the plus signs and to a_L by using the minus signs. With small numbers the iterative technique may fail, since it is possible that a_i may be negative, or may be greater than n_1 or m_1. One must then choose a different starting value for a_0 (Gart 1971).

Table 7.3. Iterative Calculation of a_L and a_U Based on Cornfield's Method for Approximate Confidence Limits on ψ^1

Iteration	a_L	a_U
1	47.766	62.234
2	47.237	61.275
3	47.211	61.437
4	47.209	61.410
5	47.209	61.415
6		61.414
7		61.414

1. Taking $z_\alpha = 1.96$ for approximate 95 percent confidence limits, equation (7.10) is applied to Table 7.2 using the starting value $a_0 = 55$.

Table 7.3 shows the iterative procedure applied to the data in Table 7.2. Using $a_L = 47.21$ and $a_U = 61.41$, approximate 95 percent confidence limits for ψ are calculated from equation (7.9) as

$$\hat{\psi}_L = 47.21(183 - 74 + 47.21)/(74 - 47.21)(183 - 47.21) = 2.03$$

$$\hat{\psi}_U = 61.41(183 - 74 + 61.41)/(74 - 61.41)(183 - 61.41) = 6.84.$$

Had one used only two iterations in this example, taking $a_L = 47.24$ and $a_U = 61.28$, approximate limits for ψ would be (2.03, 6.74). The iterative technique coverges quite rapidly. Equations (7.9) and (7.10) can be easily programmed on a programmable pocket calculator, so that in practice, computation of confidence limits based on Cornfield's method can be just as simple to calculate as those based on Woolf's method.

Confidence intervals based on either Woolf's or Cornfield's method can be interpreted as tests of significance for a range of null hypotheses. A null hypothesis corresponding to any value of ψ falling outside a $1 - \alpha$ confidence interval would be rejected at the α-level of significance. Because of the discreteness of the distribution of the exact test, the confidence coefficient for limits based on Cornfield's method will be greater than or equal to the nominal $1 - \alpha$ level. In this regard, the limits are conservative, providing an unconditional coverage probability that exceeds the nominal level. Confidence limits based on Woolf's method will be too narrow from the perspective of Fisher's exact test. In repeated large samples, however, their unconditional coverage probability will correspond to the nominal level $1 - \alpha$.

Under the null hypothesis of no association ($\psi = 1$), the expected counts in the i-jth cell of Table 7.1 are given by $(n_i m_j/n)$. If the minimum expectation exceeds 1, Cornfield's method provides good estimates of the 95 percent limits corresponding to Fisher's exact test. For 99 percent limits, this minimum should exceed 3 (Gart and Thomas 1972), otherwise one should use the iterative procedure for computing "exact" confidence limits given by Thomas (1975).

Approximate Tests of Significance

The standard chi-square test for association in a 2×2 table provides an approximate test of the null hypothesis of no association, $H_0 : \psi = 1$. The chi-square test is computed from Table 7.1 as

$$\chi^2 = [(ad - bc)^2 n]/[n_1 n_2 m_1 m_2]. \tag{7.11}$$

Under the null hypothesis, the statistic χ^2 has an approximate chi-square distribution with one degree of freedom. The approximate unit normal deviate $z = \pm \sqrt{\chi^2}$ can be used for a one-sided test of significance. The sign is chosen by the direction of the alternative hypothesis, $(+)$ for $H_A : \psi > 1$ and $(-)$ for $H_A : \psi < 1$.

The Yates continuity corrected chi-square test is given by

$$\chi_c^2 = [(|ad - bc| - \tfrac{1}{2} n)^2 n]/[n_1 n_2 m_1 m_2]. \tag{7.12}$$

The p-value associated with χ_c^2, as opposed to χ^2, better approximates the p-value based on Fisher's exact test. From the perspective of repeated tests of significance based on a comparison of χ_c^2 with the chi-square distribution, use of the continuity correction results in an overly conservative test, rejecting the null hypothesis too infrequently with respect to the nominal level of significance. The appropriateness of the continuity correction has been extensively discussed with much disagreement among statisticians (Grizzle 1967, Mantel and Greenhouse 1968, Conover 1974, Garside and Mack 1976, Barnard 1979, Kempthorne 1979).

The value of χ^2 for the data in Table 7.2 is calculated from (7.11) to be $\chi^2 = 21.95$, with a corresponding two-sided p-value of $p = 2.8 \times 10^{-6}$. The continuity corrected chi-square is $\chi_c^2 = 20.75$, giving a two-sided p-value of $p = 5.4 \times 10^{-6}$. Both tests indicate that the sample odds ratio ($\hat{\psi} = 3.71$) is significantly greater than unity.

Tests of Significance and Confidence Intervals Based on the Exact Conditional Distribution

An exact, one-sided test of significance of the null hypothesis $H_0:\psi = \psi_0$ against the alternative $H_A:\psi > \psi_0$ can be directly calculated from the distribution of the number of exposed cases (a), conditional on all marginal totals being fixed. Let $r_2 = \min(n_1, m_1)$, $r_1 = \max(m_1 - n_2, 0)$, and define the function

$$g(x\,|\,m_1;\,\psi_0) = \binom{n_1}{x}\binom{n_2}{m_1-x}\psi_0^x \Big/ \sum_{j=r_1}^{r_2}\binom{n_1}{j}\binom{n_2}{m_1-j}\psi_0^j. \quad (7.13)$$

A one-sided p-value is then calculated from (e.g. Gart 1971)

$$p = \sum_{x=a}^{m_1} g(x\,|\,m_1;\,\psi_0). \quad (7.14)$$

The p-value corresponding to an exact, one-sided test of $H_0:\psi = \psi_0$ against the alternative $H_A:\psi < \psi_0$ is given by

$$p = \sum_{x=0}^{a} g(x\,|\,m_1;\,\psi_0). \quad (7.15)$$

The term "exact" refers only to the fact that, conditional on the marginal totals, the distribution of a on the null hypothesis is free from any unknown parameter (Barnard 1979). Equations (7.14) and (7.15) give the probability of observing an outcome as extreme or more so than the a exposed cases observed in the sample, assuming that the marginal totals in the 2×2 table are fixed and that under the null hypothesis the odds ratio is ψ_0.

A confidence interval for ψ may be based on the exact conditional distribution of a (Cornfield 1956, Fisher 1962, Stenhouse 1963). Consider a set of hypothetical values of ψ such that $\psi_L < \psi < \psi_U$, where the values of ψ_L and ψ_U are approximate solutions to the following two equations:

$$\sum_{x=0}^{a} g(x\,|\,m_1;\,\psi_U) = \alpha/2 \quad (7.16)$$

$$\sum_{x=a}^{m} g(x\,|\,m_1;\,\psi_L) = \alpha/2. \quad (7.17)$$

Since $g(x\,|\,m_1;\,\psi)$ is the probability function of a discrete distribution, there are generally no values of ψ_U and ψ_L that solve (7.16) and (7.17) exactly. The value for ψ_L is taken to be the largest such that the expression in (7.17) is $\leq \alpha/2$, whereas the value for $\psi_U > \psi_L$ is taken to be the smallest such that the expression in (7.16) is $\leq \alpha/2$. Thomas (1975) has published computer programs that provide iterative techniques for the numerical solution of these equations. The confidence interval (ψ_L, ψ_U) derived from the solution of (7.16) and (7.17) has a coefficient $\geq 1 - \alpha$. The term "exact confidence limits" is often applied to this procedure. This is somewhat confusing, because "exact" does not refer to the confidence coefficient being exactly $1 - \alpha$, but rather to the fact that the limits, which only approximate a $1 - \alpha$ confidence interval, are based on the exact conditional distribution of a.

Conditional Point Estimate of the Odds Ratio

Conditional on all marginal totals being fixed, the maximum likelihood estimate of the odds ratio is obtained by maximizing the function $g(a \mid m_1; \psi)$ with respect to the parameter ψ. This is performed by the computer program of Thomas (1975). Mantel and Hankey (1975) have emphasized that this estimate is generally not equal to $\hat{\psi} = ad/bc$. Refer to Birch (1964) and Gart (1971) for additional details.

7.2 ADJUSTMENT FOR CONFOUNDING

A mistaken assessment of risk may result from uncontrolled confounding. The study exposure, by virtue of its association with some other variable, may appear to elevate or reduce the risk of disease when in fact it has no effect. A related consequence of confounding is that the effect of an exposure may be distorted. The apparent relative risk, estimated by the odds ratio, may correctly indicate whether an exposure truly increases or reduces the risk of disease, but the magnitude of the effect may be over-estimated or underestimated. Section 2.10 of Chapter 2 gives an example in which the apparent effect of an exposure is diminished by failure to control for confounding by age.

Stratification provides a direct method for eliminating biased comparisons that result from confounding (Mantel and Haenszel 1959). To return to an example discussed in Chapter 2, suppose that one wants to investigate a postulated causal connection between alcohol consumption and myocardial infarction (MI). Smoking is known to be a cause of MI, and alcohol intake and smoking are known to be correlated. Suppose that alcohol consumption in fact is *not* a cause of MI. By virtue of its association with smoking, however, alcohol intake would be found to be associated, apparently increasing the risk of this disease. One might even find an apparent dose response between alcohol and MI due to heavy drinkers being heavy smokers. To disentangle the effect of smoking from the effect (if any) of alcohol, one may stratify subjects (both cases and controls) into a smoking group and a nonsmoking group. Within each subgroup, one may look for an association between alcohol consumption and MI. Insofar as cases and controls are similar with respect to smoking habits within subgroups, a subgroup-specific association between alcohol and MI cannot be explained in terms of differences in smoking habits. Table 7.4 gives a hypothetical example in which an apparent association between alcohol and MI is explained entirely in terms of confounding due to smoking. The statistically significant elevation in risk ($\hat{\psi} = 2.26$, $p \simeq$

Table 7.4. Relationship of Alcohol Consumption to
Myocardial Infarction[1]

A. *Apparent Association Between Alcohol Consumption and*
   Myocardial Infarction (MI), Ignoring Smoking

	MI	Control
Alcohol:		
Yes	71	52
No	29	48
Total	100	100

$\hat{\psi} = 2.26$, $\chi^2 = 7.62$, $p \simeq .006$ (two-sided)

B. *Association Between Alcohol Consumption and MI, by*
   Smoking Status

	Nonsmokers		Smokers	
	MI	Control	MI	Control
Alcohol:				
Yes	8	16	63	36
No	22	44	7	4
Total	30	60	70	40
	$\hat{\psi} = 1.0$		$\hat{\psi} = 1.0$	

1. Hypothetical data.

.006, two-sided) in the analysis that ignores smoking is spurious. Among
nonsmokers, the estimated relative risk (odds ratio) of an MI associated
with alcohol consumption is $\hat{\psi} = 1.0$, with an identical estimate among
smokers. Table 7.4 shows that pooling the data, by summing the entires
across subgroups of a confounder to form a single 2 × 2 table, can produce misleading results, as effect known as Simpson's paradox (Simpson
1951, Edwards 1963).

One may regard the subgroup-specific odds ratios in Table 7.4 as representing the effect of alcohol, "adjusted for smoking," on the risk of MI.
Conceptually, the effect of smoking has been "held constant," although
not in an experimental sense. When an analysis has been stratified on the
basis of one or more variables, each of the subgroup-specific disease-
exposure odds ratios may be regarded as representing the effect of the
study exposure on the risk of disease when the joint effect of the stratification variables has been held constant. In the event that the odds ratios
are relatively constant across subgroups, being consistently elevated or
reduced, one may combine them to form a summary estimate. One refers
to the summary estimate as having been "adjusted" for the effects of those
variables used in the stratification. A variety of methods have been proposed for obtaining point estimates, tests of significance, and confidence

intervals for a summary odds ratio based on stratified data (e.g. Cochran 1954, Woolf 1955, Mantel and Haenszel 1959, Gart 1962, Birch 1964, Cox 1966, Goodman 1969). The following sections present the two most widely used methods.

Mantel-Haenszel Method

Mantel and Haenszel (1959) proposed on heuristic grounds a highly efficient method for estimating a summary odds ratio from a series of 2×2 tables. Their technique is remarkably easy to apply and requires no iterative calculations.

Suppose that cases and controls are stratified on the basis of one or more variables into k subgroups. Let the observations in the ith subgroup be written as in Table 7.5. The Mantel-Haenszel estimate of the odds ratio, adjusted for the effects of the stratification variables, is calculated as

$$\hat{\psi}_{mh} = \sum_{i=1}^{k} (a_i d_i / n_i) / \sum_{i=1}^{k} (b_i c_i / n_i). \qquad (7.18)$$

An approximate test of the hypothesis of no association ($H_0: \psi = 1$) is calculated as follows. For the ith subgroup, the conditional (all margins fixed) mean and variance of a_i, calculated under H_0, is given by

$$E(a_i) = n_{1i} m_{1i} / n_i$$

and

$$V(a_i) = n_{1i} n_{2i} m_{1i} m_{2i} / n_i^2 (n_i - 1).$$

The Mantel-Haenszel test of $H_0: \psi = 1$ against the two-sided alternative $H_A: \psi \neq 1$ is then given by

$$\chi^2_{mh} = [|\Sigma a_i - \Sigma E(a_i)| - \tfrac{1}{2}]^2 / \Sigma V(a_i). \qquad (7.19)$$

Table 7.5. Frequency of Exposure Among Cases and Controls in the i-th Subgroup

	Cases	Controls	Total
Exposure:			
Yes	a_i	b_i	m_{1i}
No	c_i	d_i	m_{2i}
Total	n_{1i}	n_{2i}	n_i

The ½ correction for continuity is used so that the p-value based on χ^2_{mh} more closely approximates the value based on the exact conditional test (Li, Simon, and Gart 1979). The statistic χ^2_{mh} has an approximate chi-square distribution with one degree of freedom under H_0. For a one-sided test, one may use the approximate unit normal deviate $z = \pm \sqrt{\chi^2_{mh}}$, the sign being chosen by the direction of the alternative hypothesis.

Mantel and Fleiss (1980) give a rule for determining when the chi-square approximation to the exact p-value should be adequate. Bennett and Kaneshiro (1974) have reported some Monte Carlo studies on the small-sample power and size of the Mantel-Haenszel test without the continuity correction. Birch (1964) has shown that χ^2_{mh} is asymptotically the uniformly most powerful unbiased test of H_0 against the logistic alternative (see Day and Byar 1979).

If one assumes that the subgroup odds ratios are constant, being equal to ψ, a small-sample confidence interval may be calculated from the exact conditional test (Gart 1970). Thomas (1975) gives a computer program for the iterative calculations. Miettinen (1974b, 1976a) has proposed an approximate method which is discussed in Section 7.5.

Hauck (1979) has given an estimate of the variance of $\ln \hat{\psi}_{mh}$ that is appropriate when the case and the control sample sizes within each subgroup are large. For the ith subgroup, let

$$w_i = b_i c_i / n_i \qquad (7.20)$$

and

$$v_i = (a_i + c_i)/a_i c_i + (b_i + d_i)/b_i d_i. \qquad (7.21)$$

One sees from equation (7.5) that the term v_i represents an estimate of the variance of $\ln \hat{\psi}_i$. A large sample estimate of the variance of $\ln \hat{\psi}_{mh}$ is given by

$$\mathrm{var}(\ln \hat{\psi}_{mh}) \simeq \Sigma w_i^2 v_i / (\Sigma w_i)^2 \qquad (7.22)$$

where the summation on the subscript i is taken over the k subgroups. An approximate $1 - \alpha$ confidence interval for $\ln \psi$ is thus given by

$$\ln \hat{\psi}_{mh} \pm z_\alpha \sqrt{\mathrm{var}(\ln \hat{\psi}_{mh})}$$

Approximate lower and upper confidence limits for ψ, adjusted for the stratification variables, are found by taking antilogs of the lower and upper limits for $\ln \psi$:

$$\hat{\psi}_L = \hat{\psi}_{mh} \exp[-z_\alpha \sqrt{\mathrm{var}(\ln \hat{\psi}_{mh})}]$$
$$\hat{\psi}_U = \hat{\psi}_{mh} \exp[+z_\alpha \sqrt{\mathrm{var}(\ln \hat{\psi}_{mh})}]. \qquad (7.23)$$

Mantel (1977) and McKinlay (1978) discuss alternative approaches to setting approximate confidence limits which in large samples should give results equivalent to equation (7.23).

The Mantel-Haenszel estimate $\hat{\psi}_{mh}$ can be regarded as a weighted average of the subgroup-specific odds ratios, provided that none of the values of b_i or c_i are equal to zero. In the i-th subgroup the disease-exposure odds ratio is estimated as

$$\hat{\psi}_i = a_i d_i / b_i c_i. \tag{7.24}$$

Using the weights w_i given by (7.20), one can write

$$\hat{\psi}_{mh} = \Sigma w_i \hat{\psi}_i / \Sigma w_i. \tag{7.25}$$

The rationale of stratification as a method for the removal of bias is that within each subgroup the ranges of the stratification variables are restricted. Thus, within subgroups, cases and controls cannot differ much on the stratification variables, so that $\hat{\psi}_i$ should be relatively free from potential bias due to these variables. As a consequence, a weighted average $\Sigma w_i \hat{\psi}_i / \Sigma w_i$ will also be free of bias.

The weights w_i are approximately proportional to the reciprocals of the variances of the $\hat{\psi}_i$, so that the Mantel-Haenszel estimate $\hat{\psi}_{mh}$ is an average of odds ratios that are weighted approximately according to their precision (reciprocal of variance). This may be shown as follows. The asymptotic variance of $\hat{\psi}_i$ is equal to

$$\psi^2[(n_{1i}p_{1i}q_{1i})^{-1} + (n_{2i}p_{2i}q_{2i})^{-1}], \tag{7.26}$$

where p_{1i} and p_{2i} are respectively the proportions of exposed cases and exposed controls within the ith subgroup of the target population, and $q_{1i} = 1 - p_{1i}$ and $q_{2i} = 1 - p_{2i}$. A sample estimate of the term in brackets in (7.26) is given by

$$[(a_i + c_i)/a_i c_i + (b_i + d_i)/b_i d_i]. \tag{7.27}$$

Rearranging terms, expression (7.27) may be written as

$$[(a_i + d_i)/a_i d_i + (b_i + c_i)/b_i c_i]. \tag{7.28}$$

If $\psi_i \simeq 1$, then $a_i d_i \simeq b_i c_i$, so that (7.28) is approximately equal to

$$[(a_i + d_i) + (b_i + c_i)]/b_i c_i = 1/w_i.$$

Thus, w_i is approximately proportional to the reciprocal of the variance of $\hat{\psi}_i$. Dayal (1978) has commented on related properties of the weighting in (7.25).

AN EXAMPLE OF THE MANTEL-HAENSZEL METHOD

As an application of the Mantel-Haenszel procedure, consider the data in Table 7.6 from a case-control study (Shapiro et al. 1979) of oral contraceptive use in relation to myocardial infarction (MI). Taking recent

Table 7.6. Relation of Myocardial Infarction (MI) to Recent Oral Contraceptive (OC) Use[1] According to Age and Cigarette Smoking

Cigarette smoking	OC use	25–29 MI	Ctl[2]	30–34 MI	Ctl	35–39 MI	Ctl	40–44 MI	Ctl	45–49 MI	Ctl
None	Yes	0	25	0	13	0	8	1	4	3	2
	No	1	106	0	175	3	153	10	165	20	155
1–24 (per day)	Yes	1	25	1	10	1	11	0	4	0	1
	No	0	79	5	142	11	119	21	130	42	96
≥25 (per day)	Yes	3	12	8	10	3	7	5	1	3	2
	No	1	39	7	73	19	58	34	67	31	50

1. Last use within the month before admission.
2. Ctl: Control.

Source: Shapiro et al. 1979.

use of oral contraceptives (OC) as the study factor of primary interest, the investigators used logistic regression to control for the potential confounding effects of age, cigarette smoking, weight, diabetes, lipid abnormality, hypertension, angina pectoris, pre-eclamptic toxemia and hospital of admission (Boston, New York, Philadelphia). Our analysis, in order to simplify the presentation, considers age and smoking as the only variables in addition to oral contraceptive use. This example will be further discussed in Chapter 8 as an application of logistic regression.

Suppose that one first concentrates on oral contraceptive use as the exposure of interest, and ignores information on age and smoking. One would then have a single 2 × 2 table showing OC use among cases and controls, as in Table 7.7A. A crude estimate (i.e. not adjusted for age or smoking) of the MI-OC odds ratio is given by $\hat{\psi} = 1.68$, calculated from equation (7.1). An approximate 95 percent confidence interval is (1.10, 2.57), computed by Woolf's method from (7.5) and (7.7). This suggests that oral contraceptive use is associated with a statistically significant 1.7 times increased risk of MI. However, if one stratifies on age, as shown in Table 7.7B, a different assessment emerges. The age-specific odds ratios $\hat{\psi}$ all exceed the crude estimate of 1.7, apart from the value $\hat{\psi}_i = 1.5$ for the 35–39 year age group. The Mantel-Haenszel estimate of the odds ratio, adjusted for age, is $\hat{\psi}_{mh} = 3.97$, calculated from (7.18). This estimate is more than two times higher than the crude estimate 1.68, and even falls outside its 95 percent confidence interval. An approximate 95 percent confidence interval for the age-adjusted odds ratio is (2.28, 6.93), calculated from equation (7.23).

Smoking is known to be a risk factor for MI. If smoking were associated with oral contraceptive use conditional on age, then further adjustment of the MI-OC odds ratio would be prudent. In this example, smoking and OC use are associated. If one calculates the odds of OC use within each of the 15 age-smoking subgroups in Table 7.6, one finds that

Table 7.7. Relation of Myocardial Infarction to Recent Use of Oral Contraceptives

A. *Relation of Myocardial Infarction (MI) to Recent Oral Contraceptive (OC) Use, Ignoring Age and Smoking*

OC	MI	Control
Yes	29	135
No	205	1607
Total	234	1742

$$\hat{\psi} = (29 \times 1607)/(205 \times 135) = 1.68$$

$$\text{var}(\ln \hat{\psi}) \simeq (29^{-1} + 205^{-1} + 135^{-1} + 1607^{-1}) = 0.0474$$

$$\hat{\psi}_L = 1.68 \exp[-1.96 \sqrt{.0474}] = 1.10$$

$$\hat{\psi}_U = 1.68 \exp[+1.96 \sqrt{.0474}] = 2.57$$

B. *Relation of Myocardial Infarction (MI) to Recent Oral Contraceptive (OC) Use According to Age, Ignoring Smoking*

OC	25–29		30–34		35–39		40–44		45–49	
	MI	Ctl[1]	MI	Ctl	MI	Ctl	MI	Ctl	MI	Ctl
Yes	4	62	9	33	4	26	6	9	6	5
No	2	224	12	390	33	330	65	362	93	301
$\hat{\psi}_i$	7.2		8.9		1.5		3.7		3.9	
n_i	292		444		393		442		405	
w_i	.425		.892		2.183		1.324		1.148	
v_i	.771		.227		.322		.296		.381	

$$\hat{\psi}_{mh} = [\Sigma(a_i d_i/n_i)]/[\Sigma(b_i c_i/n_i)] = 23.71/5.97 = 3.97$$

$$\text{var}(\ln \hat{\psi}_{mh}) \simeq \Sigma(w_i^2 v_i)/(\Sigma w_i)^2 = 2.876/(5.972)^2 = .0806$$

$$\hat{\psi}_L = 3.97 \exp[-1.96 \sqrt{.0806}] = 2.28$$

$$\hat{\psi}_U = 3.97 \exp[+1.96 \sqrt{.0806}] = 6.93$$

1. Ctl: Control.

for each age group, the odds of OC use increase with increasing levels of cigarette smoking.

Stratifying cases and control on the basis of 5 age groups and 3 smoking categories results in fifteen 2×2 tables (see Table 7.6) to which the Mantel-Haenszel technique is applied in order to adjust the MI-OC odds ratio for both age and smoking. The estimated relative risk (odds ratio) of an MI associated with oral contraceptive use, adjusted for both age and smoking, is calculated to be $\hat{\psi}_{mh} = 20.95/6.29 = 3.33$. Thus, some of the apparent effect of OC use in the age-adjusted estimate ($\hat{\psi}_{mh} = 3.97$) is actually due to an effect of smoking.

Six of the fifteen 2×2 tables comprising the age-smoking subgroups have zero entries. Thus, one cannot calculate a confidence interval directly from equation (7.23), because the evaluation of v_i in (7.21) would involve division by zero in these six tables. One approach that avoids this problem is a *test-based confidence interval* using the Mantel-Haenszel statistic χ^2_{mh} (Section 7.5). Letting a_i denote number of cases who were OC users in the ith age-smoking subgroup, the Mantel-Haenszel test statistic χ^2_{mh} is calculated from equation (7.19) to be $\chi^2_{mh} = (|29 - 14.23| - \frac{1}{2})^2/10.03 = 20.03$. Using equation (7.44) in Section 7.5, an approximate 95 percent confidence interval is then given by the term $\exp[(1 \pm 1.96/\sqrt{20.03})\ln 3.33] = (1.97, 5.62)$.

An alternative approach, which also avoids division by zero, uses

$$v'_i = [(a_i + \frac{1}{2})^{-1} + (b_i + \frac{1}{2})^{-1} + (c_i + \frac{1}{2})^{-1} + (d_i + \frac{1}{2})^{-1}]$$

in place of v_i in equation (7.22). The expression for v'_i, is an estimate of $\mathrm{var}(\ln \hat{\psi}_i)$ which has smaller bias than v_i (Gart and Zweifel 1967). One thus calculates $\Sigma w_i^2 v'_i/(\Sigma w_i)^2 = .0935$. Using equation (7.23), an approximate 95 percent confidence interval for the MI-OC odds ratio, adjusted for age and smoking, is (1.83, 6.06).

A third approach uses the exact conditional test. Using the program of Thomas (1975) to compute approximate confidence limits based on asymptotic theory for the exact conditional test (Gart 1970), a 95 percent confidence interval for the MI-OC odds ratio, adjusted for age and smoking, is (1.90, 5.76).

As indicated earlier, smoking itself is a risk factor for myocardial infarction. Suppose that one now wants to estimate the effect of smoking on the risk of an MI. To simplify the discussion for the moment, let us combine the two smoking categories 1–24 and ≥ 25 cigarettes per day, and consider only smoking (≥ 1 cigarettes per day) vs. nonsmoking (none). Table 7.8A shows the relation of smoking to MI, ignoring both age and recent oral contraceptive use. The estimated odds ratio $\hat{\psi} = 4.44$

Table 7.8. Relation of Myocardial Infarction to Cigarette Smoking

A. *Relation of Myocardial Infarction (MI) to Smoking, Ignoring Recent Oral Contraceptive Use and Age*

Smoking:	MI	Control
Yes	196	936
No	38	806
Total	234	1742

$\hat{\psi} = (196 \times 806)/(38 \times 936) = 4.44$

B. *Relation of Myocardial Infarction (MI) to Smoking According to Age, Ignoring Recent Oral Contraceptive Use*

	25–29		30–34		35–39		40–44		45–49	
	MI	Ctl	MI	Ctl	MI	Ctl	MI	Ctl	MI	Ctl
Smoking:										
Yes	5	155	21	235	34	195	60	202	76	149
No	1	131	0	188	3	161	11	169	23	157
n_i	292		444		393		442		405	

$\hat{\psi}_{mh} = \Sigma(a_i d_i/n_i)/\Sigma(b_i c_i/n_i) = 79.02/15.51 = 5.09$

suggests that smoking one or more cigarettes per day is associated with a 4.4 times increase in the risk of an MI. Table 7.8B shows that the MI-smoking odds ratio, adjusted for age, is $\hat{\psi}_{mh} = 5.09$. Further adjustment for both age and OC use results in an MI-smoking odds ratio of $\hat{\psi}_{mh} = 4.98$. Confidence intervals may be calculated by any one of the previously cited methods.

This example shows that for a set of variables, each in its turn might be taken as the exposure of interest. By forming the appropriate sub-tables, one can estimate any disease-exposure odds ratio, adjusting for one or more of the remaining variables. The choice of which variables (if any) should be used for adjustment and in what order they should be introduced are issues that cannot be decisively resolved by appeal to any statistical method. Variables that are known from other studies to be associated with the risk of disease should certainly be considered for inclusion. One's knowledge of the disease process and hypotheses about causal paths and potential sources of confounding should guide the analysis.

One is often concerned that an apparent association is in fact spurious, being due entirely or in part to one or more extraneous factors. If one takes the approach of adjusting only for those factors that reduce the apparent association, then one's estimated odds ratio will be biased toward unity (Day, Byar, and Green 1980). Adjustment for confounding should not be regarded solely as a method for explaining away apparent associations, but rather as a technique for eliminating a biased comparison of cases and controls. The removal of bias may increase the estimated effect just as well as reduce it. However, by analogy with multiple regression analysis, one expects that unnecessary adjustments will increase the sampling variance of the estimated effect of exposure without contributing to a reduction in bias. Day, Byar, and Green (1980) have given some of the mathematical and numerical details that are pertinent to this issue in case-control studies.

The analysis of the data in Table 7.6 has thus far considered individually the effects of recent oral contraceptive use and smoking on the risk of myocardial infarction. The estimated odds ratio, adjusted for age and the effect of the other variable, were $\hat{\psi}_{mh} = 3.33$ (MI-OC odds ratio, adjusted for age and smoking) and $\hat{\psi}_{mh} = 4.98$ (MI-smoking odds ratio, adjusted for age and OC use). Thus, smoking is estimated to increase the risk of an MI nearly five times, whereas recent oral contraceptive use is estimated to increase the risk 3.3 times. One might next inquire about the joint effect of smoking and oral contraceptive use, an issue that shall be taken up in Section 7.3.

Woolf's Method

Assuming that the subgroup-specific odds ratios are constant, $\psi_i = \psi$, Woolf (1955) proposed an adjusted estimate of ψ that is based on the log odds ratio. An estimate of the variance of $\ln \hat{\psi}_i$ is given by v_i in (7.21). Taking a weighted average of the log odds ratios, with weights being the reciprocals of the estimated variances, $\ln \psi$ may be estimated by the quantity $\Sigma v_i^{-1} \ln \hat{\psi}_i / \Sigma v_i^{-1}$. Thus, an estimate of ψ is given by

$$\hat{\psi}_w = \exp[\Sigma v_i^{-1} \ln \hat{\psi}_i / \Sigma v_i^{-1}], \qquad (7.29)$$

where the index i is summed over the k subgroups.

Tests of significance and confidence intervals assume that $\ln \hat{\psi}_w$ is approximately normally distributed. Letting

$$W = \Sigma v_i^{-1}, \qquad (7.30)$$

an approximate chi-square test of the null hypothesis $H_0: \psi = \psi_0$ against the two-sided alternative $H_A: \psi \neq \psi_0$ may be based on the statistic

$$\chi_w^2 = W(\ln \hat{\psi}_w - \ln \psi_0)^2. \tag{7.31}$$

Under the null hypothesis, χ_w^2 has an approximate chi-square distribution with one degree of freedom. For $H_0:\psi = 1$, equation (7.31) becomes $\chi_w^2 = W(\ln \hat{\psi}_w)^2$. Equation (7.31) gives approximate $1 - \alpha$ confidence limits of

$$
\begin{aligned}
\hat{\psi}_L &= \hat{\psi}_w \exp(-z_\alpha / \sqrt{W}) \\
\hat{\psi}_U &= \hat{\psi}_w \exp(+z_\alpha / \sqrt{W}).
\end{aligned}
\tag{7.32}
$$

As an example of Woolf's method, consider the data in Table 7.7B, to which the Mantel-Haenszel procedure was previously applied. One calculates $W = \Sigma v_i^{-1} = 14.8$ and $\Sigma v_i^{-1} \ln \hat{\psi}_i = 21.4$. Thus $\hat{\psi}_w = \exp(21.4/14.8) = 4.2$ from (7.29). An approximate 95 percent confidence interval is calculated from equation (7.32) to be (2.5, 7.0). A test of significance of $H_0:\psi = 1$, is calculated from (7.31) as $\chi_w^2 = 14.8(\ln 4.2 - \ln 1.0)^2 = 30.48$ ($p \simeq 10^{-7}$, one-sided).

Gart (1962) has shown that the weighted arithmetic mean of the $\hat{\psi}_i$ and the weighted harmonic mean are asymptotically as efficient as $\hat{\psi}_w$. Gart and Zweifel (1967) and Cox (1970, pp. 79–80) have also given modifications of $\hat{\psi}_w$ based on adding ½ correction factors to the cell entries.

Point and Interval Estimates of the Odds Ratio Based on the Exact Conditional Distribution of the Number of Exposed Cases (a_i)

Assuming that the marginal totals are fixed at the observed outcomes for each of the subgroup 2×2 tables, inference on a common odds ratio ψ may be based on the joint distribution of a_i, conditional on m_{1i} (Cornfield 1956, Gart 1970). Let $r_1 = \max(m_{1i} - n_{2i}, 0)$ and $r_2 = \min(n_{1i}, m_{1i})$. The conditional distribution of a_i in the ith 2×2 table is

$$g_i(\psi) = \binom{n_{1i}}{a_i} \binom{n_{2i}}{m_{1i}-a_i} \psi^{a_i} \Big/ \sum_{j=r_1}^{r_2} \binom{n_{1i}}{j} \binom{n_{2i}}{m_{1i}-j} \psi^j.$$

Assuming that the 2×2 tables are independent, the joint conditional distribution of the a_i is

$$g(\psi) = \prod_{i=1}^k g_i(\psi). \tag{7.33}$$

The value of ψ that maximizes equation (7.33), which we shall denote by $\hat{\psi}_c$, is the *exact conditional estimate*. The program by Thomas (1975) performs the computations. Birch (1964) and Goodman (1969) have given approximate solutions that are valid when $\psi \simeq 1$. In practice, the Mantel-Haenszel estimate $\hat{\psi}_{mh}$ and $\hat{\psi}_c$ will often have similar values (Armitage 1975, McKinlay 1978).

A second approach to the estimation of ψ, which requires the iterative solution of a system of k quadratic equations, is based on maximizing the asymptotic likelihood. For any given value of ψ, let $\hat{a}_i$ be the solution to the quadratic equation

$$\psi = a_i(n_{2i} + a_i - m_{1i})/[(n_{1i} - a_i)(m_{1i} - a_i)].$$

The *asymptotic conditional maximum likelihood estimate* of ψ, denoted $\hat{\psi}_a$, is the value of ψ that solves the equation

$$\sum_{i=1}^{k} \hat{a}_i = \sum_{i=1}^{k} a_i. \tag{7.34}$$

Gart (1971) gives an explicit algorithm that was suggested by Cornfield (1956) for solving (7.34). The program by Thomas (1975) performs these calculations as well as the computation of the corresponding exact and asymptotic conditional confidence limits. Asymptotic methods are used with large samples because the calculation of the "exact" estimate and confidence limits may require very large amounts of computer time and yield answers almost identical to those based on the asymptotic approach.

Discussion

An adjusted odds ratio estimated from a stratified analysis represents the constant component of an association across subgroups. Even though the subgroup-specific odds ratios may be heterogeneous, one often wants a summary measure. Of course, a combined odds ratio estimate should not be based on individual odds ratios that differ substantially in direction, some being less than and others greater than unity (McKinlay 1978).

An estimate of the disease-exposure odds ratio that is "adjusted" for one or more variables does not necessarily represent the effect of exposure in the *absence* of those variables. The latter odds ratio would be based on the comparison of exposure between cases and controls within the subgroup of individuals who have no exposure to the other variables involved in the analysis. However, if the disease-exposure odds ratio is constant across subgroups, indicating no interaction on a multiplicative scale between exposure and the other variables, then the two estimates will be the same.

The Mantel-Haenszel estimate was intended to be a weighted average of the individual odds ratios (Mantel 1977). In fact, Mantel and Haenszel (1959) indicated their disbelief in the constancy of the odds ratio, stating that the assumption of a constant relative risk is usually untenable. By contrast, the odds ratio estimates derived by Woolf (1955), Gart (1962, 1970), Birch (1964) and Goodman (1969) were based on the assumption of a constant odds ratio across the subgroup 2×2 tables. Despite this assumption, these estimates may be regarded as a summary odds ratio if there is heterogeneity. In addition to the estimate $\hat{\psi}_{mh}$, Mantel and Haenszel (1959) have given four other summary estimates of an adjusted odds ratio. One was based on the direct method of standardizing mortality ratios, and the other three were based on procedures of direct adjustment of the proportions exposed, using as a standard the distribution of the cases, the distribution of the controls, or the combined distribution of the cases and controls.

Odds ratios estimated from different studies may vary because of underlying differences in extraneous variables (confounders) among the case-control series. Stratification can be used to reduce the effects of confounding by establishing comparable odds ratios within subgroups defined by strata of the confounders. One may then compare adjusted odds ratios in which the effects of the confounders have been removed.

Breslow (1981) has investigated the bias and precision of $\hat{\psi}_{mh}$, $\hat{\psi}_w$ (with ½ correction factors), $\hat{\psi}_a$ and $\hat{\psi}_c$. For a limiting model in which the numbers of cases and controls in each subgroup remain small while the total sample size increases as a result of an increase in the number of subgroups, neither $\hat{\psi}_w$ nor $\hat{\psi}_a$ converged to the true odds ratio. As a consequence, these methods were not recommended for "sparse" data. Both $\hat{\psi}_{mh}$ and $\hat{\psi}_c$ converged to the true odds ratio. For a wide range of values of ψ and exposure probabilities among controls, the Mantel-Haenszel estimate $\hat{\psi}_{mh}$ was nearly fully efficient, its asymptotic variance infrequently exceeding that of $\hat{\psi}_c$ by more than 10 percent. In an extensive Monte Carlo study, McKinlay (1978) found that $\hat{\psi}_c$ was no less biased nor more precise than $\hat{\psi}_{mh}$. In view of the simplicity of computation of $\hat{\psi}_{mh}$ in comparison with $\hat{\psi}_c$, the Mantel-Haenszel estimate is preferred as a general technique. An accurate but simply computed approximation for the standard error of $\hat{\psi}_{mh}$ in small samples remains to be found.

Test for Heterogeneity of Odds Ratios

Suppose that one has two comparably adjusted estimates of an odds ratio derived from independent studies or from independent subgroups within the same study. Let x_1 and x_2 denote the logarithms of the two respective Mantel-Haenszel estimates, $\ln \hat{\psi}_{mh}$, and let y_1 and y_2 denote the corresponding estimated variances of $\ln \hat{\psi}_{mh}$ calculated from equation (7.22). A test of whether the two Mantel-Haenszel estimates differ significantly may be based on

$$\chi^2 = (x_1 - x_2)^2/(y_1 + y_2), \qquad (7.35)$$

which has an approximate chi-square distribution with one degree of freedom under the null hypothesis of no difference. In effect, equation (7.35) provides a test of whether there is interaction on a multiplicative scale between the exposure variable and the variable used for the stratification.

In some instances one may be interested in whether a set of subgroup odds ratios are constant across strata formed by one or more confounding variables. Let $\hat{\psi}_w$ be given by equation (7.29) and let v_i be defined by (7.21). Woolf's (1955) test for heterogeneity of two or more subgroup odds ratios is calculated as

$$\chi_w^2 = \sum_{i=1}^{k} v_i^{-1} (\ln \hat{\psi}_i - \ln \hat{\psi}_w)^2. \tag{7.36}$$

In large samples, the statistic χ_w^2 has a chi-square distribution with $k - 1$ degrees of freedom under the hypothesis $H_0 : \psi_i = \psi$. Odoroff (1970) has given some Monte Carlo results on small sample properties of Woolf's test for heterogeneity, as well as comparisons with several alternative tests.

As an example of Woolf's test for heterogeneity, consider data from a case-control study investigating an association between lung cancer and employment in shipbuilding (Blot et al. 1978). Table 7.9 classifies 458 cases of lung cancer and 523 controls according to past employment in a shipyard and current cigarette smoking. Taking shipbuilding (which involved exposure to asbestos) as the exposure of interest, the smoking-specific estimates of the relative risk of disease (odds ratio) associated with shipbuilding increase from 1.28 to 1.69 to 2.43 as smoking varies from minimal to moderate to heavy. Although this suggests a trend in the odds ratios with increasing levels of smoking, Woolf's test for heterogeneity gives a chi-square value of $\chi_w^2 = 0.80$ with 2 degrees of freedom. This is far from significant, thereby providing no evidence of a multiplicative interaction between smoking and shipbuilding.

By closely examining Table 7.9, one can see the reason for the nonsignificant value of χ_w^2. Very small changes in the distribution of exposure among cases and controls can make the odds ratios appear homogeneous. For example, if the odds of exposure among minimal-smoking cases were 13/48 instead of the observed 11/50, the estimated odds ratio would be 1.57. Similarly, if the odds of exposure among heavy-smoking controls were 5/48 instead of the observed 3/50, the estimated odds ratio would be 1.40. Thus slight changes in the two smallest groups produce large changes in the estimated odds ratios. The test for heterogeneity accounts

Table 7.9. Cigarette Smoking and Employment in Shipbuilding Among Cases of Lung Cancer and Controls

Smoking	Shipbuilding	Cancer	Control	$\hat{\psi}_i$*
Minimal†	Yes	11	35	
	No	50	203	1.28
Moderate	Yes	70	42	
	No	217	220	1.69
Heavy	Yes	14	3	
	No	96	50	2.43

Woolf's Test for Heterogeneity

i	$\ln \hat{\psi}_i$	v_i^{-1}
1	.247	6.92
2	.525	21.16
3	.888	2.30

$\hat{\psi}_w = \exp(\Sigma v_i^{-1} \ln \hat{\psi}_i / \Sigma v_i^{-1}) = \exp(14.86/30.38) = 1.63$
$\chi_w^2 = \Sigma v_i^{-1}(\ln \hat{\psi}_i - \ln \hat{\psi}_w)^2 = 0.80$ (2 d.f.)

*Smoking-specific odds ratios.
†Minimal: nonsmoker, light smoker, or stopped smoking.

Source: Blot et al. 1978.

for the inherent large variability in assessing the significance of the differences.

One may want to compare odds ratios from two different subgroups in terms of their ratio $\hat{\psi}_i/\hat{\psi}_j$. Thus, in Table 7.9 the estimated relative risk (odds ratio) of lung cancer associated with shipbuilding is 90 percent greater in heavy smokers as compared with minimal smokers, $2.43/1.28 = 1.90$. Approximate confidence intervals on the ratio of odds ratios are easily calculated. Let ψ_i and ψ_j denote the unknown parameter values of the odds ratios in the ith and jth subgroups, sample estimates of which are given by $\hat{\psi}_i$ and $\hat{\psi}_j$. A large-sample $1 - \alpha$ confidence interval on the ratio ψ_i/ψ_j is then given by

$$(\hat{\psi}_i/\hat{\psi}_j) \exp[\pm z_\alpha \sqrt{v_i + v_j}] \qquad (7.37)$$

where v_i and v_j are defined by (7.21). Goodman (1964) provides methods for calculating simultaneous confidence intervals for a set of ratios ψ_i/ψ_j, and Heilbron (1981) considers adjustment for confounding. (See Chapter 2, Section 2.4 and 2.6 for caveats regarding the comparison of odds ratios.)

Table 7.10. Odds (in Parentheses) and Odds Ratios for Lung Cancer Associated with Various Combinations of Smoking and Employment in Shipbuilding

Smoking	Shipbuilding	
	No	Yes
Minimal	(50/203)	(11/35)
	1.0[1]	1.28
Moderate	(217/220)	(70/42)
	4.01	6.78
Heavy	(96/50)	(14/3)
	7.80	18.95

1. Reference group.

7.3 ASSESSMENT OF INDIVIDUAL AND JOINT EFFECTS OF TWO OR MORE VARIABLES

The assessment of the individual and joint effects of a set of variables in an unmatched study may be done by appropriately stratifying the data and comparing various subgroups against one that is used as a standard of reference. The reference group is generally taken to be the one with minimal levels of exposure on all of the variables under consideration as risk factors for the study disease. For example, refer again to the data in Table 7.9. Both employment in shipbuilding and smoking may be considered risk factors for the development of lung cancer. [Ship construction and repair involves contact with asbestos, which is known to induce lung cancer and mesothelioma.] For each of the six combinations of smoking and shipbuilding [(minimal, yes), (minimal, no), . . . , (heavy no)] one may compute the odds of "disease" [11/35, 50/203, . . . , 96/50]. Taking as the reference group individuals who smoked minimally and were not employed in shipbuilding, the odds of "disease" for each of the other combinations of smoking and shipbuilding may be expressed as a ratio relative to the reference, as shown in Table 7.10. Thus, heavy smokers not employed in shipbuilding are estimated to have a 7.8 times increased risk of lung cancer as compared with individuals who smoke minimally and are not employed in shipbuilding. Shipbuilders who smoked minimally are estimated to have a 1.28 times increased risk. Heavy smokers employed in shipbuilding are estimated to have a 18.95 times increased risk, etc.

One should study carefully the different analyses and interpretations of Tables 7.9 and 7.10. In Table 7.9, the odds ratios estimate the relative risk of cancer associated with employment in shipbuilding for each of three smoking groups. The odds of "disease" among shipbuilders is expressed relative to the odds of "disease" among non-shipbuilders. Since the reference group of non-shipbuilders changes for each of the three smoking categories, the odds ratios are "subgroup-specific." For example, among heavy smokers, employment in shipbuilding is estimated to increase the risk of lung cancer 2.4 times, whereas among moderate smokers, shipbuilding is estimated to result in only a 1.7 times increased risk. (The difference is not statistically significant.) Thus, in Table 7.9, the relative risk of lung cancer associated with shipbuilding is estimated in the presence of various degrees of smoking.

The Mantel-Haenszel estimate of the relative odds of lung cancer associated with shipbuilding, adjusted for smoking, is $\hat{\psi}_{mh} = 1.64$. This estimate is a weighted average of the relative effect of shipbuilding, in the presence of various levels of smoking, on the risk of lung cancer (Section 7.2).

A confidence interval or test of significance for any individual odds ratio in Table 7.10 may be calculated by the methods in Section 7.1, which apply to a single 2×2 table. Tests for heterogeneity (7.35) and (7.36), and confidence limits (7.37) on ψ_i/ψ_j, do not apply to Table 7.10, however, because the odds ratios are not independent, all being calculated relative to the same reference.

Analysis of the individual and joint effects of three or more risk factors proceeds exactly as above. One uses a single subgroup of cases and controls as the reference, expressing the odds of "disease" for all other combinations relative to it.

Test for Synergy

Table 7.10 suggests synergy (see Chapter 2, Section 2.11) between heavy smoking and shipbuilding:

$$(18.95 - 1) > (7.80 - 1) + (1.28 - 1).$$

Since all of the odds ratios are expressed relative to the same reference, one may alternatively express the above relationship in terms of the odds of "disease" in the four subgroups:

$$(14/3 - 50/203) > (96/50 - 50/203) + (11/35 - 50/203)$$

or

$$(14/3 + 50/203) - (96/50 + 11/35) > 0.$$

An approximate chi-square test of significance for synergy may thus be made as follows. First, define the following odds of "disease"; a_0/b_0

(reference group), a_1/b_1 (presence of first variable only), a_2/b_2 (presence of second variable only), a_3/b_3 (joint presence of first and second variables). Let

$$S = (a_3/b_3 + a_0/b_0) - (a_1/b_1 + a_2/b_2). \qquad (7.38)$$

Values of S which are greater than zero suggest synergy. [The index S is derived from equation (2.29) in Chapter 2 by using odds ratios as approximations to relative risks.]

Let u_i denote an estimate of the variance of a_i/b_i in large samples (a_i and b_i large),

$$u_i = \mathrm{var}(a_i/b_i) \simeq (a_i/b_i)^2 (a_i + b_i)/(a_i b_i) \qquad (7.39)$$

and let

$$U = u_0 + u_1 + u_2 + u_3. \qquad (7.40)$$

A large sample chi-square test (1 d.f.) of whether S is significantly greater than zero is then given by

$$\chi^2 = S^2/U. \qquad (7.41)$$

Rothman (1974) gives a related approach to testing a different index of synergy. Dayal (1980), using a formulation based on the multinominal distribution, derives an alternative chi-square test of significance of S. His procedure, while considerably more complex than the test given by equation (7.41), will likely have better agreement between the actual and nominal levels of significance in small samples.

The test of significance (7.41) for synergy between heavy smoking and employment in shipbuilding is calculated from Table 7.10 as follows: $a_0/b_0 = 50/203$, $a_1/b_1 = 11/35$, $a_2/b_2 = 96/50$ and $a_3/b_3 = 14/3$. Thus, from (7.39): $u_0 = .002$, $u_1 = .012$, $u_2 = .112$ and $u_3 = 8.815$. Hence, $S = 2.679$ and $U = 8.941$, giving $\chi^2 = (2.679)^2/8.941 = .80$, which is far from significant. This is due primarily to the large variance for the sample odds $14/3$.

Adjustment for Confounding

A direct application of the Mantel-Haenszel technique permits the assessment of the individual and joint effects of a set of risk factors, with adjustment for confounding by one or more other variables. As an example, refer back to Table 7.6, discussed in Section 7.2 as an application of the Mantel-Haenszel technique. Both cigarette smoking and recent use

Table 7.11. Separate and Combined
Effects of Oral Contraceptive (OC) Use
and Cigarette Smoking in Relation to
Myocardial Infarction (MI), Ignoring Age

A. *Distribution of Cases (MI) and*
   Controls (Ctl) within Subgroups of
   Smoking and Oral Contraceptive Use

Cigarette smoking	OC use	MI	Ctl	$\hat{\psi}*$
None	No	34	754	1.0†
None	Yes	4	52	1.7
1–24	No	79	566	3.1
1–24	Yes	3	51	1.3
25+	No	92	287	7.1
25+	Yes	22	32	15.3

*Odds ratio relative to no smoking and no OC use.
†Reference group.

B. *Estimated Odds Ratios*

Cigarette smoking	OC use No	OC use Yes
None	1.0	1.7
1–24	3.1	1.3
25+	7.1	15.3

of oral contraceptives were found to be associated with an increased risk
of myocardial infarction. First, suppose that one ignores age as a potential
confounder and sums the individual 2 × 2 tables in Table 7.6 over the
age strata. The result is shown in Table 7.11A. Taking as a reference
group individuals who neither smoked nor were recent oral contraceptive
users, Table 7.11B gives the crude (i.e. unadjusted for age) odds ratios
for various combinations of smoking and OC use.

Next, consider adjusting the crude odds ratios in Table 7.11B for the
effect of age. This is accomplished by retaining the age stratification of
Table 7.6, and computing a Mantel-Haenszel estimate $\hat{\psi}_{mh}$ for each of
the OC-smoking combinations relative to the reference group of individuals who neither smoked nor were recent users of oral contraceptives.
Table 7.12A shows the rearrangement of Table 7.6 from which the age-
adjusted Mantel-Haenszel estimates are calculated. Table 7.12B shows
the age-adjusted odds ratios which are refinements of the crude estimates
in Table 7.11B. Failure to adjust for confounding by age results in sub-

Table 7.12. Relation of Myocardial Infarction to Recent Use of Oral Contraceptives and Cigarette Smoking

A. *Separate and Combined Effects of OC Use and Cigarette Smoking in Relation to Myocardial Infarction, Stratified by Age*

Cigarette smoking	OC use	Age										$\hat{\psi}_{mh}$*
		25–29		30–34		35–39		40–44		45–49		
		MI	Ctl	MI	Ctl	MI	Ctl	MI	Ctl	MI	Ctl	
None	No	1	106	0	175	3	153	10	165	20	155	1.0†
None	Yes	0	25	0	13	0	8	1	4	3	2	4.5
1–24	No	0	79	5	142	11	119	21	130	42	96	3.4
1–24	Yes	1	25	1	10	1	11	0	4	0	1	3.7
25+	No	1	39	7	73	19	58	34	67	31	50	7.8
25+	Yes	3	12	8	10	3	7	5	1	3	2	39.3

B. *Mantel-Haenszel Age-Adjusted Odds Ratios*

Cigarette smoking	OC use	
	No	Yes
None	1.0	4.5
1–24	3.4	3.7
25+	7.8	39.3

*Odds ratios relative to no smoking and no OC use.
†Reference group.

stantial underestimates of the effect of oral contraceptive use. This occurs for each of the three smoking categories.

7.4 TEST FOR DOSE RESPONSE

Dose (intensity) and duration are two components of exposure that should often be considered in an analysis. For example, Table 7.13A shows data on maternal smoking for mothers of children with congenital malformations and mothers of controls (Kelsey et al. 1978). A trend in the odds of "disease" with increasing levels of cigarette smoking is suggested. Taking as the reference group women who did not smoke during the third month of pregnancy (a critical time of fetal development), the estimated relative risk of a malformation increases with higher levels of cigarette smoking during that month, up to a maximum of $\hat{\psi} = 1.86$. (The trend is statistically significant.) Had one ignored the differing levels of smoking by dichotomizing this variable as simply yes (≥ 1 cig/day) or no (0 cig/day), as shown in Table 7.13B, one would have found a nonsignificant association. The crude odds ratio $\hat{\psi} = 1.10$ is not sig-

Table 7.13.   Relation of Maternal Cigarette Smoking to Congenital Malformations

A. *Cigarette Smoking in Mothers of Infants with Congenital Malformations and in Mothers of Controls, According to Average Number of Cigarettes Smoked per Day During Third Month of Pregnancy*

Cig/day	Malformations (a_i)	Controls (b_i)	Odds (a_i/b_i)	Odds ratio* $\hat{\psi}_i$
0	889	1988	.447	1.0†
1–10	182	426	.427	0.96
11–20	203	420	.483	1.08
21–30	55	86	.640	1.43
≥ 31	40	48	.833	1.86

Chi-square test for trend (7.42): $\chi^2 = 9.34$ ($p \simeq 0.002$, two-sided)

B. *Presence of Cigarette Smoking During Third Month of Pregnancy in Mothers of Infants with Congenital Malformations and Controls*

Smoking	Malformations	Controls	Odds ratio
Yes‡	480	980	$\hat{\psi} = 1.10$
No	889	1988	

Chi-square test for association (7.11): $\chi^2 = 1.75$ ($p \simeq 0.19$, two-sided)

*$\hat{\psi}_i = (a_i/b_i) \div (a_0/b_0)$
†Reference group.
‡Yes (≥ 1 cig/day)

Source: Kelsey et al. 1978.

nificantly different from unity ($p \simeq 0.19$, two-sided). This points out the importance of the definition of "exposure," and shows the value of assessing dose-response relationships.

A general test of trend (either a progressive increase or decrease in the odds of "disease") can be computed in the following way (Mantel 1963). Let the data be arranged as in Table 7.14. The term x_i in this table is a score that represents the ith level of exposure. The terms a_i and b_i denote respectively the numbers of cases and controls at the ith exposure level, their total being $m_i = (a_i + b_i)$. First compute

$$T_1 = \sum_{i=0}^{t} a_i x_i \qquad T_2 = \sum_{i=0}^{t} m_i x_i \qquad T_3 = \sum_{i=0}^{t} m_i x_i^2$$

and then

$$V = n_1 n_2 (n T_3 - T_2^2) / n^2 (n-1).$$

A one-degree-of-freedom chi-square test for trend is then calculated by

$$\chi^2 = [T_1 - (n_1 T_2/n)]^2 / V. \qquad (7.42)$$

Table 7.14. Data Layout for Test of Dose Response in a
Case-Control Study

Exposure levels	Cases	Controls	Total
x_0	a_0	b_0	m_0
x_1	a_1	b_1	m_1
.	.	.	.
.	.	.	.
.	.	.	.
x_t	a_t	b_t	m_t
Total	n_1	n_2	n

If the exposure levels have a scale of measurement, one method of assigning scores objectively takes x_i to be the midpoint of the exposure category. Another method takes $x_i = i$ for the ith exposure level. Mantel (1963) discusses these and alternative scoring methods.

Applied to the data in Table 7.13A, the test for trend is calculated as follows. Let the exposure levels of smoking in each of the five subgroups be represented by $x_0 = 0$, $x_1 = 5$, $x_2 = 15$, $x_3 = 25$ and $x_4 = 35$. Then $T_1 = 6730$, $T_2 = 18990$, $T_3 = 351300$, $V = 57955.97$ and $\chi^2 = 9.34$. The value of chi-square indicates a significant ($p \simeq 0.002$, two-sided) trend in the odds of "disease" with increasing levels of cigarette smoking and points to the existence of a dose-response relationship between maternal cigarette smoking and the risk of congenital malformations in the offspring.

One may also want to test whether the odds ratio shows a trend with severity of disease or certainty of diagnosis. As an example, Table 7.15 shows data on the use of estrogens during the menopause among cases of endometrial cancer, grouped according to stage of disease, and usage among controls. The odds of exposure among controls are 0.139 (33/238). Among the cases, the odds of exposure decrease with increasing stage of disease. Taking the odds of exposure among controls as the reference, the odds ratios are reported by increasing severity of disease in the last column. The chi-square test for trend (7.42) may be applied by letting the "level of exposure" variable x_i denote the four categories: controls ($x_0 = 0$), stage 0 ($x_1 = 1$), stage I ($x_2 = 2$) and stage II, III, IV ($x_3 = 3$). The calculations are $T_1 = 224$, $T_2 = 556$, $T_3 = 1224$, $V = 130.53$, giving $\chi^2 = 38.78$. Thus, the odds ratios show a significant decline ($p < 10^{-8}$, two-sided) with increasing severity of disease, suggesting that the effect of menopausal estrogens is most pronounced in the earlier stages of endometrial cancer.

Yates (1948), Cochran (1954), and Armitage (1955) have given tests of trend in proportions which are closely related to that proposed by Mantel (1963). Considering the proportion of cases at each level of exposure, $p_i = a_i/(a_i + b_i)$ from Table 7.14, a trend in p_i implies a trend in the odds p_i/q_i. That is, $p_i < p_j$ if and only if $p_i/q_i < p_j/q_j$. Although one may test specifically whether the trend in p_i is a linear, quadratic, or some other function of x_i, an assessment is often unnecessary in practice, since the precise relationship between p_i and x_i is not frequently of direct interest. Mantel (1963) has also described a test for trend when both the disease and exposure variables occur at several levels. Snedecor and Cochran (1980, pp. 204–208) and Fleiss (1981, pp. 143–149) give detailed discussions and further references for tests of trend in proportions.

Adjustment for Confounding

The test for dose-response given by equation (7.42) has been extended by Mantel (1963) to the situation in which cases and controls have been stratified into subgroups in order to eliminate confounding by one or more variables. A test for dose response, adjusted for those factors on which the stratification is based, is calculated as follows.

For each subgroup, arrange the data as in Table 7.14. For the jth subgroup, one computes the quantities

$$T_{1j} = \sum_{i=0}^{t} a_i x_i \qquad T_{2j} = \sum_{i=0}^{t} m_i x_i \qquad T_{3j} = \sum_{i=0}^{t} m_i x_i^2.$$

Table 7.15. Use of Estrogens During the Menopause Among Cases of Endometrial Cancer, According to Stage, and Among Controls

	Estrogen use		Odds of exposure	Odds ratio
	Yes	No		
Controls	33	238	0.139	1.00*
Cases:				
Stage 0	24	11	2.182	15.70
Stage I	76	111	0.685	4.93
Stage II, III, IV	16	33	0.484	3.48

*Reference group.

Source: Antunes et al. 1979.

(Although the values of a_i, b_i, and m_i in Table 7.14 differ for each of the subgroups, we avoid a double subscript on them for simplicity.) Let n_{1j} and n_{2j} represent respectively the total numbers of cases and controls in the jth subgroup, and let $n_j = n_{1j} + n_{2j}$. One next computes the quantity

$$V_j = n_{1j}n_{2j}(n_j T_{3j} - T_{2j}^2)/n_j^2(n_j - 1).$$

A test for dose response, adjusted for confounding, is then given by

$$\chi^2 = \left\{ \sum_{j=1}^{k} [T_{1j} - (n_{1j}/n_j)T_{2j}] \right\}^2 / \sum_{j=1}^{k} V_j \qquad (7.43)$$

where the summation is over the k subgroups formed by the stratification. The statistic χ^2, which has been called the *extended Mantel-Haenszel test*, has an approximate chi-square distribution with one degree of freedom under the null hypothesis of no trend in the odds of "disease."

As an application of the extended Mantel-Haenszel test, consider the data in Table 7.16 on cigarette smoking and age among female controls and cases of myocardial infarction. This table, based on Table 7.6, ignores oral contraceptive use as a risk factor. The relationship of smoking to MI was previously discussed in Section 7.2, but the analysis dichotomized the smoking variables as yes (≥ 1 cig/day) or no (none) for simplicity, thereby ignoring the potential to analyze the data for a dose response. The age-adjusted relative odds of disease associated with smoking appear to increase with higher levels of cigarette smoking. Compared with nonsmokers, the age-adjusted odds of "disease" are three times higher in women who smoke 1–24 cigarettes per day, $\hat{\psi}_{mh} = 3.16$. Taking nonsmokers as the reference, the age-adjusted odds of "disease" are over eight times higher among women who smoke 25 or more cigarettes per day, $\hat{\psi}_{mh} = 8.57$. Computation of the extended Mantel-Haenszel test is shown at the bottom of Table 7.16. The resulting chi-square test with one degree of freedom, $\chi^2 = 129.87$, is highly significant ($p < 0.001$), indicating a definite trend of increasing risk of myocardial infarction with increasing numbers of cigarettes smoked per day.

The data in Table 7.16 have been collapsed over a fourth variable, recent use of oral contraceptives. The estimated MI-smoking odds ratios in Table 7.16, although adjusted for age, are not adjusted for oral contraceptive use. If one wanted to adjust for age and usage of oral contraceptives (OC) simultaneously, one would stratify the smoking data for cases and controls into 10 subgroups, resulting from the 2 × 5 strata formed by the cross-classification of age (5 groups) and use of oral con-

Table 7.16. Frequency of Cigarette Smoking Among Female Cases of Myocardial Infarction (MI) and Controls (Ctl), According to Age

Cig/day	(x_i)	Age (years)									
		25–29		30–34		35–39		40–44		45–49	
		MI	Ctl	MI	Ctl	MI	Ctl	MI	Ctl	MI	Ctl
None	(0)*	1	131	0	188	3	161	11	169	23	157
1–24	(1)	1	104	6	152	12	130	21	134	42	97
≥25	(2)	4	51	15	83	22	65	39	68	34	52

Computation of Mantel-Haenszel Estimates of MI-Smoking Odds Ratios, Adjusted for Age

Smoking	Age-adjusted odds ratio
1–24 vs. none	$\hat{\psi}_{mh} = 41.39/13.1 = 3.16$
≥ 25 vs. none	$\hat{\psi}_{mh} = 69.81/8.15 = 8.57$

Computation of Age-Adjusted Test for Trend in the Odds of "Disease" with Increasing Levels of Smoking†

	25–29	30–34	35–39	40–44	45–49
T_{1j}	9	36	56	99	110
T_{2j}	215	354	316	369	311
T_{3j}	325	550	490	583	483
V_j	3.3664	12.0924	20.1709	37.1548	45.2101

$\chi^2 = (4.5822 + 19.2568 + 26.2494 + 39.7262 + 33.9778)^2/117.9946 = 129.87$

*Reference group.
†Test for trend based on equation (7.43).

Source: Shapiro et al. 1979.

traceptives (2 groups). The extended test for trend (7.43) and the Mantel-Haenszel estimates of the MI-smoking odds ratios could then be computed across the 10 subgroups of age and oral contraceptive use. In the present circumstance, additional adjustment for OC use makes little difference in the analysis. The MI-smoking odds ratios, adjusted for both age and OC use, are $\hat{\psi}_{mh} = 3.25$ (1–24 vs. none) and $\hat{\psi}_{mh} = 8.22$ (≥ 25 vs. none).

In summary, stratification on the basis of one or more variables to adjust for confounding will result in k subgroups. Within each subgroup one may compare cases and controls with respect to the odds of exposure at each exposure level x_i relative to a fixed reference level x_0. The Mantel-Haenszel estimate $\hat{\psi}_{mh}$ of the relative odds of disease associated with each level x_i vs. the reference level x_0 may then be computed over the k subgroups. The test for dose response (7.43) may be regarded as a test of whether there is a progressive increase or decrease in these adjusted odds ratios. The test may also be used to determine whether the odds ratio, adjusted for confounding variables, shows a trend among the cases when they are grouped by severity of disease or certainty of diagnosis.

Tarone and Gart (1980) have shown that the test given by equation (7.43) is an optimal test of trend when the log odds of disease is a linear function of the exposure scores x_i, $\ln p/q = \alpha_j + \beta x_i$, where the slope parameter β is constant and the intercept parameter α_j varies across subgroups. Use of the extended Mantel-Haenszel procedure as a general test for trend is a good choice, even though the dose-response function may not follow the above logistic form. In practice, it is likely to be highly efficient, even in comparison with tests that are designed to be optimal in special situations (Tarone and Gart 1980).

7.5 TEST-BASED CONFIDENCE LIMITS

Miettinen (1974b, 1976a) has suggested a procedure called the *test-based method* for setting approximate confidence limits on the odds ratio. This approach applies not only to a single 2 × 2 table, but also to the combination of a series of them, including data from matched or unmatched studies. In general, let $\hat{\psi}_{mh}$ be the Mantel-Haenszel estimate of the disease-exposure odds ratio, and χ^2_{mh} the corresponding continuity corrected chi-square test of the null hypothesis $H_0: \psi = 1$. An approximate $1 - \alpha$ confidence interval for ψ is calculated from

$$\exp[(1 \pm z_\alpha / \sqrt{\chi^2_{mh}}) \ln \hat{\psi}_{mh}]. \tag{7.44}$$

For a single 2 × 2 table, one uses $\hat{\psi}$ and χ^2_c, given by equations (7.1) and (7.12) respectively, in place of $\hat{\psi}_{mh}$ and χ^2_{mh}. The test-based method is related to Woolf's (1955) approach to setting confidence limits on $\ln \psi$ (Miettinen 1977, Fleiss 1979, Gart and Thomas 1982).

Test-based limits for the odds ratio in Table 7.2 are calculated as follows. From $\hat{\psi} = 3.71$ and $\chi^2_c = 20.75$, approximate 95 percent limits for ψ are

$$\exp[(1 \pm 1.96/\sqrt{20.75}) \ln(3.71)] = (2.11, 6.52).$$

The interval (2.11, 6.52) is slightly narrower than the corresponding intervals calculated by Woolf's method (2.10, 6.55) or Cornfield's method (2.03, 6.84). The discussion of the Mantel-Haenszel technique in Section 7.2 gives another application of test-based confidence limits based on the data in Table 7.6.

The attractive feature of test-based limits is their computational simplicity. Given a point estimate of the odds ratio and a chi-square test of H_0, an approximate confidence interval is easily calculated. Test-based limits are controversial, however. Halperin (1977) has shown that the asymptotic confidence coefficient of the interval based on equation (7.44) approaches zero as the true relative odds depart increasingly from unity. For $0.25 < \psi < 4$, the asymptotic coverage probability for nominal 95 percent confidence limits is between 0.93 and 0.95 (Halperin 1977); however, in small samples the coverage probability in the unconditional sample space may be as low as 0.86 (Gart and Thomas 1982). Although test-based limits are likely to provide a reasonable approximation in practice, computer simulations of the conditional (Brown 1981) and unconditional (Gart and Thomas 1982) coverage probabilities indicate that Cornfield's method should be used for definitive results.

7.6 MATCHED ANALYSIS WITH ONE CONTROL PER CASE

Point Estimation of the Odds Ratio

The correct analysis of a properly matched study retains the pairing of cases and controls (Chapter 4). To begin, suppose that one has matched a single control to each case, and that the exposure under study is dichotomous. Denoting the presence or absence of exposure by $+$ or $-$ respectively, the four possible outcomes for each pair (case, control) are: $(++), (+-), (-+)$ and $(--)$. Table 7.17 shows the data layout for the analysis. The term A denotes the number of pairs $(++)$ in which both the case and the control were exposed to the study factor. The term B denotes the number of pairs $(+-)$ in which only the case was exposed, and so forth. The marginal totals $A + B$ and $C + D$ represent respectively the numbers of exposed and unexposed cases, whereas the marginal totals $A + C$ and $B + D$ represent the corresponding numbers of exposed and unexposed controls. The term N denotes the total number of *pairs*, so that the total number of cases and controls is $2N$. The reader should carefully compare Table 7.17 and Table 7.1 to clearly understand their differences.

In a comparison of the proportion of exposed cases $(A + B)/N$ versus the proportion of exposed controls $(A + C)/N$, the case-control difference is simply $(B - C)/N$. Thus, information regarding differential exposure to a study factor is revealed by the discordant pairs. McNemar

Table 7.17. Frequency of Exposure
Among N Case-Control Pairs[1]

		Control		
		+	−	Total
Case	+	A	B	$A + B$
	−	C	D	$C + D$
Total		$A + C$	$B + D$	N

1. Exposed (+), non-exposed (−).

(1947) proposed that inference regarding the difference in proportions derived from matched pairs be made solely on the basis of B and C. This conditional form of statistical inference has also been proposed for estimation of the odds ratio. (See Cox 1958, 1970 for the theoretical rationale.) The maximum likelihood estimate of the odds ratio, conditional on the number of discordant pairs $B + C$, is given by (Kraus 1960; also see Cox 1958)

$$\hat{\psi} = B/C. \qquad (7.45)$$

Basing the analysis of a pair-matched study solely on discordant pairs can be further explained intuitively. A study factor can distinguish pair members only if they differ on it. For example, suppose that a case-control study of thromboembolic disease and oral contraceptive use were carried out in three areas: area A, where no women take the pill, area B, where some do and some do not, and area C, where all do. Area B is obviously the only one that can contribute to our knowledge of whether taking oral contraceptives alters the risk of thromboembolic disease, since within areas A and C the cases and controls are perfectly matched on exposure (Pike and Morrow 1970).

Interestingly, the Mantel-Haenszel combined estimate of the odds ratio ($\hat{\psi}_{mh}$) computed over the N subgroups defined by the case-control pairs gives precisely the estimate (7.45). To see this, consider each pair as a subgroup with a corresponding 2×2 table, as in Table 7.5. In this situation, the frequencies a_i, b_i, c_i, and d_i can only take the values 1 or 0, and $n_i = 2$. A simple check on the computation of $\hat{\psi}_{mh}$ from equation (7.18) shows that $\hat{\psi}_{mh} = B/C$ (Mantel and Haenszel 1959). The consideration of each pair as a separate subgroup has a useful application to the logistic analysis of paired data (Chapter 8), and to the analysis of matched studies with multiple or variable numbers of controls per case (Sections 7.7, 7.8).

Throughout the remainder of this section, computational examples are

Table 7.18. Frequency of Exposure to Oral Conjugated Estrogens among 183 Cases of Endometrial Cancer and their Matched Controls[1]

		Control		
		+	−	Total
Cancer	+	12	43	55
	−	7	121	128
	Total	19	164	183

1. Exposed (+), non-exposed (−).

based on a subset of data from a case-control study of oral conjugated estrogens and endometrial cancer (Antunes et al. 1979). This is the same set of data (Table 7.2) that was used in Section 7.1 as an example of analysis for an unmatched case-control study. Now we account for the fact that cases and controls were matched on age, race, date of admission, and hospital of admission. Table 7.18 shows the frequency of exposure to oral conjugated estrogens (ever-use) among cases and their matched controls. Note that the marginal totals in the paired table correspond to the cell values in the unpaired table (Table 7.2).

From the paired data in Table 7.18, the odds ratio is estimated from equation (7.45) as $\hat{\psi} = 6.14$ (43/7). This differs considerably from the estimate based on an unmatched analysis of the same data, $\hat{\psi} = 3.71$ (Section 7.1). The estimate of the odds ratio that ignores the matching is biased toward unity. This occurs because age and race are confounders, both being related to the risk of an MI and to the use of oral contraceptives. (Chapter 4 indicates that ignoring the matching on a variable that is related to exposure results in an odds ratio estimate that is biased toward unity.)

Approximate Tests of Significance and Confidence Intervals

Among the exposure-discordant pairs, the probability of an exposed case is *estimated* by $\hat{p} = B/(B + C)$. The underlying *parameter* p, representing the conditional probability of an exposed case occurring among the exposure-discordant pairs, may be expressed in terms of the odds ratio ψ as

$$p = \psi/(1 + \psi) \qquad (7.46)$$

(Cox 1958, 1970).

The normal approximation to the binomial distribution provides a basis for approximate tests of significance using the chi-square distribution. A two-sided test of the null hypothesis $H_0: \psi = \psi_0$ against the alternative $H_A: \psi \neq \psi_0$ may be calculated as follows. Let $p_0 = \psi_0/(1 + \psi_0)$, $\hat{p} = B/(B + C)$ and

$$n = B + C.$$

Then the statistic

$$\chi^2 = n[\ |\hat{p} - p_0| - 1/(2n)]^2/[p_0(1 - p_0)] \qquad (7.47)$$

provides a continuity corrected chi-square test with one degree of freedom. For the special case of testing the null hypothesis that the odds ratio is unity $H_0: \psi = 1$, equation (7.47) reduces to McNemar's (1947) test,

$$\chi^2 = (\ |B - C| - 1)^2/(B + C). \qquad (7.48)$$

One sided tests of significance may be based on the approximate normal deviate $z = \pm \sqrt{\chi^2}$.

An approximate confidence interval for ψ can be based on equation (7.47). One first calculates confidence limits for p, from which limits for ψ are determined from equation (7.46). Let χ_α^2 be the point of the chi-square distribution with one degree of freedom that is exceeded with probability α. [The value of χ_α^2 may be determined from the normal tables by using the relationship $\chi_\alpha^2 = (z_\alpha)^2$, where z_α is the point of the normal distribution that is exceeded with probability $\alpha/2$. Thus, for $\alpha = .05$, $\chi_\alpha^2 = (1.96)^2 = 3.84$.] Approximate lower and upper $1 - \alpha$ confidence limits for p, denoted by p_L and p_U respectively, are given by the roots of the following equation

$$(\ |np - B| - 1)^2 = np(1 - p)\,\chi_\alpha^2\,, \qquad (7.49)$$

where $n = B + C$ (Johnson and Kotz 1969, p. 60). The two solutions to equation (7.49) are calculated as follows. Let

$$a = n[n + \chi_\alpha^2], \quad b = n[2(B + 1) + \chi_\alpha^2], \quad c = (B + 1)^2,$$
$$d = n[2(B - 1) + \chi_\alpha^2], \quad e = (B - 1)^2.$$

Then

$$p_U = [b + (b^2 - 4ac)^{1/2}]/2a \qquad (7.50)$$
$$p_L = [d - (d^2 - 4ae)^{1/2}]/2a.$$

Confidence limits for ψ are determined by applying the inverse transformation $\psi = p/(1 - p)$ to the limits for p. Lower and upper $1 - \alpha$ confidence limits for ψ are thus given by

$$\psi_L = p_L/(1 - p_L)$$
$$\psi_U = p_U/(1 - p_U). \qquad (7.51)$$

As an application of the preceding methods, consider again the data in Table 7.18. A test of whether the estimated odds ratio ($\hat{\psi} = 43/7$) differs significantly from unity is calculated from (7.48) as $\chi^2 = (\,|43 - 7| - 1)^2/50 = 24.5$, ($p < .0001$, two-sided). Approximate 95 percent confidence limits for ψ are determined from (7.50) and (7.51) as follows: $n = 50$, $B = 43$ and $\chi^2_{.05} = 3.84$. Thus $a = 2692$, $b = 4592$, $c = 1936$, $d = 4392$ and $e = 1764$. Using (7.50), one calculates $p_L = 0.7149$ and $p_U = 0.9438$. From (7.51) an approximate 95 percent confidence interval for ψ is (2.51, 16.79). The transformation $\psi = p/(1 - p)$ is sensitive to small changes in p for values of p near 0 or 1. Thus one should take care to minimize rounding errors in the calculations.

For large values of B and C, an approximate confidence interval for ψ can be calculated from a matched study in the following way. First, the variance of $\ln \hat{\psi}$ may be estimated as

$$\text{var}(\ln \hat{\psi}) \simeq 1/B + 1/C.$$

Approximate $1 - \alpha$ confidence limits for $\ln \psi$ are thus given by

$$\ln(B/C) \pm z_\alpha \sqrt{1/B + 1/C}.$$

Taking exponentials of the limits for $\ln \psi$, one may directly calculate the approximate $1 - \alpha$ confidence limits for ψ as

$$(B/C) \exp[\pm z_\alpha \sqrt{1/B + 1/C}].$$

Exact Tests and Confidence Intervals

Conditional on the total number of discordant pairs, $n = B + C$, the distribution of B is binomial with parameter $p = \psi/(1 + \psi)$. The exact p-value for a one-sided test of $H_0: \psi = \psi_0$ against $H_A: \psi > \psi_0$ is therefore given by

$$\alpha_1 = \sum_{x=B}^{n} \binom{n}{x} p_0^x (1 - p_0)^{n-x},$$

where $p_0 = \psi_0/(1 + \psi_0)$. For $\psi_0 = 1$, $p_0 = \frac{1}{2}$. The exact p-value for a one-sided test of $H_0: \psi = \psi_0$ against $H_A: \psi < \psi_0$ is given by

$$\alpha_2 = \sum_{x=0}^{B} \binom{n}{x} p_0^x (1 - p_0)^{n-x}.$$

Exact confidence limits for p are similarly based on standard procedures for the binomial distribution (Johnson and Kotz 1969, pp. 58–61). Charts of 95 percent and

Table 7.19 Sex and Age of Case-Control Pairs

A. *Three Case-Control Pairs Matched Solely on Age*

Pair	Case	Control
1	M 20[1]	F 20[1]
2	M 30	F 30
3	F 40	M 40

1. M 20 (male, 20 years of age), F 20 (female, 20 years of age).

B. *Ages of Cases and Controls According to Sex*[1]

Male		Female	
Case	Control	Case	Control
20	40	40	20
30			30

1. Pairing in Table 7.19A is broken.

99 percent confidence limits for p are given by Pearson and Hartley (1966). Confidence limits for ψ are derived from limits for p by application of (7.51).

Discussion

Matching controls to cases assures that the members of each pair are comparable with respect to each of the matching variables. The balance obtained by matching, however, depends on the way in which additional unmatched variables are controlled in the analysis. If one stratifies the analysis of a matched study on the basis of an unmatched variable, then one must either (1) break the pairing in order to retain all individuals in the analysis, or (2) use only a subset of the matched pairs in which the pair members are similar on the stratification variables.

For example, suppose that one matched cases and controls only on the basis of age. Then a subsequent comparison of cases and controls that is stratified only by sex would not necessarily be balanced on age. Table 7.19A shows three case-control pairs matched solely on age. (The sex and age of each pair member are shown, but exposure is not indicated.) Stratification by sex alone results in the two tables shown in Table 7.19B. Among males, the cases are younger than the controls, whereas the reverse is true among females. This example shows that to control for unmatched variables by means of stratification, one should also stratify the analysis on the basis of each of the matching variables in order to assure that comparability is maintained for them. In the example of Table 7.19, one should stratify on both age *and* sex in order to allow for further adjustment by sex.

An alternative to stratification for the control of unmatched variables is the use of a statistical model, such as the logistic, which retains the pairing and permits adjustment for variables that were not matched in the study design (Prentice 1976, Holford et al. 1978, Breslow et al. 1978). This latter approach is discussed in Chapter 8.

The usual approach to deriving the estimate of the odds ratio in matched studies assumes that ψ is constant across levels of the matching variables (Cox 1958, 1970; Egijou and McHugh 1977b). This assumption may be checked by comparing the matched estimates of ψ within strata of the matching variables. For example, having matched on sex, one may estimate $\hat{\psi}_i = B_i/C_i$ separately for males and females. In large samples ($B_i + C_i$ large), the variance of $\hat{\psi}_i$ may be estimated by

$$\text{var}(\hat{\psi}_i) \simeq (B_i/C_i)^2 \, (B_i + C_i)/(B_i C_i).$$

Even though the odds ratio may vary across levels of the matching variables, the estimate $\hat{\psi} = B/C$ may be regarded as a summary measure of association. Refer to Kraus (1960) for another approach to this problem.

Although the simplest analysis considers exposure to be dichotomous, it often occurs at various levels: $x_0, x_1, \ldots, x_t$. In this instance, one may directly apply the extended Mantel-Haenszel procedure (Section 7.4) by regarding each pair as a separate stratum. This approach can also be used with a multiple or variable number of controls matched to each case. Pike, Casagrande, and Smith (1975) describe another approach.

7.7 MATCHED ANALYSIS WITH TWO CONTROLS PER CASE

Point Estimation of the Odds Ratio

With two controls matched to each case, the observations may be represented as matched case-control triplets (case, control 1, control 2). There are eight possible outcomes for a triplet when the exposure is dichotomous. Denoting the presence or absence of exposure by + or − respectively, these eight outcomes and their corresponding sample frequencies are shown in Table 7.20. The term n_1, for example, denotes the total number of sample triplets in which the case and the first control are exposed and the second control is not. The ordering of the two controls will be shown to be immaterial to the analysis.

Table 7.20. Sample Frequencies of Eight Possible
Outcomes[1] for Matched Triplets (Case, Control 1, Control 2)

Outcome[2]	Frequency	Outcome[3]	Frequency
$+++$	n_0	$-++$	n_4
$++-$	n_1	$-+-$	n_5
$+-+$	n_2	$--+$	n_6
$+--$	n_3	$---$	n_7

1. Exposed $(+)$, non-exposed $(-)$.
2. Case $(+)$.
3. Case $(-)$.

Table 7.21. Possible 2×2 Tables for a Case-Control Triplet, Ignoring the
Ordering of the Two Matched Controls

	1		2		3	
	Case	Control	Case	Control	Case	Control
Exposure:						
$+$	1	2	1	1	1	0
$-$	0	0	0	1	0	2
$a_i d_i$:		0		1		2
$b_i c_i$:		0		0		0
Freq[1]:		n_0		$n_1 + n_2$		n_3

	4		5		6	
	Case	Control	Case	Control	Case	Control
Exposure:						
$+$	0	2	0	1	0	0
$-$	1	0	1	1	1	2
$a_i d_i$:		0		0		0
$b_i c_i$:		2		1		0
Freq:		n_4		$n_5 + n_6$		n_7

1. Frequency with which table occurs in the sample (from Table 7.20).

Table 7.22. Frequency of Eight Possible Exposure Outcomes
among Case-Control Triplets[1]

Outcome	Frequency	Outcome	Frequency
$+++$	31 (n_0)	$-++$	11 (n_4)
$\left.\begin{array}{l}++- \\ +-+\end{array}\right\}$	42 $(n_1 + n_2)$	$\left.\begin{array}{l}-+- \\ --+\end{array}\right\}$	23 $(n_5 + n_6)$
$+--$	17 (n_3)	$---$	12 (n_7)

1. Exposure $(+)$ corresponds to smoking ≥ 20 cigarettes per day. Each
triplet (case, control 1, control 2) consisted of a case of bladder cancer
matched to two controls on the basis of sex and age within 10 years
(Miller et al. 1978).

By regarding each triplet as a separate subgroup, the Mantel-Haenszel estimate of the odds ratio may be written (Miettinen 1970b)

$$\hat{\psi}_{mh} = (n_1 + n_2 + 2n_3)/(2n_4 + n_5 + n_6).$$ (7.52)

Equation (7.52) is derived as follows. By ignoring the ordering of the two matched controls, one may write the resulting six possible 2×2 tables for each triplet as in Table 7.21. Only tables numbered 2 and 3 contribute to the numerator of $\hat{\psi}_{mh}$, which is $\Sigma a_i d_i / T_i$ from (7.18). Summed over all triplets, $\Sigma a_i d_i / T_i = [1(n_1 + n_2) + 2(n_3)]/3$. Only tables numbered 4 and 5 contribute to the denominator of $\hat{\psi}_{mh}$, which is $\Sigma b_i c_i / T_i$. Summed over all triplets, $\Sigma b_i c_i / T_i = [2(n_4) + 1(n_5 + n_6)]/3$. Thus $\hat{\psi}_{mh}$ reduces to (7.52).

Approximate Tests of Significance and Confidence Intervals

The Mantel-Haenszel test of the null hypothesis $H_0 : \psi = 1$ against the two-sided alternative $H_A : \psi \neq 1$ has a particularly simple form when two controls are matched to each case (Pike and Morrow 1970). Let

$$N_1 = [n_1 + n_2 + 2(n_3 - n_4) - (n_5 + n_6)]/3$$

and

$$N_2 = 2[n_1 + n_2 + n_3 + n_4 + n_5 + n_6]/9.$$

Then χ^2_{mh} in equation (7.19) can be written

$$\chi^2_{mh} = (|N_1| - \tfrac{1}{2})^2 / N_2.$$ (7.53)

Under the null hypothesis, χ^2_{mh} has a chi-square distribution with one degree of freedom. Test-based confidence limits calculated from equation (7.44) can be used for an approximate confidence interval for ψ.

Equation (7.53) is derived from (7.19) by the same principles used in the derivation of equation (7.52). Note that only the discordant triplets are used in (7.52) and (7.53). The outcomes $+++$ and $---$ with respective sample frequencies n_0 and n_7 are ignored.

Data from a matched case-control study of various risk factors for human bladder cancer (Miller et al. 1978) will now be used as an example of the preceding techniques. Two controls were matched to each case on the basis of sex and age within ten years. Defining exposure ($+$) to be smoking twenty or more cigarettes per day, Table 7.22 shows the frequencies with which the possible triplet outcomes occurred. The odds ratio is estimated from (7.52) as $\hat{\psi}_{mh} = 1.69 \ (76/45)$. Thus, heavy smoking is estimated to increase the risk of bladder cancer by 70 percent. The chi-square test (7.53) indicates that the estimated odds ratio is significantly elevated: $N_1 = 31/3$, $N_2 = 186/9$, $\chi^2_{mh} = 4.68$ ($p \simeq .03$, two-sided). An approximate 95 percent confidence interval for ψ is estimated from (7.44) to be $\exp[(1 \pm 1.96/\sqrt{4.68}) \ln 1.69] = (1.05, 2.72)$.

Taube and Hedman (1969) have derived a minimum chi-square estimate of ψ and a chi-square test of significance for matched studies with multiple controls per case. Miettinen (1970b) has given an estimate based on conditional maximum likelihood, as well as alternative procedures for calculating exact and approximate tests of significance and confidence intervals.

7.8 MATCHED ANALYSIS WITH THREE OR MORE CONTROLS PER CASE

c Controls per Case

The Mantel-Haenszel procedure for obtaining a point estimate of the odds ratio and a test of significance may be directly applied to matched case-control studies with c (≥ 3) controls per case. As in applications to $1:1$ and $1:2$ matching, each case and its corresponding set of matched controls is regarded as a separate subgroup with a 2×2 table indicating the number of exposed $(+)$ controls and whether or not the case is exposed $(+)$.

Let $n_j(+)$ denote the number of matched sets in which the case is $(+)$ and exactly j of the controls are $(+)$. Similarly, let $n_j(-)$ denote the number of matched sets in which the case is $(-)$ and exactly j of the controls are $(+)$. By a direct extension of the method used for determining the Mantel-Haenszel estimate with two matched controls per case, detailed in Section 7.7, the corresponding estimate with c matched controls per case is given by (Miettinen 1970b)

$$\hat{\psi}_{mh} = \sum_{j=0}^{c} (c - j)n_j(+) / \sum_{j=0}^{c} jn_j(-). \qquad (7.54)$$

Equation (7.54) shows that only discordant matched sets are used to estimate the odds ratio.

With c controls matched to each case, the Mantel-Haenszel test (7.19) of the null hypothesis $H_0:\psi = 1$ may be calculated as follows. Let

$$m_j = n_{j-1}(+) + n_j(-) \qquad (7.55)$$

denote the number of matched sets with exactly j persons $(+)$, where

$n_{-1}(+) = 0$. Then one can show that the terms in χ^2_{mh} in (7.19) may be expressed as (Pike and Morrow 1970)

$$\sum a_i = \sum_{j=0}^{c-1} n_j(+) = T_1$$

$$\sum E(a_i) = \sum_{j=0}^{c} jm_j/(c + 1) = T_2$$

$$\sum V(a_i) = \sum_{j=0}^{c} j(c + 1 - j)m_j/(c + 1)^2 = T_3.$$

Thus

$$\chi^2_{mh} = (|T_1 - T_2| - \tfrac{1}{2})^2/T_3 \qquad (7.56)$$

provides a test of $H_0: \psi = 1$ which is approximately distributed as chi-square with one degree of freedom under H_0. Test-based confidence limits calculated from equation (7.44) can be used for an approximate confidence interval for ψ.

A case-control study of risk factors for vaginal cancer in young women, conducted by Herbst et al. (1971), used four matched controls per case. Table 7.23A reports the occurrence of "any prior pregnancy loss" among mothers of the cases and the matched controls. Table 7.23B reports the frequencies $n_j(+)$ and $n_j(-)$ based on the matched sets, and displays the computations for the matched analysis. For example, $n_0(+) = 3$ indicates that in three matched sets, the case's mother experienced a prior pregnancy loss, whereas none of the control mothers did; $n_1(-) = 2$ indicates that in 2 matched sets, the case's mother had no prior pregnancy loss, but 1 of the 4 matched control mothers did. From (7.54) the estimated odds ratio is $\hat{\psi}_{mh} = 10.5$. The chi-square test for association (7.56) gives $\chi^2_{mh} = 7.16$ ($p \simeq .0074$, two-sided), indicating that $\hat{\psi}_{mh}$ is significantly greater than unity. An approximate 95 percent confidence interval for ψ is (1.88, 58.8), using (7.44). Thus, prior pregnancy loss in the mother and adenocarcinoma of the vagina in the daughter are significantly associated. [Prior pregnancy loss consistently led to the administration of diethylstilbestrol (DES), which in turn was identified as the likely causative agent.]

Variable Number of Controls per Case

The Mantel-Haenszel procedure and test-based confidence limits may be applied directly to matched data with a variable number of controls per case. In fact, this approach is also applicable to frequency matching, in

Table 7.23. Frequency of Any Prior Pregnancy Loss among Mothers of Daughters with Vaginal Cancer and Mothers of Matched Controls[1]

A. *Prior Pregnancy Loss in Mothers of Cases and Matched Controls*[1]

Case No.	Case	Controls
1	Yes	1/4
2	Yes	1/4
3	No	1/4
4	Yes	0/4
5	No	1/4
6	Yes	0/4
7	Yes	1/4
8	Yes	0/4

B. *Computations for Matched Analysis* $(c = 4)$

j	$n_j(+)$	$n_j(-)$	m_j	$(c - j)n_j(+)$	$jn_j(-)$	jm_j	$j(c + 1 - j)m_j$
0	3	0	0	12	0	0	0
1	3	2	5	9	2	5	20
2	0	0	3	0	0	6	18
3	0	0	0	0	0	0	0
4		0	0	0	0	0	0
Total	6			21	2	11	38

$\hat{\psi}_{mh} = 21/2 = 10.5$ from (7.54)

$\chi^2_{mh} = (|6 - 11/5| - \frac{1}{2})^2/(38/25) = 7.16$ from (7.56)

$\exp[(1 \pm 1.96/\sqrt{7.16}) \ln 10.5] = (1.88, 58.8)$ from (7.44)

1. Four controls matched to each case (Herbst, Ulfelder, and Poskanzer 1971).

which several cases are "matched" to a set of controls. In family studies of genetic diseases, the use of all sibs as controls for index cases will result in a variable matching ratio. Similarly, in studies that plan for a fixed number of controls per case, the occurrence of refusals, interim analyses, or insufficient time or resources to obtain a full compliment of controls for each case will also result in variable numbers of controls per case (Walter 1979). In these situations, a matched analysis is performed by regarding each matched set as a separate subgroup with a corresponding 2×2 table indicating the numbers of exposed and unexposed cases and controls. The odds ratio can be estimated by $\hat{\psi}_{mh}$ in equation (7. 18).

Woolf's method, or an analysis based on the exact conditional distribution (7.33), can also be applied to matched analyses with a variable matching ratio. The program by Thomas (1975) calculates maximum likelihood estimates based on the exact conditional distribution, and can be used to perform matched analyses with either fixed or variable numbers of controls per case. Applied to the data in Table 7.23A, the conditional maximum likelihood estimate of the odds ratio is computed to be $\hat{\psi} = 8.80$. A 95 percent confidence interval based on the exact conditional distribution is (1.50, 98.10), and the exact conditional test of $H_0:\psi = 1$ against $H_A:\psi \neq 1$ gives a two-sided p-value of 0.0058. The point estimate and p-value are close to those obtained by the Mantel-Haenszel procedure. The discrepancy in the confidence limits based on the exact test and the test-based method is due partly to the exact distribution giving a conditional coverage probability exceeding 95 percent because of the discreteness of its distribution.

Discussion

In some situations, the number of cases may be limited relative to the number of available controls, so that one might consider pairing several controls to each case in order to increase the precision with which the odds ratio is estimated. Given a fixed number of cases, the efficiency of the Mantel-Haenszel test χ^2_{mh} with c controls matched per case, relative to McNemar's test with one control matched per case, is $E = 2c/(c + 1)$ (Ury 1975). Thus, for $c = 1, 2, 3, 5$ and 10, one has respectively $E = 1.0, 1.33, 1.5. 1.67$ and 1.8. The unit increase in efficiency per unit increase in c declines appreciably for $c \geq 5$. As c becomes infinitely large, E approaches a maximum of 2. Walter (1979) has described maximum likelihood estimation, tests of hypotheses, cost efficiency, power, and sample size considerations for case-control studies with variable numbers of controls per case, thus extending the work of Miettinen (1969, 1970b), Pike and Morrow (1970) and Ury (1975). Assuming that c controls are matched to each case, Ejigou and McHugh (1981) derive a noniterative, asymptotically efficient odds ratio estimate that is based on an unconditional likelihood approach.

In some situations, matched or unmatched analyses of the odds ratio may result in an estimate of ψ that is infinite as a consequence of division by zero. Although one can use the artificial device of adding ½ to the cells of the 2 × 2 table(s) from which the estimate is derived, a better approach is to simply report a lower limit for ψ based on a confidence interval.

Table 7.24 provides an example from a matched case-control study of diethylstilbestrol (DES) and vaginal cancer (Herbst, Ulfelder, and Poskanzer 1971). The Mantel-Haenszel estimate of the odds ratio may be

Table 7.24. Use of Diethylstibestrol During Pregnancy Among Mothers of Daughters with Vaginal Cancer and Mothers of Matched Controls[1]

Case no.	Case	Controls
1	Yes	0/4
2	Yes	0/4
3	Yes	0/4
4	Yes	0/4
5	No	0/4
6	Yes	0/4
7	Yes	0/4
8	Yes	0/4

$\hat{\psi}_{mh} = 28/0$
$\chi^2_{mh} = 23.2$ ($p \simeq .7 \times 10^{-6}$, one sided)

1. Four controls matched to each case (Herbst, Ulfelder, and Poskanzer 1971).

directly calculated from equation (7.18), or equivalently from (7.54). In either case, one has a matched estimate of $\hat{\psi} = 28/0$. Tests of significance and confidence limits based on the exact conditional distribution (7.33) are computed for the matched data by regarding each matched set as a separate subgroup and using the program of Thomas (1975). A one-sided lower 95 percent confidence limit is $7.49 < \psi$. Thus, loosely speaking, one is "95 percent certain" that the relative risk of vaginal cancer associated with the maternal use of DES during pregnancy exceeds 7.5. A one-sided p-value based on the exact test is $p \simeq 1.3 \times 10^{-5}$. The corresponding Mantel-Haenszel test (7.19) or (7.56) gives $\chi^2_{mh} = 23.2$ ($p \simeq .7 \times 10^{-6}$, one-sided). For practical purposes, the tests are equivalent, and indicate a significantly elevated risk.

7.9 ESTIMATION OF THE ETIOLOGIC FRACTION

Unmatched Case-Control Study with Dichotomous Exposure

The *etiologic fraction,* representing the proportion of all cases in the target population that are attributable to exposure, may be estimated from a case-control study, provided that the exposure rate in the control group can be regarded as approximately representative of the target population.

In Chapter 2, the etiologic fraction, denoted by λ (lamda), was shown to be equal to

$$\lambda = p_e(R - 1)/[p_e(R - 1) + 1],$$

where R is the relative risk, and p_e is the proportion of exposed individuals in the target population. Suppose that one estimates p_e by the proportion of exposed controls and uses the odds ratio as an approximation to the relative risk (Chapter 2). Then the etiologic fraction may be estimated from an unmatched case-control study of a dichotomous exposure as

$$\hat{\lambda} = \hat{p}_e(\hat{\psi} - 1)/[\hat{p}_e(\hat{\psi} - 1) + 1], \tag{7.57}$$

where $\hat{\psi} = ad/bc$ and $\hat{p}_e = b/n_2$ from Table 7.1. Equation (7.57) may be expressed in the equivalent form as

$$\hat{\lambda} = 1 - (cn_2/dn_1). \tag{7.58}$$

Approximate confidence limits for λ may be determined from the asymptotic normal approximation to the distribution of $\ln(1 - \hat{\lambda})$. Estimating the variance of $\ln(1 - \hat{\lambda})$ by

$$\hat{V} = a/cn_1 + b/dn_2, \tag{7.59}$$

an approximate $1 - \alpha$ confidence interval (λ_L, λ_U) for λ is calculated from (Walter 1975)

$$\begin{aligned}\lambda_L &= 1 - (1 - \hat{\lambda}) \exp(+z_\alpha \sqrt{\hat{V}}) \\ \lambda_U &= 1 - (1 - \hat{\lambda}) \exp(-z_\alpha \sqrt{\hat{V}}).\end{aligned} \tag{7.60}$$

To avoid problems arising from zero values of c or d, one may alternatively estimate λ by (Walter 1975)

$$\hat{\lambda}' = 1 - (c + \tfrac{1}{2})(n_2 + \tfrac{1}{2})/(d + \tfrac{1}{2})(n_1 + \tfrac{1}{2}). \tag{7.61}$$

As an estimate of the variance of $\ln(1 - \hat{\lambda}')$ one may use (Walter 1976)

$$\hat{V}' = a/(c + 1)n_1 + b/(d + 1)n_2. \tag{7.62}$$

A confidence interval for λ may then be calculated from (7.60), replacing $\hat{\lambda}$ and $\hat{V}$ by $\hat{\lambda}'$ and $\hat{V}'$ respectively.

As an example of the preceding analysis, consider data on the association between estrogen use and endometrial cancer shown in Table 7.2. One calculates $\hat{\lambda} = 1 - (128)(183)/(164)(183) = .22$ from (7.58). An approximate 95 percent confidence interval for λ is calculated as follows. From (7.59), one has $\hat{V} = .002981$. Thus, with $z_{.05} = 1.96$, expression

(7.60) gives the interval (.132, .299). Ignoring the fact that these data are from a matched study, one estimates that approximately 22 percent of endometrial cancer would be eliminated by the removal of exogenous estrogens. Lower and upper 95 percent confidence limits on this point estimate are 13.2 percent and 29.9 percent respectively. (The analysis of matched studies will be discussed under the topic of adjustment for confounding.)

An alternative approach (Walter 1978) to setting confidence limits estimates the variance of $\hat{\lambda}$ directly:

$$\text{var}(\hat{\lambda}) \simeq (cn_2/dn_1)^2(a/cn_1 + b/dn_2). \tag{7.63}$$

Approximate confidence limits for λ are thus given by

$$\hat{\lambda} \pm z_\alpha \sqrt{\text{var}(\hat{\lambda})}. \tag{7.64}$$

Leung and Kupper (1981) give a related method.

From the data in Table 7.2, one calculates $\text{var}(\hat{\lambda}) = .001816$ using (7.63). Thus an approximate 95 percent confidence interval for λ is estimated from (7.64) as $.22 \pm 1.96\sqrt{.001816} = (.136, .304)$.

Multiple Exposure Levels

An exposure often occurs at various levels. For instance, a drug may be given at several strengths, and the duration of use may vary considerably among users. One can extend the concept of etiologic fraction to represent the proportion of cases in the target population that are attributable to exposure at a given level.

Suppose that cases and controls from an unmatched study are classified by various levels of exposure, as in Table 7.14. If one takes level x_0 as the reference category, an estimate of the etiologic fraction at level x_i ($i = 1, 2, \ldots, t$) is given by (Miettinen 1974a, Walter 1976)

$$\hat{\lambda}_i = (a_ib_0 - b_ia_0)/(n_1b_0). \tag{7.65}$$

The term $\hat{\lambda}_i$ estimates the fraction of all cases in the target population that are attributable to exposure at level x_i.

By summing the etiologic fractions $\hat{\lambda}_i$ over the exposure levels x_1 to x_t, one obtains the estimate $\hat{\lambda}$ in (7.58) corresponding to a dichotomous exposure, "exposed" (levels x_1 to x_t) vs. "unexposed" (level x_0):

$$\sum_{i=1}^{t} \hat{\lambda}_i = \hat{\lambda}. \tag{7.66}$$

If one therefore defines

$$\hat{\lambda}_0 = 1 - \sum_{i=1}^{t} \hat{\lambda}_i , \qquad (7.67)$$

then $\hat{\lambda}_0$ estimates the proportion of cases attributable to all other factors, whatever they may be. The estimates $\hat{\lambda}_i$ depend on the choice of the reference level. If x_0 does not correspond to "unexposed," then the preceding interpretations of $\hat{\lambda}_i$ must be accordingly altered.

Confidence limits and tests of significance for each $\hat{\lambda}_i$ may be based on the following approximation to the asymptotic variance (n_1 and n_2 large) of $\hat{\lambda}_i$ (Denman and Schlesselman 1981):

$$\text{var}(\hat{\lambda}_i) \simeq \frac{1}{n_1} \left[\frac{a_i(n_1 - a_i)}{n_1^2} + \frac{a_0(n_1 - a_0)}{n_1^2} \left\{ \frac{b_i^2}{b_0^3} + \frac{b_i}{b_0^2} + \frac{b_i^2}{b_0^2} \right\} \right.$$
$$\left. + \frac{a_0^2}{n_1} \left\{ \frac{b_i^2}{b_0^3} + \frac{b_i}{b_0^2} \right\} + 2 \frac{a_i a_0}{n_1^2} \frac{b_i}{b_0} \right]. \qquad (7.68)$$

An approximate $1 - \alpha$ confidence interval for $\hat{\lambda}_i$ is given by $\hat{\lambda}_i \pm z_\alpha [\text{var}(\hat{\lambda}_i)]^{1/2}$. An approximate chi-square test (1 d.f.) of $H_0 : \lambda_i = 0$ is calculated from $\chi^2 = (\hat{\lambda}_i)^2 / \text{var}(\hat{\lambda}_i)$.

As an example, refer to Table 7.16 and consider the association between cigarette smoking and myocardial infarction (MI) within the subgroup of women 35 to 39 years of age. There are three levels of cigarette smoking. Using "none" as the reference level, one estimates from (7.65) the following etiologic fractions:

$$\hat{\lambda}_1 = [12(161) - 130(3)]/[37(161)] = 0.259$$
$$\hat{\lambda}_2 = [22(161) - 65(3)]/[37(161)] = 0.562.$$

Thus, in women aged 35–39 years, an estimated 25.9 percent of the cases of MI are attributable to smoking 1–24 cigarettes per day, and 56.2 percent are attributable to smoking 25 or more cigarettes per day. Since an estimated 82.1 percent of the cases of MI are attributable to smoking cigarettes, 17.9 percent are apparently attributable to other factors ($\hat{\lambda}_1 + \hat{\lambda}_2 = .821$ and $\hat{\lambda}_0 = 1 - .821 = .179$).

Using equation (7.68), one estimates the variance of $\hat{\lambda}_1$ and $\hat{\lambda}_2$ respectively as $\text{var}(\hat{\lambda}_1) \simeq .008461$ and $\text{var}(\hat{\lambda}_2) \simeq .007925$. Thus, approximate 95 percent confidence intervals for λ_1 and λ_2 are (.079, .439) and (.387, .737) respectively.

Adjustment for Confounding

To adjust for confounding, one may stratify cases and controls on the basis of one or more confounders. If the exposure under study occurs at various levels, then within each stratum one will have a distribution of cases and controls as in Table 7.14. With matched studies, one may disregard the pairing and stratify cases and controls into subgroups on the basis of the matching variables. Further stratification by unmatched variables can also be done. Thus our discussion is applicable to matched or unmatched studies.

To indicate that the values of a_i and b_i in Table 7.14 vary across the strata, we use a double subscript. The terms a_{ij} and b_{ij} shall denote respectively the numbers of cases and controls in the jth stratum at exposure level x_i. The terms n_{1j} and n_{2j} shall denote the corresponding total numbers of cases and controls within the jth stratum. From equation (7.63), the estimated proportion of cases within the jth stratum that are attributable to exposure at level x_i is given by (Walter 1976)

$$\hat{\lambda}_{ij} = (a_{ij}b_{0j} - b_{ij}a_{0j})/(n_{1j}b_{0j}). \qquad (7.69)$$

Suppose that exposure level x_0 represents "no exposure." Then

$$\sum_{i=1}^{t} \hat{\lambda}_{ij} = \hat{\lambda}_{+j} \qquad (7.70)$$

estimates the fraction of cases within the jth stratum attributable to exposure at any level x_1 to x_t. By taking a weighted average of the $\hat{\lambda}_{+j}$ across strata, one obtains a standardized estimate of the overall proportion of cases that are attributable to exposure at any level. For this purpose, suppose that cases are selected at random, so that the expected number occurring in each stratum is proportional to the corresponding stratum-specific number of cases in the target population. A standardized estimate of the etiologic fraction is then given by the weighted average

$$\hat{\lambda}_s = \sum_j n_{1j} \hat{\lambda}_{+j} / \sum_j n_{1j} . \qquad (7.71)$$

The summation on the subscript j is taken over all of the strata. If a stratified sample of cases has been taken, then the weights n_{1j} should be adjusted by the sampling fractions to be proportional to the expected number of cases in the target population. Cochran (1977) discusses the type of adjustment that is needed with stratified sampling.

The quantity $\hat{\lambda}_s$ in (7.71) estimates the overall proportion of cases in

Table 7.25. Estimated Proportion of Cases of Myocardial Infarction Attributable to Smoking at Various Levels, by Age of Woman[1]

| Cig/day | Age-specific etiologic fractions ($\hat{\lambda}_{ij}$) | | | | | Age-Adjusted $\hat{\lambda}_{i.}$ |
	25–29	30–34	35–39	40–44	45–49	
1–24	.034	.286	.259	.173	.281	.239
≥ 25	.602	.714	.562	.487	.266	.429
$\hat{\lambda}_{+j}$	.636	1.000	.821	.660	.547	.668

1. Estimates based on data in Table 7.16.

the target population that are attributable to exposure at any level x_1 to x_t. One may also want to estimate the overall proportion of cases that are attributable to exposure at a specific level, x_i. This is accomplished by taking the weighted average

$$\hat{\lambda}_{i.} = \sum_j n_{1j} \hat{\lambda}_{ij} / \sum_j n_{1j} . \qquad (7.72)$$

By summing the $\hat{\lambda}_{i.}$ over exposure levels x_1 to x_t, one obtains the overall standardized estimate $\hat{\lambda}_s$, in equation (7.71): $\sum_i \hat{\lambda}_{i.} = \hat{\lambda}_s$.

As an example of adjustment for confounding, consider again the data in Table 7.16, which shows the age-specific frequency of cigarette smoking at three levels among female cases of myocardial infarction and among controls. Taking "no smoking" as the reference level, the estimated etiologic fractions of MI attributable to smoking 1–24 cigarettes per day and 25 or more cigarettes per day are shown in Table 7.25 for each of the five age groups. For example, among women 25–29 years of age, an estimated 3.4 percent of the cases of MI are attributable to smoking 1–24 cigarettes per day, and 60.2 percent of the cases are estimated to be attributable to smoking 25 or more cigarettes per day:

$$\hat{\lambda}_{11} = [1(131) - 104(1)]/[6(131)] = .034$$
$$\hat{\lambda}_{21} = [4(131) - 51(1)]/[6(131)] = .602.$$

Among women 25–29 years of age, an estimated 63.6 percent of the cases of MI are attributable to some degree of smoking ($\hat{\lambda}_{+1} = .636$). Overall, an estimated 23.9 percent of cases of MI among women aged 25 to 49 are attributable to smoking 1–24 cigarettes per day:

$$\hat{\lambda}_{1.} = [6(.034) + 21(.286) + 37(.259)$$
$$+ 71(.173) + 99(.281)]/234 = .239$$

Among all cases of MI occuring in women aged 25–49, an estimated 66.8 percent are attributable to some degree of smoking ($\hat{\lambda}_{1.} + \hat{\lambda}_{2.} = .668$).

In view of equation (7.66), confidence limits for $\hat{\lambda}_{+j}$ may be based on methods appropriate for a 2×2 table, in which exposure in the jth stratum is regarded as a dichotomous variable, unexposed (level x_0) and exposed (levels x_1 to x_l). The variance of $\hat{\lambda}_s$, the standardized estimate of the etiologic fraction, follows from

$$\text{var}(\hat{\lambda}_s) = \sum_j n_{1j}^2 \, \text{var}(\hat{\lambda}_{+j}) / \left(\sum_j n_{1j} \right)^2.$$

Similarly, the variance of $\hat{\lambda}_{i.}$ may be determined from

$$\text{var}(\hat{\lambda}_{i.}) = \sum_j n_{1j}^2 \, \text{var}(\hat{\lambda}_{ij}) / \left(\sum_j n_{1j} \right)^2,$$

where $\text{var}(\hat{\lambda}_{ij})$ may be estimated in the jth stratum from equation (7.68).

Discussion

If the study exposure were causal and independent of other causal risk factors, then the etiologic fraction would indicate the reduction in the rate of the study disease that would occur if the exposure were removed. Even though the exposure may be a cause of the disease, however, the estimated etiologic fraction may not accurately reflect the actual change that would result from the elimination of the exposure. First, it may not be possible to alter the level of exposure to one risk factor independently of others. For example, reduction in the incidence of myocardial infarction anticipated by the cessation of cigarette smoking may be partially offset by the weight gains that tend to accompany its discontinuation. Second, an analysis which considers an individual risk factor, but ignores potential confounding or interactions with other major risk factors, can result in a substantially biased estimate of an individual factor's effect (Walter 1980b). Third, a factor may have beneficial as well as harmful effects, so that the full impact of altering exposure should be assessed by considering the spectrum of consequent benefits as well as risks. Cornfield (1969), Miettinen (1974a) and Walter (1976, 1978, 1980b) give further discussion of these and other points. Walter (1976, 1978) has also shown how to estimate the effect of changes in the exposure distribution, and has indicated how one may combine estimates of the etiologic fraction obtained from different studies.

8 Multivariate Analysis

8.0 INTRODUCTION

A case-control study may focus either on a specific factor thought to affect the risk of disease, or attempt to explore the individual and joint effects of a number of variables. Even though a study may emphasize a single factor, one often needs to control or adjust for numerous others. In this circumstance, methods of analysis based on multiple cross-classification become infeasible as the number of variables increases.

Consider, for example, a study of whether the administration of hormones during pregnancy affects the risk of major malformations at birth. Variables relating to the mother that may either confound an association between hormone use and malformations, or that may otherwise alter the estimate of relative risk, include age, parity, ethnicity, relative weight, smoking, alcohol consumption, prior spontaneous abortion, prior low-birthweight infant, bleeding in current or past pregnancy, difficulty in conception, prior treatment for infertility, and socioeconomic status. It is unlikely that all of these variables would need to be included in an analysis. Nonetheless, if only seven were required, a total of 128 subgroups would result from a multiple cross-classification based on a simple dichotomy of each factor. Thus, if one desired only 10 cases and 10 controls per subgroup, a minimum of 1280 cases and 1280 controls would be needed if all of the separate and joint effects of seven dichotomous variables on the risk of disease were to be investigated.

Logistic Model

In the early 1960s, the *logistic model* was proposed for the analysis of the individual and joint effects of a set of variables on the risk of disease

(Cornfield, Gordon, and Smith 1961, Cornfield 1962). The logistic model specifies that the probability of disease depends on a set of variables x_1, $x_2, \ldots, x_p$ in the following way:

$$p_x = p(d = 1 \mid x) \tag{8.1}$$
$$= 1/\{1 + \exp[-(\beta_0 + \beta_1 x_1 + \cdots + \beta_p x_p)]\}.$$

The variable d denotes either the presence ($d = 1$) or absence ($d = 0$) of disease, and x denotes a set of p variables, $x = (x_1, x_2, \ldots, x_p)$. The variables $x_1, \ldots, x_p$ may represent any potential risk factor or confounding variable, functions of them, or interactions of interest. The βs, which will be explained more fully in Section 8.1, are parameters that represent the effects of the xs on the risk (probability) of disease. Although this model is formulated in terms of the analysis of cohort studies, it may be applied directly to the analysis of case-control data. Furthermore, the interpretation of the model parameters is the same for both study designs.

Figure 8.1 shows the general shape of the logistic function, which may be considered as a basic model for dose-response relationships (Cornfield, Gordon, and Smith 1961). The higher the blood pressure (dose), for instance, the greater the incidence of coronary heart disease (response). In addition to simply postulating a logistic dose-response relationship between a set of variables and the probability of disease (Cox 1966, Walker and Duncan 1967), several different assumptions about the variables $x_1, \ldots, x_p$ in diseased and nondiseased individuals have been shown to lead to the logistic model. These include the assumption that the variables are: (1) multivariate normally distributed with equal covariance matrices (Cornfield, Gordon, and Smith 1961); or (2) multivariate independent dichotomous variables (Anderson 1972); or (3) discrete variables following a loglinear model with second and higher-order effects the same in each population (Birch 1963); or (4) a combination of (1) and (3).

Two common alternatives to the logistic model are the *linear regression model*

$$p_x = \beta_0 + \beta_1 x_1 + \ldots + \beta_p x_p$$

and the *probit model*

$$p_x = \frac{1}{\sqrt{2\pi}} \int_{-\infty}^{\beta_0 + \beta_1 x_1 + \cdots + \beta_p x_p} e^{-u^2/2} \, du.$$

The probit model, based on the *probability integral transformation*, has been commonly used to represent dose-response relationships in biologi-

Figure 8.1. General shape of the logistic function; $p = 1/(1 + e^{-x})$.

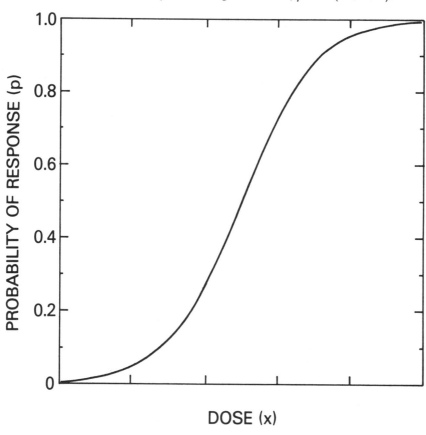

PROBABILITY OF RESPONSE (p)

DOSE (x)

cal assay (Finney 1971). Feldstein (1966) gives details of the application of the linear regression model.

The major objection to the linear regression model is that the parameters have a limited interpretation and range of validity due to the restriction that $0 \le p_x \le 1$. Although a linear function may provide a satisfactory approximation to p_x over a restricted range of x, extrapolation would be suspect, since it is certain that the linear relation will fail outside some range of values of x. Cox (1970, pp. 16–18) discusses these and other important points.

There is no overriding biological rationale for general use of the logistic model, and its widespread application to the analysis of epidemiologic studies can only be supported on grounds of mathematical convenience, much like the extensive use of multiple linear regression analysis in various fields. Preference for the logistic model as opposed to the probit model is based on the existence of simpler computational methods for parameter estimation (Cox 1970, Grizzle 1971). Furthermore, letting $t = \Sigma\beta_i x_i$, the logistic and probit models, regarded as functions of t, agree closely over a wide range (see Cox, 1970, pp. 26–28). Thus, one generally expects that an analysis in terms of either of the two models will give similar results.

Proportional Hazards Model

Cox's (1972) *proportional hazards model* assumes that the risk of disease is a time-dependent function of a set of variables $x_1, \ldots, x_p$, which themselves may change with time. The instantaneous probability of disease occurrence at time (age) t in an individual initially free of disease is represented by

$$\lambda(t \mid x) = \lambda_0(t) \exp[\Sigma\beta_i x_i]$$

where $\lambda_0(t)$ is an unknown function giving the instantaneous risk at $x_i = 0$. Using the terminology of Chapter 2, Section 2.1, the λ terms represent person-time incidence rates. This model, which has wide applications to the analysis of follow-up data, including clinical trials and cohort studies (Breslow 1975, 1978), is also applicable to the analysis of case-control studies (Prentice and Breslow, 1978). Sheehe (1962) discusses an early application of a proportional hazards model to the analysis of pair-matched case-control studies.

Sections 8.1 and 8.2 give a discussion of the algebraic properties of the logistic model and an interpretation of the parameters. This is followed by an explanation of methods for parameter estimation and an application of logistic regression to the analysis of data from a case-control study. The analysis of matched studies and the use of loglinear models are taken up later.

Throughout this chapter, the following properties of the logarithmic function and the exponential function are used repeatedly: (1) $\ln a/b = \ln a - \ln b$; (2) $\ln ab = \ln a + \ln b$; (3) $\exp(a + b) = \exp(a)\exp(b)$; (4) $\exp(-a) = 1/\exp(a)$; (5) $\exp[\ln a] = a$; (6) $\ln[\exp(a)] = a$ (Apostol 1961).

8.1 INTERPRETATION OF LOGISTIC PARAMETERS

Cohort Study

Truett, Cornfield, and Kannel (1967) provide an application of the logistic model (8.1) to a cohort study of 12-year incidence of coronary heart

Table 8.1. Maximum Likelihood Estimates of Logistic Parameters Relating Seven Potential Risk Factors at Initial Examination to the 12-Year Risk of Coronary Heart Disease in Men 40 to 49 Years of Age

Variable	Parameter	Estimate ($\hat{\beta}_i$)	Standard error of $\hat{\beta}_i$	Standardized parameter ($\hat{\beta}'_i$)
x_0 intercept	β_0	−13.2573		
x_1 age (yr)	β_1	.1216	.0437	.3376
x_2 cholesterol (mg/dl)	β_2	.0070	.0025	.3034
x_3 systolic BP (mm Hg)	β_3	.0068	.0060	.1320
x_4 relative weight	β_4	.0257	.0091	.3458
x_5 hemoglobin (g%)	β_5	−.0010	.0098	−.0012
x_6 cigarettes (coded 0, 1, 2, 3)	β_6	.4223	.1031	.4952
x_7 ECG abnormality (coded 0, 1)	β_7	.7206	.4009	.1750

Source: Halperin, Blackwelder, and Verter 1971, Table 2.

disease (CHD) in 2187 men and 2669 women aged 30–62 and found free of coronary disease at first examination. Seven different factors measured at initial exam were studied for their effects on the 12-year incidence of CHD. The variables were:

x_1: age (years)
x_2: serum cholesterol (mg/dl)
x_3: systolic blood pressure (mm Hg)
x_4: relative weight (100 × actual weight ÷ median for sex-height group)
x_5: hemoglobin (g/dl)
x_6: cigarettes per day (coded 0 = never, 1 = less than one pack, 2 = one pack, 3 = more than one pack)
x_7: ECG (coded 0 normal, 1 abnormal)

Table 8.1 gives estimates of the logistic parameters derived from a subset of the data, consisting of 12-year follow-up of 742 men aged 40–49 years at initial exam, 88 of whom developed CHD within the 12-year period. Although the analysis was done separately for men and women within several age strata, age was included as a variable in the logistic model to allow for the coarse grouping on age. Since our immediate objective is the interpretation of the logistic model, we defer discussion of parameter estimation to Section 8.4.

Using the estimated coefficients in Table 8.1, the probability of developing CHD within 12 years of an initial exam for a man aged 40–49 years is thus represented by

$$p_x = 1/\{1 + \exp[-(-13.2573 + 0.1216x_1 + \ldots + 0.7206x_7)]\}.$$

Consider, for example, a man with the following characteristics: age (45), cholesterol (210), systolic blood pressure (130), relative weight (100), hemoglobin (120), cigarette smoking (0), and ECG (0):

$$x = (45, 210, 130, 100, 120, 0, 0).$$

From these values one calculates

$$\hat{\beta}_0 + \hat{\beta}_1 x_1 + \ldots + \hat{\beta}_7 x_7$$
$$= -13.2573 + 0.1216(45) + \ldots + 0.7206(0) = -2.9813$$

and

$$p_x = 1/[1 + \exp(2.9813)] = 0.048.$$

Thus, for every 1000 men with the preceding characteristics, one expects 48 to develop CHD within twelve years.

The effect of each variable x_i included in the risk function may be interpreted in terms of its regression coefficient β_i, which represents the effect of x_i "adjusted" for the effects of the other variables. To directly estimate the effect of a change in one or more variables on the risk of disease, one substitutes their values into equation (8.1). For example, suppose that one wanted to compare the risk of disease for two men who are 45 years of age, with cholesterols of 210 mg/dl, systolic blood pressures of 130 mm Hg, relative weights of 100, hemoglobins of 120 percent and normal ECG, the only difference between the two being that one was a nonsmoker, $x_6 = 0$, and the other smoked more than one pack of cigarettes per day, $x_6 = 3$. The estimated probability of a coronary event within 12 years for each of the two men is calculated as follows:

$$x = (45, 210, 130, 100, 120, 0, 0) \quad x^* = (45, 210, 130, 100, 120, 3, 0)$$
$$\hat{\beta}_0 + \ldots + \hat{\beta}_7 x_7 = -2.9813 \qquad \hat{\beta}_0 + \ldots + \hat{\beta}_7 x_7^* = -1.7144$$
$$\hat{p}_x = 1/[1 + \exp(2.9813)] \qquad \hat{p}_x = 1/[1 + \exp(1.7144)]$$
$$= 0.0483 \qquad\qquad\qquad = 0.1526$$

Thus, for every 1000 men with characteristics similar to the smoker, 153 are estimated to experience a coronary event within 12 years. An event rate of 48 per thousand is expected among the nonsmokers, so that an excess of 105 coronary events per thousand men per 12 years is estimated to be associated with smoking more than one pack of cigarettes per day among men aged 40–49 years. The 12-year risk of disease for the smoker relative to the risk for the nonsmoker is 3.16 (0.1526/0.0483).

Although the logistic parameters β_i do not have a simple relationship to differences in risk, they can be easily interpreted in terms of odds and odds ratios. From equation (8.1), the odds of disease for an individual with the value $x = (x_1, x_2, \ldots, x_p)$ is seen to be

$$p_x/q_x = \exp(\beta_0 + \beta_1 x_1 + \ldots + \beta_p x_p), \qquad (8.2)$$

where

$$q_x = 1 - p_x = p(d = 0 \mid x). \qquad (8.3)$$

Using algebra, one can show that a unit change in a particular variable x_j, from x_j to $x_j + 1$, multiplies the odds of disease by the factor $\exp(\beta_j)$. A unit change occurring jointly in two variables, x_j and x_k, from x_j to $x_j + 1$ and x_k to $x_k + 1$, is similarly seen to change the odds of disease by the factor $\exp(\beta_j + \beta_k) = \exp(\beta_j) \exp(\beta_k)$.

Returning to the example in Table 8.1, smoking one or more packs of cigarettes per day is estimated to increase the odds of disease, relative to nonsmoking, by the factor $\exp[0.4223(3)] = 3.55$. Since the twelve-year incidence of CHD is low for the reference group, 48 cases per 1000 at risk, the relative odds 3.55 is a close approximation to the relative risk 3.16.

In general, the relative odds of disease for an individual with variable value $x^* = (x_1^*, x_2^*, \ldots, x_p^*)$ as compared with an individual with the value $x = (x_1, x_2, \ldots, x_p)$ is given by the odds ratio:

$$\psi(x^* : x) = \frac{p(d = 1 \mid x^*)\, p(d = 0 \mid x)}{p(d = 0 \mid x^*)\, p(d = 1 \mid x)} = \exp[\Sigma \beta_i (x_i^* - x_i)]. \qquad (8.4)$$

Equation (8.4) derives algebraically from equation (8.2). The odds ratio $\psi(x^* : x)$ depends only on those factors for which two individuals *differ*. That is, if the value $x_j^* = x_j$, then the term $\beta_j(x_j^* - x_j)$ is equal to zero. Thus, if one of the variables, say x_1, represents an exposure of particular interest, the disease-exposure odds ratio for two individuals who are equal on the remaining variables is simply $\psi = \exp[\beta_1(x_1^* - x_1)]$. In particular, if the variable x_1 is coded 1 (present) and 0 (absent), then $\psi = \exp(\beta_1)$. The general formulation of the odds ratio in equation (8.4), however, does not designate any particular variable as the "study exposure," but treats all variables on an equal footing.

Logits

The logistic model (8.1), which relates the log odds *(logits)* to a set of variables, is often expressed directly in terms of logits, $\ln p_x/q_x$. From equation (8.2), one has

$$\ln p_x/q_x = \beta_0 + \beta_1 x_1 + \ldots + \beta_p x_p. \tag{8.5}$$

Equation (8.5) has the familiar form of a multiple linear regression model, and it is appropriate and useful to think in terms of regression when performing a multivariate analysis based on the logistic model. The parameters β_i are called *logistic regression coefficients*. The term "logistic model" is used to refer to either expression (8.1) or (8.5), which are algebraically equivalent. Equation (8.5) is also called a *logit model*. Expressed in terms of logits, a unit change in the variable x_j changes the logit of risk ($\ln p_x/q_x$) by the amount β_j. The logit model (8.5) is a linear function of the variables $x_1, \ldots, x_p$ indicating that the "effect" of x_j does not depend on the values of the other variables. By introducing transformed variables such as $x_1 x_2$ or x_1^2 in equation (8.1) or (8.5), one may allow for logistic interaction and nonlinearity, which is discussed in Section 8.2.

Relative Importance of Variables

In Table 8.1 the coefficient for age $\hat{\beta}_1 = 0.1216$ is larger than the coefficient for cholesterol $\hat{\beta}_2 = 0.0070$. This does not mean that age is a "more important" risk factor for coronary heart disease. One interprets $\hat{\beta}_1$ as indicating that a one-year increase in age is associated with an increase of 0.1216 in the logit of risk, or equivalently, that the odds of disease are increased by 13 percent [exp(0.1216) = 1.13]. To obtain an equivalent effect from serum cholesterol, an increase of 17.4 mg/dl (0.1216/0.0070) is required.

The relative importance of variables may be compared in terms of *standardized coefficients*. The coefficient $\hat{\beta}_i$ may be expressed as a multiple of the standard deviation of x_i in order to obtain a coefficient in "standard units" (Truett, Cornfield, and Kannel 1967),

$$\hat{\beta}_i' = \hat{\beta}_i \sqrt{\mathrm{var}(x_i)}. \tag{8.6}$$

Each standardized coefficient $\hat{\beta}_i'$ measures the change in the logit of risk resulting from a change of one standard deviation in the variable x_i.

Expressed in these terms, age and cholesterol are of equal "importance" for the development of coronary heart disease among men aged 40–49 years, both variables having standardized coefficients approximately equal to 0.3.

If individuals are selected in a way that increases or diminishes the variation in a particular variable x_j, then the standardized coefficient $\hat{\beta}'_j$ will be affected, as well as the assessment of the relative importance of x_j. This caveat applies particularly to matched studies.

A second approach to assessing the relative importance of variables considers the reduction in the logit of risk as an objective. One first estimates the magnitude of the changes $\Delta x_1, \ldots, \Delta x_p$ in each of the p variables that can be effected with a given expenditure of resources. One then ranks the variables in order of the sizes of $\hat{\beta}_i \Delta x_i$, these being the estimated amounts of change that will be produced in the logit of risk (Snedecor and Cochran 1980, pp. 357–358).

A problem with both of the preceding methods is that variables are often correlated, so that a change in one is accompanied by a corresponding change in the others. Thus, the change in the logit of risk estimated to result from a postulated change in any particular variable may be misleading (Box 1966, Snedecor and Cochran 1980, pp. 352–357, Gordon 1972).

8.2 LOGISTIC REGRESSION FOR CASE-CONTROL STUDIES

Although initial applications of the logistic model (8.1) involved the analysis of data from cohort studies, this model can be applied directly to the analysis of data from case-control studies (Anderson 1972, 1973, Mantel 1973, Seigel and Greenhouse 1973b). Only the coefficient β_0 differs in a logistic model based on the cohort as opposed to the case-control sampling scheme. The remaining logistic parameters β_i are unaffected, and their interpretation is identical for both study designs. Mantel (1973) has provided the following rationale.

Suppose that one takes a random sample of cases and controls, with sampling fractions π_1 and π_2 respectively. The possible outcomes for an individual with variable $x = (x_1, \ldots, x_p)$ are: (1) he can develop disease and *be in the sample*, with probability $\pi_1 p_x$; (2) he can develop disease and not be in the sample, with probability $(1 - \pi_1)p_x$; (3) he can remain disease free and *be in the sample*, with probability $\pi_2 q_x$; (4) he can remain disease free and not be in the sample, with probability $(1 - \pi_2)q_x$. Therefore, in the sample of cases and controls, the probability of the outcome $d = 1$ (disease), given the value x, is simply

$$p'_x = \pi_1 p_x / [\pi_1 p_x + \pi_2 q_x].$$

In the sample of cases and controls, the odds of disease associated with the variable x may thus be written

$$p'_x / q'_x = \pi_1 p_x / \pi_2 q_x \qquad (8.7)$$

where

$$q'_x = 1 - p'_x.$$

Using equations (8.7) and (8.5), the log odds of disease in a case-control study is related to the log odds of disease in a cohort study by the following equation:

$$\ln p'_x / q'_x = \ln \pi_1 / \pi_2 + \ln p_x / q_x \qquad (8.8)$$
$$= \beta'_0 + \beta_1 x_1 + \ldots + \beta_p x_p$$

where

$$\beta'_0 = \ln \pi_1 / \pi_2 + \beta_0.$$

The logistic model (8.8) for the case-control study shows the same dependence on the variables $x_1, \ldots, x_p$ as the logistic model (8.5) for the cohort study. This indicates that the joint and individual effects of the variables x_i on the risk of disease, as measured by their coefficients β_i, can be estimated from either the cohort or the case-control design.

A case-control study provides estimates of the logistic parameters β'_0, $\beta_1, \ldots, \beta_p$. Since the parameter β'_0 depends on the sampling fraction ratio π_1 / π_2, the incidence rate p_x, which depends on the parameter β_0, cannot be estimated unless one knows the value of π_1 / π_2, which is not typical of most applications. If one knew π_1 / π_2, however, then the parameter β_0 could be estimated from a case-control study by taking $\hat{\beta}_0 = \hat{\beta}'_0 - \ln(\pi_1 / \pi_2)$.

One application in which the sampling proportions π_1 and π_2 will be known is in a "synthetic retrospective study," which involves a case-control study applied to cohort data. Mantel (1973) describes a situation in which 165 cases of a particular condition arose from a cohort study of 4000 individuals. Logistic regression using maximum likelihood estimation of the parameters β_i was too expensive when all of the subjects were included. Using the analogy that little precision is gained by letting the size of the control group become arbitrarily large when the size of the experimental group must remain fixed, Mantel suggested that analyses be done on all of the cases ($\pi_1 = 1$) and a random sample of the noncases ($\pi_2 = .15$). This approach considerably reduced the computational burden and permitted a more comprehensive analysis than would have been possible on the entire data set.

The term p'_x/q'_x represents, for a given value of x, the odds of disease in the *sample* of cases and controls. Equation (8.7) indicates that this quantity is related to the odds of disease in the target population (p_x/q_x) by the factor π_1/π_2, the case-control sampling ratio (see Chapter 2). In practice π_1/π_2 will be large, since a very small proportion of potential controls are selected for study, whereas a comparatively large proportion of cases are chosen. Upon taking odds ratios, the factor π_1/π_2 cancels. Equivalently, the term β'_0 in equation (8.8) cancels when one considers log odds ratios. Substitution of (8.8) into (8.4) shows that the odds ratio for x^* vs. x, $\psi(x^*:x)$, determined from either a case-control or a cohort study, is equal to

$$\psi(x^*:x) = \exp[\beta_1(x_1^* - x_1) + \ldots + \beta_p(x_p^* - x_p)].$$

Thus, estimates of β_0 or β'_0 are irrelevant for the estimation of odds ratios.

The logistic regression model (8.1) or (8.5) is formulated in terms of a prospective study. It relates the probability of disease developing in a defined period of time to a set of variables representing individuals' characteristics. One might refer to such a model as a logistic "disease incidence" model. The argument of Mantel (1973) provides a heuristic rationale for the direct application of logistic disease incidence models to case-control data. Prentice and Pyke (1979) have given a rigorous mathematical justification, with a discussion of matched designs and multiple disease outcomes. Farewell (1979) gives some efficiency comparisons for estimates of the βs based on conditional and unconditional maximum likelihood estimation.

Nonrepresentative Samples

If one takes random samples of cases and controls, then they are "representative" in the sense that the probability of an individual's being selected for study does not depend on the factors under investigation (see Chapter 2). The preceding section indicates that except for β_0, the estimates of the βs derived from a case-control study, based on a random sample of cases and controls, will agree, apart from sampling variation, with the estimates based on an analysis of the entire population.

Under certain forms of nonrepresentative sampling, the dependence of

In p'_x/q'_x on the variable x can still be the same for the cohort and the case-control designs (Mantel 1973). Suppose that instead of taking a random sample of cases and controls, one sampled in a way that depended on the value of x, with $\pi_1(x)$ and $\pi_2(x)$ denoting respectively the sampling dependence on x among potential cases and controls. If $\pi_1(x)$ and $\pi_2(x)$ factor into $\pi_1 f(x)$ and $\pi_2 f(x)$ respectively, then the common factor $f(x)$ would cancel in equation (8.7), resulting again in the logistic model (8.8). Thus, the case-control method does not require random sampling, but only sampling that is *unbiased* in the sense that the nonrandomness with respect to x should be the same for both cases and controls (also see Chapter 2 and Chapter 5). If a 100 percent sample of cases is taken, however, then the sample of controls should be random with respect to x.

Confounding

Thus far, the variables $x_1, \ldots, x_p$ have been treated on an equal footing. Suppose for the moment that one particular factor, say x_1, coded $x_1 = 1$ for *exposed* and $x_1 = 0$ for *unexposed*, is of primary interest. Let $\mathbf{x}_2 = (x_2, \ldots, x_p)$ denote the remaining variables. The odds ratio estimate of the effect of x_1 for two individuals who are identical on the variable $\mathbf{x}_2$ but differ on x_1 is then given by

$$\psi = \frac{p(d = 1 | x_1 = 1, \mathbf{x}_2) \, p(d = 0 | x_1 = 0, \mathbf{x}_2)}{p(d = 0 | x_1 = 1, \mathbf{x}_2) \, p(d = 1 | x_1 = 0, \mathbf{x}_2)}. \tag{8.9}$$

Substitution of (8.1) in the above expression for ψ gives $\psi = \exp(\beta_1)$.

With respect to the assessment of the effect of x_1, the remaining variables $x_2, \ldots, x_p$ which have nonzero coefficients β_i are *potential confounding variables*. That is, if the exposed individual as compared with the unexposed individual differed on any of the variables $x_2, \ldots, x_p$, then the odds ratio ψ would depend not only on the presence or absence of exposure, but also on the particular values of the variables $x_2, \ldots, x_p$ on which they differed. This can be shown as follows.

Suppose that one wanted to assess the effect of x_1 by calculating the odds ratio for two individuals who differed only on the variable x_1. The correct odds ratio is $\psi = \exp(\beta_1)$. If in fact the individuals also differed on any of the other variables $x_2, \ldots, x_p$, the exposed individual having the values $x_2^*, \ldots, x_p^*$, and the unexposed individual having the values $x_2', \ldots, x_p'$, then the calculated odds ratio would be biased, being

$$\exp[\beta_1 + \beta_2(x_2^* - x_2') + \ldots + \beta_p(x_p^* - x_p')]$$

from equation (8.4). The bias component $\Sigma\beta_i(x_i^* - x_i')$ depends on the regression coefficients β_i and on the magnitude of the individual differences $x_i^* - x_i'$. If either $\beta_i = 0$ or if $x_i^* - x_i' = 0$, then the ith variable does not affect the odds ratio estimate of the effect of x_1. If $\beta_i \neq 0$, then the variable x_i is only *potentially* confounding, since the estimate of ψ is unaffected if $x_i^* = x_i'$. In general, the bias component $\Sigma\beta_i(x_i^* - x_i')$ can be either positive or negative, thereby resulting in an overestimate or an underestimate of the odds ratio.

Estimates of each of the logistic parameters in equation (8.1) are interpreted as being "adjusted" for the effects of the remaining variables in the equation. Thus $\exp(\hat{\beta}_1)$ estimates the odds ratio associated with exposure to x_1 for two individuals who are otherwise comparable on the remaining variables, $x_2, \ldots, x_p$. This interpretation assumes that all of the relevant variables can be related to the risk of disease by an equation such as (8.1).

Multiplicative Model

The logistic model (8.1) implies that the log odds $\ln p_x/q_x$ is a linear function of the variables $x_1, \ldots, x_p$. The linear logistic model (8.1) further implies a *multiplicative model* for odds ratios. To see this, suppose that there are two dichotomous variables of particular interest, x_1 and x_2, coded 0 (absent) and 1 (present). Suppose, furthermore, that one wants to assess the effects of x_1 and x_2 in individuals who have the same values for variables $x_3, \ldots, x_p$. Then from equation (8.4), the relative odds of disease in individuals with values $x_1^*, x_2^*, x_3, \ldots, x_p$ as compared with individuals with values $x_1', x_2', x_3, \ldots, x_p$ is

$$\psi = \exp[\beta_1(x_1^* - x_1') + \beta_2(x_2^* - x_2')].$$

Taking individuals with the values $x_1' = 0$ and $x_2' = 0$ as the reference group, the relative odds of disease associated with the presence of x_1 alone $(x_1^* = 1, x_2^* = 0)$ is $\exp(\beta_1)$; the relative odds of disease associated with the presence of x_2 alone $(x_1^* = 0, x_2^* = 1)$ is $\exp(\beta_2)$ and the relative odds of disease associated with the joint presence of x_1 and x_2 $(x_1^* = 1, x_2^* = 1)$ is $\exp(\beta_1 + \beta_2) = \exp(\beta_1)\exp(\beta_2)$. This shows that the use of the linear logistic model (8.1) or (8.5) implies that odds ratios that represent the individual effects of variables (expressed relative to a common reference group) are *multiplied* to obtain their joint effects.

Logistic Interaction

A generalization of equation (8.1) that allows for a first order interaction between the variable x_1 and *each* of the remaining variables $x_2, \ldots, x_p$ is given by

$$p_x = 1/\{1 + \exp[-(\beta_0 + \beta_1 x_1 + \sum_{i=2}^{p} \beta_i x_i + \sum_{i=2}^{p} \gamma_i (x_1 x_i))]\}. \qquad (8.10)$$

The parameter γ_i represents a statistical interaction between x_1 and the variable x_i. The effect of x_1 now depends on the values of the other variables; rearranging terms in (8.10), the coefficient of x_1 is seen to be $(\beta_1 + \sum_{i=2}^{p} \gamma_i x_i)$.

Suppose that x_1 is a dichotomous variable denoting the presence or absence of exposure. Considering the association between disease and exposure to x_1, the log odds ratio corresponding to the logistic model (8.10) is

$$\ln \psi = \beta_1 + \sum_{i=2}^{p} \gamma_i x_i, \qquad (8.11)$$

by substitution in (8.9). In this context, ψ denotes the relative odds of disease in individuals exposed to x_1 as compared with those who are not exposed to x_1. Variables with nonzero coefficients γ_i may be considered to be *effect modifiers* of the disease-exposure relationship (Prentice 1976), a term Miettinen (1974c) has used in a more general sense to refer to any dependence of the odds ratio on one or more variables. Equation (8.11) shows a specific form of dependence. Expressed directly in terms of the odds ratio, equation (8.11) may be written

$$\psi = \exp(\beta_1 + \sum_{i=2}^{p} \gamma_i x_i). \qquad (8.12)$$

In specifying a model such as (8.10), one may effectively set certain values of the βs or γs equal to zero by simply deleting these terms from the logistic equation to be fitted. From (8.10), one sees that a variable x_j can be a confounder $(\beta_j \neq 0)$ without being an effect modifier $(\gamma_j = 0)$, and vice versa (Fisher and Patil 1974, Miettinen 1974c, Prentice 1976).

An equivalent interpretation of the interaction between x_1 and the other variables in equation (8.10) is that the effect of the variables $x_2, \ldots, x_p$ on the risk of disease differs for those exposed to x_1 versus those not exposed. For example, the effect of x_j among those exposed $(x_1 = 1)$ is given by the coefficient $(\beta_j + \gamma_j)$, whereas the effect of x_j among those not exposed $(x_1 = 0)$ is given by the coefficient β_j.

Equation (8.11) shows a specific form of dependence of the log odds ratio on the variables $x_2, \ldots, x_p$. If a variable x_i is continuous, one may regard γ_i as the *slope* of the regression of $\ln \psi$ on x_i. The specification of an interaction between x_1 and x_i of the form $(x_1 x_i)$ thus implies a linear relationship between $\ln \psi$ and x_i. One may wish to specify alternative forms for the interaction, for example, by introducing additional terms $\delta_i(x_1 x_i^2)$ to allow for nonlinearities in $\ln \psi$. Transformation of variables provides additional flexibility in the logistic model. Thus, for example, if x_2 represents height and x_3 represents weight, one may consider using the *ponderal index* $x_2/\sqrt[3]{x_3}$ as a single variable in the model equation, rather than using two separate variables x_2 and x_3.

8.3 INDICATOR VARIABLES

The logistic model (8.1) implies a linear dependence of the log odds of disease on each of the variables $x_1, \ldots, x_p$. Estimates of the parameters β_i are made under the assumption that the variables in the model equation either have a scale of measurement or that the representation (8.1) makes proper allowance for the lack of one. For example, if x_3 represents age in years, then the logistic model $\ln p_x/q_x = \beta_0 + \beta_3 x_3$ implies that each one-year increase in age is associated with an increase of β_3 in the logit of risk. If one thought that $\ln p_x/q_x$ was not a linear function of age, one might transform the variable x_3, using $\sqrt{x_3}$, for example. Alternatively, one might introduce additional parameters, such as $\beta_3 x_3 + \beta_3' x_3^2$, and so forth.

Discrete variables such as occupation, religion, race, and sex do not have an ordinal scale of measurement. *Indicator* ("dummy") *variables* taking the values 1 or 0 to designate the presence or absence of an attribute must be used to correctly represent the effects of such variables in a logistic regression model. Consider, for example, four variables: x_1, a dichotomous variable coded 1 or 0 for exposure or non-exposure to a specified factor; x_2, a dichotomous variable designating sex, coded 0 (female) and 1 (male); x_3, a continuous variable representing age in years; and x_4, a discrete variable representing race, coded improperly (see below) as 1, 2, 3, and 4 for white, black, Asian, and others, respectively.

With a dichotomous variable such as sex, the indicator variable x_2, coded 0 (female) and 1 (male) is appropriate. The coefficient β_2 in the term $\beta_2 x_2$ may be interpreted as the change in the logit of risk that is associated with a change in the variable x_2 from female to male. Thus, for females, $\beta_2 x_2 = 0$, whereas for males, $\beta_2 x_2 = \beta_2$, so that $\exp(\beta_2)$

represents the relative odds of disease for males as compared with females (assuming no interactions between x_2 and any of the other variables).

With the discrete variable x_4, representing race and having four categories in our example, one needs to use three indicator variables. First, one designates one of the categories as a reference. For each of the other categories of race, one introduces a variable R_j, which is coded 1 (present) or 0 (absent). In general, if a discrete variable has k categories, one needs to use $k - 1$ indicator variables. The coefficient β_j associated with the indicator variable R_j then represents the change in the logit of risk for this category relative to the reference category. Equivalently, $\exp(\beta_j)$ represents the relative odds of disease for individuals of the racial category R_j as compared with individuals of the reference racial category.

With the discrete variable x_4 in our example, use of a term such as $\beta_4 x_4$ in a logistic model would be inappropriate, because it implies that the logit of risk increases from β_4 to $2\beta_4$ to $3\beta_4$ to $4\beta_4$ as the variable x_4 assumes respectively the arbitrary values 1, 2, 3, and 4. In this instance, one needs to recode the data on the variable x_4, introducing three indicator variables. Taking whites as the reference group, for example, one introduces three indicator variables for race: R_1, coded 1 (black) or 0 (not black); R_2, coded 1 (Asian) or 0 (not Asian); R_3, coded 1 if the individual is neither black, white, nor Asian, or 0 otherwise. The variable x_4 is thereby replaced by three indicator variables R_1, R_2, R_3, and the data input for the regression analysis must be recoded to reflect this change. Rather than estimating the parameters of a model such as

$$\ln p_x/q_x = \beta_0 + \beta_1 x_1 + \beta_2 x_2 + \beta_3 x_3 + \beta_4 x_4,$$

one should fit the model

$$\ln p_x/q_x = \beta_0 + \beta_1 x_1 + \beta_2 x_2 + \beta_3 x_3 + \beta_4 R_1 + \beta_5 R_2 + \beta_6 R_3.$$

For an individual who is white ($R_1 = 0$, $R_2 = 0$, $R_3 = 0$), the logit of risk is given by

$$\ln p_x/q_x = \beta_0 + \sum_{i=1}^{3} \beta_i x_i.$$

For an individual who is black ($R_1 = 1$, $R_2 = 0$, $R_3 = 0$), the logit of risk is

$$\ln p_x/q_x = \beta_0 + \sum_{i=1}^{3} \beta_i x_i + \beta_4.$$

Thus β_4 represents the change in $\ln p_x/q_x$ as the variable race changes from white to black, and $\exp(\beta_4)$ represents the relative odds of disease for blacks as compared with whites. Similarly $\exp(\beta_5)$ represents the relative odds of disease for Asians as compared with whites.

As another application of indicator variables, consider a multicenter case-control study conducted in several hospitals. Suppose that there are $m + 1$ hospitals, and that one designates H_0 as the reference. One may introduce the dummy variables $H_1, \ldots, H_m$, where $H_i = 1$ if an individual comes from the ith hospital, and $H_i = 0$ otherwise. One could then fit the model

$$p(d = 1 \mid x, H) = 1/\{1 + \exp[-(\beta_0 + \sum_{j=1}^{m} \alpha_j H_j + \sum_{i=1}^{p} \beta_i x_i)]\}.$$

This model allows the level of risk to vary among hospitals, but assumes that the dependence of risk on the variables $x_1, \ldots, x_p$ is the same for all hospitals. The odds of disease in the ith hospital relative to the odds of disease in the reference hospital is $\exp(\alpha_i)$. The choice of a reference is arbitrary, although for a specific application the decision may be based on substantive grounds.

In situations where cases and controls are matched only approximately, for example, matched on age to within five years, one may consider a stratified analysis as an alternative to a fully paired analysis. Thus, for example, one may form strata by five-year age groups, ignore the pairing, and introduce indicator variables in order to fit the following logistic model

$$p(d = 1 \mid x, j\text{th stratum}) = 1/\{1 + \exp[-(\alpha_j + \sum_{i=1}^{p} \beta_i x_i)]\}. \quad (8.13)$$

The parameter α_j allows the risk of disease to vary among the strata. For example, if one had three age groups (yrs), 30–34, 35–39 and 40–44, one might designate the group 30–34 as the reference and introduce two indicator variables, A_1 and A_2. One would code $A_1 = 1$ if an individual were 35–39 (0 otherwise) and $A_2 = 1$ if an individual were 40–44 (0 otherwise). Corresponding to equation (8.13) one could then write

$$p(d = 1 \mid x, A_1, A_2)$$
$$= 1/\{1 + \exp[-(\alpha_0 + \alpha_1 A_1 + \alpha_2 A_2 + \sum_{i=1}^{p} \beta_i x_i)]\}. \quad (8.14)$$

The relative odds of disease in the age group 35–39 as compared with the group 30–34 is thus $\exp(\alpha_1)$. Similarly, the relative odds of disease in the age group 40–44 as compared with the group 30–34 is $\exp(\alpha_2)$.

The approach of dropping the original pairing and forming strata on the basis of the matching variables assumes that there is some quantitative or qualitative dimension upon which the grouping can be based. The use of siblings or relatives as pair-matched controls for cases, for example, will often preclude this maneuver, although with sibling controls, it is doubtful that one would ever want to ignore the pairing. Sibship is a factor that uniquely distinguishes one pair from others. With other variables such as sex, race, age, or socioeconomic status, matching is essentially arbitrary, in the sense that any two individuals may be paired, provided they are similar on the matching variables.

Indicator variables can also be used to represent nonlinear effects of continuous variables. To do this, one stratifies on the variable in question, taking one of the strata as a reference group and using indicator variables to represent the effect of each of the remaining strata relative to the reference. For example, with individuals ranging in age from 25 to 39 years, one might stratify age into several categories and use indicator variables, rather than assume a linear or quadratic relationship between $\ln p_x/q_x$ and age.

The use of indicator variables to represent the effect of a continuous variable, such as age, requires grouping. In particular, the model (8.14) makes no distinction between individuals who differ in age but fall within the same age group. The relative odds of disease for an individual who is 35 years old (vs. 30–34) are taken to be the same as the relative odds for an individual who is 39 years old, both being equal to $\exp(\alpha_1)$ from (8.14). Thus, in using indicator variables to represent the effect of a continuous variable x_i, one should attempt to construct strata in a way that $\ln p_x/q_x$ does not vary appreciably as a function of x_i within each subgroup.

As in multiple regression, the use of indicator variables is an important technique in the application of logistic regression. The discussion by Draper and Smith (1981, pp. 241–256) and the paper by Suits (1957) should be read for further details. Taken to the extreme of stratifying all of the variables and using indicator variables to represent individual and joint effects, one arrives at an analysis that is equivalent to that based on the loglinear model for categorial data, discussed in Section 8.10.

8.4 ESTIMATION OF LOGISTIC PARAMETERS

The logistic model has been presented thus far without indicating how one estimates the parameters (β_i) from a set of data. In fact, there are two basic approaches: maximum likelihood estimation and discriminant analysis.

Discriminant Analysis

Consider two groups of individuals, one made up of cases and the other of controls. Suppose that one wanted to distinguish between them on the basis of a linear combination of the variables x_i, $y = \Sigma \beta_i x_i$, classifying an individual as a case if $y > y_0$ and as a control if $y \leq y_0$. The linear discriminant function is the linear combination of the x_i, $\Sigma \beta_i x_i$, which minimizes the probability of misclassification (Anderson 1958). Under the assumption that the variables $x_1, \ldots, x_p$ have a multivariate normal distribution with different means for cases and controls, but equal covariance matrices, the coefficients β_i in the logistic model (8.1) can be shown to be equivalent to those of the linear discriminant function (Cornfield 1962, Cornfield, Gordon, and Smith 1961). Thus, linear discriminant analysis has been used as one method for estimating the logistic parameters β_i in equation (8.1). However, maximum likelihood estimation, which is described in the following section, is the preferred approach to estimating the parameters of the logistic model.

Maximum Likelihood Estimation

Suppose that one has a sample of n individuals, and that the jth individual has values $x_{j1}, x_{j2}, \ldots, x_{jp}$ for the variables $x_1, x_2, \ldots, x_p$. Introduce a dummy variable x_0, such that $x_{j0} = 1$ for all individuals, and define

$$y_j = \sum_{i=0}^{p} \beta_i x_{ji}. \tag{8.15}$$

One may then write the logistic model (8.1) as

$$p_j = 1/[1 + \exp(-y_j)]$$
$$= \exp(y_j)/[1 + \exp(y_j)] \tag{8.16}$$

where

$$q_j = 1 - p_j = 1/[1 + \exp(y_j)]. \tag{8.17}$$

The quantity p_j denotes the probability that the jth individual develops disease in a defined interval of time, and q_j denotes the probability that he remains "disease free." Let d_j be a variable that indicates the occurrence ($d_j = 1$) or absence ($d_j = 0$) of disease in the jth individual. Thus, $d_j = 1$ with probability p_j and $d_j = 0$ with probability q_j. Assuming that the occurrence of disease is independent across individuals, the *likelihood* (probability) of the outcome $d_1, d_2, \ldots, d_n$ is given by

$$\prod_{j=1}^{n} p_j^{d_j} \, q_j^{1-d_j} = \prod_{j=1}^{n} \exp(y_j d_j) \Big/ \prod_{j=1}^{n} [1 + \exp(y_j)]. \quad (8.18)$$

The likelihood (8.18) contains the factor p_j when $d_j = 1$ and the factor q_j when $d_j = 0$.

Equation (8.18), regarded as a function of the parameters β_i, is called a *likelihood function. Maximum likelihood estimates* (mle's) of the parameters β_i are values $\hat{\beta}_i$ that maximize (8.18) for the observed sample values of d_j and x_{ji}. The computations require iterative calculations that are best done by computer. The BMDP statistical package (Dixon and Brown 1979) has a stepwise logistic regression routine for maximum likelihood estimation. Another has been written by Hosmer et al. (1978). Our analyses are based on a logistic regression program written by Brown (1980).

When using the BMDP logistic regression program PLR on data sets discussed later in this chapter, all variables such as "OC use" (= 0, 1) or "smoke 1" (= 0, 1) or age (= 27, 32, 37, 42, 47) must be specified as INTERVAL variables in the /REGRESS paragraph in order to obtain parameter estimates that correspond to fitting a logistic regression to variables that assume the values (0, 1) or (27, 32, 37, 42, 47), etc.

The preceding development of the likelihood function (8.18) is appropriate for a cohort study. Prentice and Pyke (1979) give the corresponding derivation for a case-control study, and show that in large samples, the mle's of the β-parameters are equivalent for studies based on either the cohort or the case-control design (also see Pike, Hill, and Smith 1980).

Confidence Intervals and Tests of Significance

Approximate standard errors, confidence intervals, and tests of significance based on maximum likelihood estimation of the logistic parameters are computed as follows. Let $(\hat{c}_{ik})$ denote a $(p + 1) \times (p + 1)$ matrix, the $i-k$-th element of which is defined by

$$\hat{c}_{ik} = \sum_{j=1}^{n} x_{ji} \, x_{jk} \exp(\hat{y}_j) / [1 + \exp(\hat{y}_j)]^2 \quad (8.19)$$

where

$$\hat{y}_j = \sum_{i=0}^{p} \hat{\beta}_i x_{ji}. \quad (8.20)$$

Let $\hat{\sigma}_{ik}$ denote the i-k-th element of the inverse matrix of $(\hat{c}_{ik})$,

$$(\hat{\sigma}_{ik}) = (\hat{c}_{ik})^{-1}. \tag{8.21}$$

The matrix $(\hat{\sigma}_{ik})$ is the estimated covariance matrix of the logistic parameter estimates $\hat{\beta}_0, \hat{\beta}_1, \ldots, \hat{\beta}_p$ (Cox 1970, p. 87).

A large sample estimate of the standard error of $\hat{\beta}_i$ is $\sqrt{\hat{\sigma}_{ii}}$, and an
estimate of the covariance of $\hat{\beta}_i$ and $\hat{\beta}_k$ is $\hat{\sigma}_{ik}$. An approximate $(1 - \alpha)$
confidence interval for β_i is given by

$$\hat{\beta}_i \pm z_\alpha \sqrt{\hat{\sigma}_{ii}} \tag{8.22}$$

where z_α is the value of the unit normal distribution that is exceeded with
probability $\alpha/2$.

Using the logistic model (8.16) as the basis for a statistical analysis of
data from a case-control study, an estimate of the relative odds of disease
in an individual with values $x_1^*, \ldots, x_p^*$ as compared with an individual
with values $x_1, \ldots, x_p$ is given by

$$\hat{\psi}(x^*:x) = \exp\left[\sum_{i=1}^{p} \hat{\beta}_i (x_i^* - x_i) \right]. \tag{8.23}$$

The odds ratio in equation (8.23) does not designate any particular variable as the "study exposure," but treats all variables on an equal footing.

The variance of $\ln \hat{\psi} (x^*:x)$ is estimated by

$$\hat{V} = \sum_{i=1}^{p} \hat{\sigma}_{ii}(x_i^* - x_i)^2 + \sum\sum_{i \neq j} \hat{\sigma}_{ij}(x_i^* - x_i)(x_j^* - x_j). \tag{8.24}$$

An approximate $(1 - \alpha)$ confidence interval for the odds ratio $\psi(x^*:x)$
is thus given by

$$\exp[\ln \hat{\psi}(x^*:x) \pm z_\alpha \sqrt{\hat{V}}]. \tag{8.25}$$

In particular, if the variable values x^* and x are identical, except for a
single factor, say $x_i^* \neq x_i$, then the relative odds for an individual with
the value x_i^* as compared with an individual with the value x_i is estimated simply as

$$\hat{\psi}_i = \exp[\hat{\beta}_i(x_i^* - x_i)]. \tag{8.26}$$

The corresponding approximate $(1 - \alpha)$ confidence interval for ψ_i based
on equation (8.25) reduces to

$$\exp[\hat{\beta}_i(x_i^* - x_i) \pm z_\alpha \sqrt{\hat{\sigma}_{ii} (x_i^* - x_i)^2}]. \tag{8.27}$$

If x_i is a dichotomous variable, coded 1 (exposed) and 0 (unexposed), then the relative odds of disease associated with exposure to x_i is estimated from equation (8.26) as

$$\hat{\psi}_i = \exp(\hat{\beta}_i).   \qquad (8.28)$$

An approximate $(1 - \alpha)$ confidence interval for ψ_i based on (8.27) reduces to

$$\exp[\hat{\beta}_i \pm z_\alpha \sqrt{\hat{\sigma}_{ii}}].   \qquad (8.29)$$

Likelihood Ratio Test

The logarithm of the likelihood function (8.18) may be written

$$L(\beta) = \sum_{i=0}^{p} \beta_i T_i - \sum_{j=1}^{n} \ln\left[1 + \exp\left(\sum_{i=0}^{p} \beta_i x_{ji}\right)\right] \qquad (8.30)$$

where

$$T_i = \sum_{j=1}^{n} x_{ji} d_j.$$

The likelihood ratio can be used to test the hypothesis that a specified subset of the variables $x_1, \ldots, x_p$ have regression coefficients that are equal to zero. For this purpose, let $\hat{\beta}$ denote the estimates of the logistic parameters in the model (8.1) with the full complement of variables. Let $\hat{\beta}^*$ be the parameter estimates for those variables remaining in the model when q variables have been deleted. A test of the hypothesis that the coefficients β_i corresponding to the q omitted variables are equal to zero may be based on the statistic

$$\chi_q^2 = 2[L(\hat{\beta}) - L(\hat{\beta}^*)].   \qquad (8.31)$$

If the hypothesis is true, then in large samples χ_q^2 has a chi-square distribution with q degrees of freedom. Large values of χ_q^2 indicate that one or more of the q omitted variables has a nonzero regression coefficient, thereby suggesting that one or more of the omitted variables is significantly associated with the risk of disease.

The likelihood ratio test (8.31) provides an alternative method of finding an approximate confidence interval for any particular parameter β_j, and can also be used to compute a joint confidence region for a set of parameters (see Cox 1970, p. 88).

The statistic (8.31) may be used as a one degree of freedom chi-square test of whether a particular variable, say x_p, shows a significant association with the risk of disease in the presence of the remaining variables, $x_1, \ldots, x_{p-1}$. An exact test of $\beta_p = 0$, conditional on $T_1, T_2, \ldots, T_{p-1}$, has been given by Cox (1970 pp. 46–48). Bayer and Cox (1979) have published a program that performs the computations.

Considering logistic models applicable to unmatched, matched, or stratified case-control studies, Day and Byar (1979) show that score statistics (Cox and Hinkley 1974, pp. 314–315) based on the likelihood function are identical to the Mantel-Haenszel test and its extensions (Mantel and Haenszel 1959, Mantel 1963). These results establish the asymptotic optimality of the Mantel-Haenszel approach and provide an alternative method for significance testing based on likelihood theory. The approach is expected to be more appropriate in small samples than tests based on the large sample distribution of the unconditional likelihood ratio test.

Maximum Likelihood vs. Discriminant Estimates of Logistic Parameters

Maximum likelihood estimates (mle's) of the logistic parameters are based on the *ad hoc* assumption that the logistic model (8.1) correctly describes the relationship between the variables $x_1, \ldots, x_p$ and the probability of disease (Cox 1966, Walker and Duncan 1967). If the variables $x_1, \ldots, x_p$ have a multivariate normal distribution with equal covariance matrices for the cases and controls, then the mle's are between one-half and two-thirds as efficient as the estimates based on discriminant analysis (Efron 1975). This result also applies to the less restrictive assumption that the linear function $y = \Sigma \beta_i x_i$ has a univariate normal distribution.

As a general estimation procedure, maximum likelihood is preferable to discriminant analysis, however, since it does not depend on any a priori assumption of multivariate normality. If the normality assumption is not correct, which is true of most applications, then the discriminant function estimates can result, even in large samples, in estimated coefficients $\hat{\beta}_i$ that are incorrect. Furthermore, maximum likelihood generally gives slightly better fits to the logistic model, judged by comparing the observed and expected numbers of cases per decile of risk. The maximum likelihood estimates also result in the total expected number of cases equalling the observed total, which is not a property of the discriminant estimates. In summarizing the above results and others from an extensive theoretical and empirical investigation, Halperin, Blackwelder, and Verter (1971) state that if one is fitting the logistic model in order to isolate relevant risk factors by means of tests of significance, then the discriminant function approach works reasonably well, even when the normality assumption is violated. On the other hand, if one wants to estimate the actual magnitudes of the parameters or the probabilities of events under the logistic model, then the maximum likelihood approach should be used. [Press and Wilson (1978) also discuss these points.]

8.5 DISCUSSION OF LOGISTIC MODELS

Interaction

The use of a probabilistic model, such as the logistic model (8.1), should be regarded as a provisional working basis for an analysis, rather than a rigid specification to be accepted uncritically (Cox 1970). Models "smooth" the data by requiring that the estimates conform to the relationship specified in the model equation. Although smoothing data is desirable to the extent that it removes the effects of chance variation, an incorrect specification of the relationship between the risk of disease and the variables x_i may lead to a mistaken assessment of their individual and joint effects.

In a cohort study of potential risk factors for coronary heart disease (CHD), Truett, Cornfield, and Kannel (1967) stratified their analyses by age and sex in order to allow for an interaction between these and the other variables. They fit separate logistic models involving age, cholesterol, systolic blood pressure, relative weight, hemoglobin, cigarette smoking, and ECG abnormality within each of the age-sex strata. For men 40–49 years old, the coefficient for serum cholesterol was estimated by discriminant analysis to be $\hat{\beta}_2 = 0.0074$, with a standard error of 0.0027. For men 30–39 years old, the corresponding estimate was $\hat{\beta}_2 = 0.0231$, with a standard error of 0.0040. Adjusted for the effects of the remaining six variables, serum cholesterol was estimated to have a significantly greater effect on the risk of CHD among the younger men. Had one not stratified on age, or had one not fit a model with an interaction term between age and serum cholesterol, the differential effect of serum cholesterol in the two age groups would have been missed. [A one degree of freedom chi-square test of the difference between the two coefficients for cholesterol is calculated as $\chi^2 = (.0231 - .0074)^2 / \{(.0040)^2 + (.0027)^2\}$ $= 18.4, p < .0001$ (two-sided)].

Referring back to the discussion (Section 8.1) of the analysis of seven potential risk factors for coronary heart disease in men 40–49 years of age, the maximum likelihood estimates of the logistic parameters reported in Table 8.1 are based on fitting the following model

$$p_x = 1/\{1 + \exp[-(\beta_0 + \beta_1 x_1 + \ldots + \beta_7 x_7)]\}. \quad (8.32)$$

One implication of this model is that the effect of any one variable does not depend on the values assumed by the other variables. Thus, from Table 8.1, a 10 mg/dl increase in serum cholesterol is estimated to increase the logit of risk by 0.0070(10) = 0.070, irrespective of whether systolic blood pressure is 120 mm Hg or 180 mm Hg.

One approach to investigating whether an interaction exists between serum cholesterol and blood pressure would be to stratify the data on systolic blood pressure and fit separate logistic functions involving serum cholesterol and the remaining variables to each of the blood pressure strata. If the coefficient for cholesterol were constant across the strata, there would be evidence for a lack of interaction on a logistic scale between serum cholesterol and blood pressure.

A second approach to the study of interaction between serum cholesterol (x_2) and systolic blood pressure (x_3) would be to introduce a term of the form $\gamma(x_2 x_3)$ into the model equation (8.32). Estimating γ by maximum likelihood and testing for significance would provide an assessment of an interaction taking the specific functional form $x_2 x_3$. Thus, from equation (8.32), the logit of risk would be alternatively specified as

$$\ln p_x/q_x = \beta_0 + \beta_1 x_1 + \ldots + \beta_7 x_7 + \gamma(x_2 x_3). \quad (8.33)$$

By rearranging terms in (8.33), one sees that the effect of the variable x_2 on the logit of risk is now given by the coefficient $\beta_2 + \gamma x_3$. This coefficient depends on the value assumed by x_3. Similarly, the effect of the variable x_3, given by the coefficient $\beta_3 + \gamma x_2$, depends on the value of x_2. Interactions more complicated than $\gamma(x_2 x_3)$ could also be specified and tested, although one usually begins with this simple form unless there is external evidence suggesting some alternative. Interactions involving the other variables can also be addressed by stratification or modeling.

Interpretation of Statistical Models

Frequently one wants to evaluate the effect of a single variable while making allowance for the effects of other related variables. For example, if interest lies in the relation of diabetes to the incidence of congestive heart failure, one may or may not want to control for the effect of blood pressure, which is both correlated with diabetes and also strongly associated with the development of the study disease. Entering blood pressure along with the presence or absence of diabetes as variables in a multivariate analysis will result in underestimating the effect of diabetes, to the extent that blood pressure is controlled by glucose tolerance (Gordon 1974).

As a second example, if serum cholesterol, blood pressure, and relative weight are entered as variables in a logistic model involving coronary heart disease as the dependent variable, the coefficient for relative weight, which may be statistically significant by itself, may approach zero in the multivariate equation. This does not mean that relative weight is unimportant, but suggests that its effect is mediated by blood pressure and serum cholesterol levels (Gordon 1974). Thus, knowledge of the univariate relationships is important to interpreting the results of a multivariate analysis. This problem of interpretation arises whenever two or more highly correlated variables are involved (Snedecor and Cochran 1980, pp. 352–353). An effective approach to this problem is based on a stepwise procedure, adding and deleting variables from the equation to assess their impact on the coefficients of the remaining variables (Cramer 1972). Subject matter knowledge should guide the analysis by suggesting hypotheses involving causal and noncausal paths of association.

The coefficient for any variable in a logistic regression equation depends on the entire set of variables included in the model. Thus, a variable that by itself shows a significant association with disease may have a coefficient that is indistinguishable from zero in a multivariate analysis. Similarly, the coefficient for a given variable may be significant when evaluated with one set of variables, but may become nonsignificant when included among a different set. The effect of adding a variable to a given set, however, does not always reduce the coefficients of the original variables. In judging the appropriateness of a fitted model, one should carefully examine its implications in terms of the estimated effects of the variables included in the analysis. The estimated effects should be plausible in light of current biological knowledge.

Choice of a Model

As with analyses based on stratification (Chapter 7), a multivariate analysis should be guided by a series of questions of increasing complexity derived from hypotheses based on subject matter knowledge. Invariably the first question is whether there is a crude association between a particular variable, say x_1, and the risk of disease. The corresponding linear logistic model is $\ln p_x/q_x = \beta_0 + \beta_1 x_1$. Next, one might ask whether the effect of exposure to x_1, represented by the coefficient β_1, is correctly estimated in regard to its magnitude and direction. To state the question more specifically, does an association between x_1 and some other variable alter one's assessment of the effect of x_1? Failure to control for a confounder will bias the estimate of β_1 (Snedecor and Cochran 1980, pp. 353–355). Again, using subject matter knowledge of variables likely to be associated with the study disease and exposure to x_1, one may consider models such as $\ln p_x/q_x = \beta_0 + \beta_1 x_1 + \beta_2 x_2$, or $\ln p_x/q_x = \beta_0 + \beta_1 x_1 + \beta_3 x_3$, etc. If the estimated coefficient β_1 remains unchanged from a practical point of view, then the effect of the variable x_1 is not simply explained by the existence of a confounding variable x_2 or x_3, etc. (It is not appropriate to perform a statistical test of whether the estimated coefficient β_1 differs "significantly" among the above alternative models. See, for example Miettinen 1976b.)

The next level of complexity concerns questions of interactions among the variables. For example, one might ask whether the effect of x_1 depends on the level of some other variable, say x_2. The logistic model $\ln p_x/q_x = \beta_0 + \beta_1 x_1 + \gamma(x_1 x_2)$ addresses this question. If γ differs markedly from zero, an interaction in terms of a logistic model exists between x_1 and x_2.

Estimates of the parameters in a statistical model require that the model first be stated explicitly. This gives rise to two related questions. (1) What is the proper functional form of the model? (2) Which variables should be included? These questions are fundamentally ones of scientific explanation and as such are often not amenable to a definitive resolution. An incomplete or improper formulation of a model results in what has been called "specification errors." The discrepancy that can occur between the estimated parameters based on a postulated model and those based on the correct (but unknown) model cannot be assessed definitively by statistical methods (Wold 1956).

In regard to variable selection, it is fair to say that among statisticians there is an overemphasis on stepwise selection procedures based on tests of significance. Stepwise procedures find the "best fit" within a specified functional form (Draper and Smith 1981). From the viewpoint of scientific explanation, there are at least three basic weaknesses in the approach. First, the procedures do not distinguish among associations that are causal, noncausal (but due to an associated causal factor), or artifactual (due to some source of study bias). Second, the procedures emphasize formal tests of significance, which are dependent on the size of the study sample. In large studies, variables with trivial effects on the risk of disease may be selected for inclusion in the model, because they have "highly significant" associations (i.e. small p-values), while in small studies, variables with important effects may be selected for deletion because they have "nonsignificant" associations (i.e. large p-values). Third, stepwise selection procedures are oblivious to causal paths. A variable that is affected by the development of disease could be selected for inclusion in a model intended to identify disease risk factors. Walter and Holford (1978) and Greenland (1979) discuss other important issues concerning the role of statistical models in the analysis of epidemiologic data.

8.6 APPLICATION OF LOGISTIC REGRESSION

Point Estimates and Confidence Intervals

As an application of logistic regression, consider again the data in Table 7.6 from a case-control study of oral contraceptive use in relation to myocardial infarction (Shapiro et al. 1979). Taking recent use of oral contraceptives as the study factor of primary interest, the investigators used logistic regression to control for the potential confounding effects of age, cigarette smoking, weight, diabetes, lipid abnormality, hypertension, angina pectoris, pre-eclamptic toxemia, and hospital (Boston, New York, Philadelphia). Our analysis considers only age, smoking, and oral contraceptive use in order to simplify the presentation.

Let x_1 denote the presence ($x_1 = 1$) or absence ($x_1 = 0$) of oral contraceptive use within one month prior to admission. Although the variables age and cigarette smoking need not be stratified as in Table 7.6, use of their actual values would preclude displaying all of the data, since this would require listing their individual values for the 234 cases and 1742 controls. We therefore use the midpoint of each age category (27, 32, 37, 42, 47) as values for the age variable, designated by x_2. The smoking variable has an open-ended category (25 or more cigarettes per day). To deal with this, we introduce two indicator variables for smoking. Taking the category "none" as the reference, let x_3 and x_4 be indicator variables for each of the remaining two groups. Thus, if an individual smokes 1–24 cigarettes per day, $x_3 = 1$ and $x_4 = 0$. If the individual smokes 25 or more cigarettes per day, $x_3 = 0$ and $x_4 = 1$. Finally, if the individual is a nonsmoker, $x_3 = 0$ and $x_4 = 0$.

Table 8.2. Maximum Likelihood Estimates of Logistic
Parameters[1] Relating Age, Smoking, and Recent Oral
Contraceptive Use to the Risk of Myocardial Infarction in
Women

Variable	β_i	$\hat{\beta}_i$	$SE(\hat{\beta}_i)$
x_0 intercept	β_0	−9.2834	.6328
x_1 OC use	β_1	1.1883	.2610
x_2 age	β_2	0.1521	.0141
x_3 smoke 1–24	β_3	1.1246	.2095
x_4 smoke $\geq$ 25	β_4	2.1371	.2087

Maximized log likelihood: $L(\hat{\beta}) = -582.39$

Estimated Covariance Matrix $(\hat{\sigma}_{ik})$

	β_0	β_1	β_2	β_3	β_4
β_0	.4004	−.0580	−.0086	−.0377	−.0460
β_1		.0681	.0012	.0017	−.0004
β_2			.0002	.0002	.0004
β_3				.0439	.0291
β_4					.0436

1. Logistic model: $\ln p_x/q_x = \beta_0 + \beta_1 x_1 + \beta_2 x_2 + \beta_3 x_3 + \beta_4 x_4$.

Taking case-control status ($d = 1$ or $d = 0$ respectively) as the dependent variable, the maximum likelihood estimates of the parameters of the logistic model $\ln p_x/q_x = \beta_0 + \beta_1 x_1 + \ldots + \beta_4 x_4$ are given in Table 8.2. Also shown are the standard errors and the estimated covariance-matrix $(\hat{\sigma}_{ik})$ of the $\hat{\beta}_i$, along with the maximized log likelihood $L(\hat{\beta})$. The standard errors (SE) are determined by taking the square roots of the diagonal entries in the estimated covariance matrix. Thus, $SE(\hat{\beta}_1) = (0.0681)^{1/2} = 0.2610$, and so forth. The estimated logistic regression model is (to two decimals):

$$\ln p_x/q_x = -9.28 + 1.19x_1 + 0.15x_2 + 1.12x_3 + 2.14x_4. \quad (8.34)$$

Adjusted for age and smoking, the relative odds of a myocardial infarction (MI) associated with recent use of oral contraceptives is therefore estimated to be $\hat{\psi} = \exp(1.19) = 3.29$. An approximate 95 percent confidence interval is (1.97, 5.48), calculated from (8.29) as $\exp[1.19 \pm 1.96(0.0681)^{1/2}]$.

From the analysis of Section 7.2, the corresponding Mantel-Haenszel estimate of the MI-OC odds ratio, adjusted for age and smoking, is $\hat{\psi}_{mh} = 3.33$. The asymptotic mle (Gart 1971) based on equation (7.34) is $\hat{\psi} = 3.31$, determined by using the program of Thomas (1975).

Table 8.3. Maximum Likelihood Estimates for Logistic Models Relating Various Combinations of Risk Factors to Myocardial Infarction in Women

Variable	Estimated Model[1]					
	(1)	(2)	(3)	(4)	(5)	(6)
x_0 intercept	−2.0075	−2.0591	−7.7640	−9.2834	−7.0187	−8.5804
x_1 OC use (yes, no)		0.5211	1.3364	1.1883		
x_2 age (yrs)			0.1418	0.1521	0.1264	0.1373
x_3 smoke 1–24				1.1246		1.1086
x_4 smoke ≥ 25				2.1357		2.1703
Maximized log likelihood $L(\hat{\beta})$	−718.80	−716.19	−644.21	−582.39	−657.00	−591.78

1. The estimated logistic coefficients in columns (1)–(6) result from fitting different models. For example, column (2) is based on the model $\ln p_x/q_x = \beta_0 + \beta_1 x_1$, whereas column (3) is based on the model $\ln p_x/q_x = \beta_0 + \beta_1 x_1 + \beta_2 x_2$, etc.

The relative odds of an MI associated with recent OC use is estimated to be $\hat{\psi} = 3.29$ by a logistic model that allows for adjustment for the effects of both age and smoking. Table 8.3 (column 2) shows that the crude odds ratio (no adjustment for age or smoking) is $\hat{\psi} = \exp(0.5211) = 1.68$. Adjusted for age (column 3), the MI-OC odds ratio is $\hat{\psi} = \exp(1.3364) = 3.81$. Thus, the estimated effect of OC use on the risk of an MI depends on which variables are included for adjustment in the model equation (Section 8.5).

Next, consider smoking as the risk factor of interest. Taking nonsmokers as the reference group, the relative odds of a myocardial infarction associated with smoking 1–24 cigarettes per day is determined from equation (8.34) as $\hat{\psi} = \exp(1.12) = 3.06$. This estimate is adjusted for both age and recent oral contraceptive use. The corresponding relative odds of an MI associated with smoking 25 or more cigarettes per day is $\hat{\psi} = \exp(2.14) = 8.50$. Approximate 95 percent confidence intervals, calculated from equation (8.29), are (2.03, 4.62), and (5.64, 12.80) respectively.

From Section 7.4, the corresponding Mantel-Haenszel estimates of the MI-smoking odds ratios, adjusted for both age and OC use are $\hat{\psi}_{mh} = 3.25$ (1–24 vs. none) and $\hat{\psi}_{mh} = 8.22$ (≥ 25 vs. none). For practical purposes, these are in close agreement with the estimates based on the logistic regression model (8.34).

Finally, consider estimating the combined effect of recent oral contraceptive use and smoking 25 or more cigarettes per day. Taking women who neither use OCs nor smoke as the reference group ($x_1 = 0$, $x_3 = 0$, $x_4 = 0$), the age-adjusted estimate of the relative odds of an MI associated with the combined use of OCs and smoking 25 or more cigarettes per day ($x_1^* = 1$, $x_3^* = 0$, $x_4^* = 1$) is $\hat{\psi} = \exp(1.19 + 2.14) = \exp(3.33) = 27.9$. This result follows from the application of equation (8.4) to the parameter estimates in (8.34). A corresponding approximate 95 percent confidence interval for the odds ratio is calculated as follows. From equation (8.24), the variance of $\ln \psi$ is estimated as

$$\hat{V} = 0.0681 + 0.0436 + 2(-0.0004) = 0.1109.$$

Thus, using equation (8.25), $\exp[3.33 \pm 1.96(0.1109)^{1/2}]$ gives the approximate 95 percent confidence interval (14.5, 53.7) corresponding to the point estimate $\hat{\psi} = 27.9$.

The odds ratio $\hat{\psi} = 27.9$ is estimated by logistic regression. Table 7.12B shows that the corresponding age-adjusted estimate calculated by the Mantel-Haenszel method is $\hat{\psi}_{mh} = 39.3$. Table 7.12B also gives the Mantel-Haenszel estimates of the age-adjusted odds ratios associated with various other combinations of smoking and oral contraceptive use, a topic to which we shall return after a brief digression.

Likelihood Ratio Tests

If a parameter β_i in the logistic model (8.1) equals zero, then the variable x_i is not associated with the risk of disease. Section 8.2 shows that this statement applies to logistic analyses of data from either cohort or case-control studies. The likelihood ratio test (8.31) may be used to assess whether an apparent association ($\hat{\beta}_i \neq 0$) is statistically significant. For example, consider fitting the logistic model $\ln p_x/q_x = \beta_0 + \beta_1 x_1$ to the data in Table 7.6. From Table 8.3 (column 2), the parameter estimates are $\hat{\beta}_0 = -2.0591$ and $\hat{\beta}_1 = 0.5211$. A test of whether OC use shows a crude association with the risk of an MI is thus made by comparing the log likelihoods in columns 1 and 2. Application of equation (8.31) gives

$$\chi_1^2 = 2[-716.19 - (-718.80)] = 5.22.$$

The likelihood ratio test indicates that the association is significant ($p \simeq .02$, two-sided). If $\hat{\beta}_i$ differs significantly from zero, then $\exp(\hat{\beta}_i)$ differs significantly from unity. Thus, the above likelihood ratio test of $\hat{\beta}_1$ implies that the crude relative odds of an MI associated with recent OC use [$\hat{\psi} = \exp(.5211) = 1.68$] is significantly greater than unity.

Consider next a test of whether the effect of OC use, adjusted for age, is significantly related to the risk of an MI. The likelihood ratio test of $\beta_1 = 0$, based on the logistic model $\ln p_x/q_x = \beta_0 + \beta_1 x_1 + \beta_2 x_2$, is made by comparing log likelihoods from columns 3 and 5 in Table 8.3. One calculates

$$\chi_1^2 = 2[-644.21 - (-657.00)] = 25.58,$$

which indicates that the coefficient $\hat{\beta}_1 = 1.3364$ is significantly ($p <$ .0001, two-sided) greater than zero. Adjusted for age, the MI-OC odds ratio [$\hat{\psi} = \exp(1.34) = 3.81$] is therefore significantly greater than unity. Failure to adjust the crude odds ratio for the effect of age, which is a confounding variable because of its association with both oral contraceptive use and myocardial infarction, results in an underestimate of the effect of OC use on the risk of an MI.

A comparison of log likelihoods in columns 4 and 6 of Table 8.3 shows that OC use, adjusted for both age and smoking, is also significantly associated with the risk of an MI

$$\chi_1^2 = 2[-582.39 - (-591.78)] = 18.78. \ (p < .0001, \text{two-sided})$$

An alternative test based on a comparison of $\hat{\beta}_1$ with its standard error gives

$$\chi_1^2 = (1.1883/0.2610)^2 = 20.73$$

($p < .0001$, two-sided) from Table 8.2. For practical purposes, the above two tests give equivalent results in this instance.

Suppose that one now considers smoking (variables x_3 and x_4) as a potential risk factor for myocardial infarction, and that one wants to adjust for potential confounding by age (x_2). Maximum likelihood estimation of the logistic model $\ln p_x/q_x = \beta_0 + \beta_2 x_2 + \beta_3 x_3 + \beta_4 x_4$ applied to the data in Table 7.6 results in the parameter estimates given in column 6 of Table 8.3. The likelihood ratio test of the null hypothesis $\beta_3 = \beta_4 = 0$, which states that there is no age-adjusted effect of smoking on the risk of an MI, is made by comparing the log likelihoods in columns 5 and 6. Using equation (8.31), a chi-square test with 2 degrees of freedom is given by

$$\chi_2^2 = 2[-591.78 - (-657.00)] = 130.44.$$

This test rejects the null hypothesis at the $p < .001$ level (two-sided), thereby indicating an age-adjusted association between cigarette smoking and the risk of an MI in women.

Tests of significance based on likelihood ratios supplement an analysis that reports point estimates and confidence intervals. In large samples, a one degree of freedom chi-square test of significance based on $\chi^2 = [\hat{\beta}_i/\text{SE}(\hat{\beta}_i)]^2$ is equivalent to the corresponding likelihood ratio test. The

Table 8.4. Estimated Parameters and Covariances for a Logistic Interaction Model[1] that Relates Various Risk Factors to the Occurrence of Myocardial Infarction in Women

Variable	Parameter	Estimate	Standard error
x_0 intercept	β_0	-9.2760	.6360
x_1 OC use	β_1	1.2756	.5784
x_2 age	β_2	0.1517	.0142
x_3 smoke 1-24	β_3	1.1977	.2182
x_4 smoke ≥ 25	β_4	2.0828	.2211
x_1x_3	γ_1	-1.1709	.8492
x_1x_4	γ_2	0.3392	.6651

Maximized log likelihood: $L(\hat{\beta}) = -579.61$

Estimated Covariance Matrix $(\hat{\sigma}_{ik})$

	β_0	β_1	β_2	β_3	β_4	γ_1	γ_2
β_0	.4045	$-.0676$	$-.0087$	$-.0387$	$-.0470$	.0140	.0072
β_1		.3345	.0008	.0324	.0332	$-.3294$	$-.3287$
β_2			.0002	.0002	.0004	.0004	.0006
β_3				.0476	.0321	$-.0471$	$-.0313$
β_4					.0489	$-.0310$	$-.0472$
γ_1						.7212	.3322
γ_2							.4424

1. Logistic model: $\ln p_x/q_x = \beta_0 + \beta_1 x_1 + \beta_2 x_2 + \beta_3 x_3 + \beta_4 x_4 + \gamma_1(x_1 x_3) + \gamma_2(x_1 x_4)$.

likelihood ratio method is more general, however, since it permits simultaneous tests of sets of parameters, as shown by the above test for an age-adjusted effect of smoking.

Assessment of Interaction

Now consider the possibility of an age-adjusted interaction between OC use and smoking. The logistic model is

$$\ln p_x/q_x = \beta_0 + \beta_1 x_1 + \beta_2 x_2 + \beta_3 x_3 + \beta_4 x_4 + \gamma_1(x_1 x_3) + \gamma_2(x_1 x_4).$$

The maximum likelihood estimates of the logistic parameters and their covariances are given in Table 8.4. The likelihood ratio test of the null hypothesis $\gamma_1 = \gamma_2 = 0$ is

$$\chi_2^2 = 2[-579.61 - (-582.39)] = 5.56$$

($p \simeq 0.07$, two-sided) using the log likelihoods in Table 8.3 (column 4) and Table 8.4. Although one cannot reject the null hypothesis at the tra-

Table 8.5. Age-Adjusted Odds Ratios Estimated From Logistic Models with and without an Interaction Between Smoking and Oral Contraceptive Use

Cig/day	No interaction model[1] OC use		Interaction model[2] OC use	
	No	Yes	No	Yes
None	1.0^3	3.3 (2.0, 5.5)	1.0^3	3.6 (1.2, 11.1)
1–24	3.1 (2.0, 4.6)	10.1 (5.2, 19.5)	3.3 (2.2, 5.1)	3.7 (1.04, 13.0)
≥ 25	8.5 (5.6, 12.8)	27.8 (14.4, 53.5)	8.0 (5.2, 12.4)	40.4 (19.4, 84.1)

1. $\ln p_x/q_x = \beta_0 + \beta_1 x_1 + \ldots + \beta_4 x_4$ (See Table 8.3, column 4 for mle's).
2. $\ln p_x/q_x = \beta_0 + \beta_1 x_1 + \ldots + \beta_4 x_4 + \gamma_1(x_1 x_3) + \gamma_2(x_1 x_4)$ (See Table 8.4 for mle's).
3. Reference group. Approximate 95 percent confidence intervals are given in parentheses.

ditional $\alpha = 0.05$ level, there is a suggestion that smoking and OC use have an interactive effect on the risk of an MI.

More important than the test of significance are the estimates of the odds ratio for various combinations of smoking and oral contraceptive use. The age-adjusted estimates based on logistic models with and without interaction terms are given in Table 8.5. One should refer back to Table 7.12B for the corresponding Mantel-Haenszel estimates.

As an example of the calculation of point estimates and confidence intervals in Table 8.5, consider the age-adjusted relative odds of an MI for OC users who smoke 25 or more cigarettes per day as compared with women who neither use OCs nor smoke. The odds ratio, estimated from the logistic model with interaction terms, is $\hat{\psi} = 40.4$, and is calculated as follows. For OC users who smoke 25 or more cigarettes per day, one has $x_1 = 1$, x_2, $x_3 = 0$, $x_4 = 1$, $x_1 x_3 = 0$, $x_1 x_4 = 1$. (The value of the variable x_2, which represents age, is arbitrary in this example, and is therefore designated simply as x_2.) Using the logistic parameters in Table 8.4, the corresponding log odds is estimated to be

$$\ln p_x/q_x = -9.2760 + 1.2756 + .1517 x_2 + 2.0828 + .3392.$$

For women who neither use OCs nor smoke, $x_1 = 0$, x_2, $x_3 = 0$, $x_4 = 0$, $x_1 x_3 = 0$, $x_1 x_4 = 0$. Thus, the log odds for this group is estimated as

$$\ln p_x/q_x = -9.2760 + .1517 x_2.$$

The difference in logits estimates the log odds ratio. Hence, $\ln \hat{\psi} = 1.2756 + 2.0828 + .3392$. Finally,

$$\hat{\psi} = \exp(1.2756 + 2.0828 + .3392) = 40.4.$$

Confidence intervals are calculated from equations (8.24) and (8.25).

For example, consider again the estimate $\hat{\psi} = 40.4$. Since $\ln \hat{\psi} = \hat{\beta}_1 + \hat{\beta}_4 + \hat{\gamma}_2$ (see above), the variance of $\ln \hat{\psi}$ involves terms $\hat{\sigma}_{ik}$ in equation (8.24) that correspond to $(\beta_1 + \beta_4 + \gamma_2)^2$. Using the estimated covariance matrix in Table 8.4, one calculates

$$\hat{V} = .3345 + .0489 + .4424 + 2(.0332)$$
$$+ 2(-.3287) + 2(-.0472) = .1404.$$

Thus an approximate 95 percent confidence interval corresponding to the estimate $\hat{\psi} = 40.4$ is (19.4, 84.1), calculated from equation (8.25) as $\exp(3.6976 \pm 1.96 \sqrt{.1404})$.

Among all three analyses, there is a single discrepancy that has a substantive effect on the interpretation. It occurs for OC users who smoke 1–24 cigarettes per day. Both the Mantel-Haenszel estimate and that based on the logistic model with interactions suggest that among moderate smokers (1–24 cigarettes per day) OC use has a negligible effect on the risk of disease. This is inconsistent with the substantial effect of OC use that is estimated to occur among nonsmokers and among women who smoke 25 or more cigarettes per day.

Comparing the odds ratios for OC-yes vs. OC-no among smokers of 1–24 cigarettes per day, one estimates the age-adjusted relative odds of an MI associated with OC use to be $\hat{\psi} = 3.7/3.4 = 1.09$ (Mantel-Haenszel, Table 7.12B) or $\hat{\psi} = 3.7/3.3 = 1.12$ (logistic interaction, Table 8.5). [Within each smoking category, the ratio of odds ratios is an estimate of the effect of OC use, because all of the category-specific odds ratios are expressed relative to the same reference group, namely, women who neither smoke nor use OCs.]

By contrast with the apparent lack of an effect of OC use among moderate smokers, both the Mantel-Haenszel estimates and those based on the logistic interaction model indicate an approximate fourfold increase in risk associated with OC use in nonsmokers ($\hat{\psi} = 4.5/1.0$, Mantel-Haenszel; $\hat{\psi} = 3.6/1.0$, logistic interaction). In heavy smokers, these estimates suggest that OC use is associated with an approximate fivefold increased risk ($\hat{\psi} = 39.3/7.8$, Mantel-Haenszel; $\hat{\psi} = 40.4/8.0$, logistic interaction).

In comparison with the above results, the logistic model without interactions indicates that OC use produces a 3.3 times increase in the risk of an MI for each smoking category (3.3/1.0, 10.1/3.1 and 27.8/8.5 from Table 8.5).

An apparent lack of association between OC use and myocardial infarction for moderate smokers could have been caused by case-control

Figure 8.2. Relationship between log odds of "disease" and age among users of oral contraceptives.

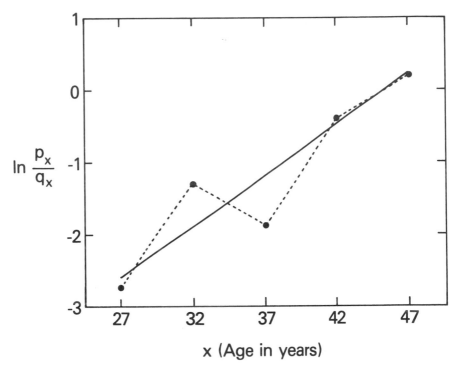

differences in variables which were not controlled in the study design or analysis. In the absence of such information, we prefer the interpretation and estimates based on the no-interaction model, because an analysis that suggests an increased risk of an MI due to OC use among nonsmokers and heavy smokers but no increase in risk among moderate smokers is biologically implausible.

In this example, the logistic interaction model and the Mantel-Haenszel procedure have "overfit" the data as a result of too many parameters being introduced. The interaction model in Table 8.4 uses 7 logistic parameters to fit the log odds. The Mantel-Haenszel procedure, in calculating an age-adjusted odds ratio for each of three smoking groups, may be compared to fitting a separate logistic regression $\ln p_x/q_x = \beta_0 + \beta_1 x_1 + \beta_2 x_2$ in each of these strata. Thus 9 parameters are effectively used. By comparison, the no-interaction logistic model (Table 8.3) uses five parameters.

Figure 8.2 illustrates the general concept of overfitting the log odds. [The data in Table 7.6 were collapsed over smoking to calculate the odds of "disease" (MI/control) among OC users in each age group.] Although the dashed line, which follows every peak and valley, may better reproduce the data than the (solid) straight line, it implies a relationship which, if taken literally, is an unlikely representation of the effect of a quantitative variable. A statistical analysis should not simply reproduce the data, but lead to an interpretation that is plausible in terms of knowledge of the subject matter. [The straight line in Figure 8.2 is based on the fitted logistic regression equation $\ln p_x/q_x = -7.7640 + 1.3364\,\text{OC} + 0.1418\,\text{Age}$, from Table 8.3.]

8.7 FURTHER TOPICS IN LOGISTIC REGRESSION

Goodness of Fit

Given estimated values of the logistic parameters, one may assess "goodness of fit" of a logistic model in several ways. A global assessment may be made by applying the estimated logistic model to the variable values for each individual. Thus, given values x_{j1}, x_{j2}, ..., x_{jp} for the variables x_1, x_2, ..., x_p on the jth individual, one first calculates

$$\hat{y}_j = \hat{\beta}_0 + \sum_{i=1}^{p} \hat{\beta}_i x_{ji}$$

and then

$$\hat{p}_j = 1/[1 + \exp(\hat{y}_j)].$$

The variables x_1, ..., x_p may be transformations of a set of original variables, or may represent any interactions among them. One next pools the values of $\hat{p}_j$ for the cases and the controls, and then ranks them from smallest to largest. The values of $\hat{p}_j$ are then grouped into deciles, quintiles, or in general g groups. Within each group, the observed number of cases is tallied and compared with the number of cases expected, determined by summing the calculated values of $\hat{p}_j$ for all subjects in that group (Cornfield 1962, Truett, Cornfield, and Kannel 1967).

Based on data from a cohort study, the quantity $\hat{p}_j$ may be interpreted as the estimated risk of disease for the jth individual. If the logistic model has been fitted to data from a case-control study, the quantity $\hat{p}_j$ may be interpreted as the estimated probability that the jth individual is a "case."

Table 8.6. Observed and Expected Numbers of Cases of Coronary Heart Disease by Decile of $\hat{p}_j$

Decile of $\hat{p}_j$	1	2	3	4	5	6	7	8	9	10	Total
Observed	1	4	3	8	5	9	11	6	14	27	88
Expected	2.1	3.3	4.2	5.1	6.2	7.4	8.9	11.5	15.2	24.1	88.0

Source: Halperin, Blackwelder, and Verter 1971, Table 3.

Returning to the example of Section 8.1 concerning the incidence of coronary heart disease in 742 men age 40–49 years at initial exam, Table 8.6 shows the results of the described procedure for calculating observed and expected numbers of cases falling within each decile of $\hat{p}_j$. One sees an approximate twelvefold increase in risk from the lowest to the highest decile.

Let O_i and E_i denote respectively the observed and expected number of cases in the ith group (decile, quintile, etc.), where $E_i = \Sigma \hat{p}_j$, the summation being taken over all values of $\hat{p}_j$ that fall into the ith group. A chi-square test of fit may then be calculated as

$$\chi^2_{g-2} = \Sigma (O_i - E_i)^2 / \{E_i[1 - (E_i/n_i)]\} \qquad (8.35)$$

where n_i is the total number of cases and controls in the ith group. Under the null hypothesis that the fitted model is correct, χ^2_{g-2} is well approximated in large samples by a chi-square distribution with $g - 2$ degrees of freedom (Hosmer and Lemeshow 1980). Large values of χ^2_{g-2} indicate lack of fit.

This procedure for testing lack of fit is not very powerful in discriminating between alternative parameterizations of the logistic model, because the test is based on groupings of estimates $\hat{p}_j$, which themselves combine information over a set of variables.

Applying the test of fit (8.35) to the data in Table 8.6, one calculates $\chi^2_8 = 7.84$, indicating good agreement between observed and expected. (Since the values of n_i were not reported, we have taken $n_i = 74.2$, corresponding to grouping 742 observations into deciles.) One may perform related analyses by comparing the observed and expected numbers of cases within cells of the multiple cross-classification determined by the variables in the fitted logistic model (see Cornfield 1962, Truett, Cornfield, and Kannel 1967).

A second approach to assessing the adequacy of a given logistic model is to fit a more complicated model that contains additional parameters representing particular types of departure from the initial model. The likelihood ratio test (8.31) can then be applied to determine whether the additional regression coefficients associated with the more complex model are equal to zero. Cox (1970) describes this approach, as well as other methods based on graphical analysis.

Tsiatis (1980) has given a goodness-of-fit test based on cross-classifying the variables in the logistic model and calculating a test statistic that is a quadratic form in the observed counts minus the expected counts. When the variables are discrete, the test is equivalent to the Pearson chi-square test $\Sigma(O_i - E_i)^2/E_i$, which is discussed in Section 8.10 [equation (8.58)].

Test for Dose Response Using Logistic Regression

Suppose that x denotes a quantitative variable representing an exposure of interest. The logistic model

$$\ln p_x/q_x = \beta_0 + \beta_1 x \qquad (8.36)$$

specifies that the logit of risk is a linear function of x, the parameter β_1 representing the slope of the regression line. This model implies that the relative odds of disease for individuals with exposure level $x = x_i$ as compared with individuals with exposure level $x = x_0$ is

$$\hat{\psi}_i = \exp[\hat{\beta}_1(x_i - x_0)]. \qquad (8.37)$$

Thus, compared with the reference level $x = x_0$, the relative odds of disease increases with larger values of x if $\beta_1 > 0$, the reverse being true if $\beta_1 < 0$. Equation (8.36) represents a particular type of dose-response relationship, one in which the logit of risk is a linear function of exposure. This implies a dose-response relationship in which the odds ratio is a simple exponential function of exposure [equation (8.37)]. Nonlinear relationships can be represented by transformations of x, such as $\sqrt{x}$, $\ln x$, $1/\sqrt{(x + c)}$, or by introducing polynomial functions of x, such as $\beta_1 x + \beta_2 x^2$. More complicated functions can also be fitted.

To adjust one's estimate of β_1 for the effect of a potential confounding variable (z), one may fit the model

$$\ln p_x/q_x = \beta_0 + \beta_1 x + \beta_2 z. \qquad (8.38)$$

Rather than assume a linear relationship between the logit of risk and z, one may stratify z into $k + 1$ subgroups, and introduce indicator variables to allow for nonlinear effects of z. Thus, as opposed to (8.38), one may fit the following model

$$\ln p_x/q_x = \beta_0 + \beta_1 x + \sum_{j=1}^{k} \beta_{2j} z_j \qquad (8.39)$$

where the z_j are indicator variables for the subgroups based on the variable z. By a change of notation, equation (8.39) may be expressed in the equivalent form

$$\ln p_x/q_x = \alpha_j + \beta_1 x. \qquad (8.40)$$

Both equations (8.39) and (8.40) indicate that, within each of the subgroups of z, the logit of risk has a constant slope of regression on x. The overall levels of $\ln p_x/q_x$, represented by the $k + 1$ parameters α_j, are allowed to vary across subgroups. Adjustment for more than one confounder, and allowance for interactions, follows directly from the discussion in the previous sections of this chapter.

As an example of a test for dose response based on logistic regression, reconsider the data in Table 7.16, which was analysed in Chapter 7 (Section 7.4) using the extended Mantel-Haenszel procedure. To assess whether the risk of myocardial infarction shows a dose-response relationship with cigarette smoking, the logistic model (8.38) was fit by maximum likelihood. Adjustment for potential confounding by age was made in terms of the variable z, taking the values 0, 1, 2, 3, and 4 for the five age groups. [One could just as well have let z take the values 25, 30, 35, 40, and 45, resulting in a change of scale for $\hat{\beta}_2$ and origin ($\hat{\beta}_0$), but with no effect on $\hat{\beta}_1$.] The exposure variable x took the values 0, 1, and 2 respectively for the smoking groups "none," "1–24," and "≥ 25."

Note that for $x = 0$ and $z = 1$, corresponding to nonsmokers who are 30–34 years old, the observed odds are 0/188 (Table 7.16). Thus, the observed value of $\ln p/q$ is undefined at this point, and the maximum likelihood procedure will not converge (Anderson 1974). This difficulty was avoided by taking two different approaches, both leading to virtually the same result. In the first analysis, the observation 0/188 was omitted from the data. The resulting estimated model is

$$\ln p_x/q_x = -4.7039 + 1.0374x + 0.6572z.$$

The age-adjusted estimate of the relative odds of an MI among women smoking 1–24 cigarettes per day as compared with nonsmoking women is thus computed from (8.37) as

$$\hat{\psi}_1 = \exp[1.0374(1 - 0)] = 2.82.$$

Similarly, the relative odds of an MI among women smoking 25 or more cigarettes per day as compared with nonsmoking women is estimated to be

$$\hat{\psi}_2 = \exp[1.0374(2 - 0)] = 7.96.$$

The Mantel-Haenszel estimates in Table 7.16, $\hat{\psi}_{mh} = 3.16$ and $\hat{\psi}_{mh} = 8.57$ respectively, agree reasonably well with $\hat{\psi}_1$ and $\hat{\psi}_2$.

As a second approach to fitting the logistic model (8.38), the "correction factor" $\frac{1}{2}$ was added to each of the 30 cells. The resulting fitted model is

$$\ln p_x/q_x = -4.7094 + 1.0540x + 0.6564z.$$

The corresponding age-adjusted odds ratios are $\hat{\psi}_1 = 2.87$ and $\hat{\psi}_2 = 8.23$, showing somewhat better agreement with the Mantel-Haenszel estimates. Of course, one should not expect perfect agreement between the two methods of estimation. We make the comparison primarily to assist the reader in relating the two approaches.

If one introduces indicator variables for age, fitting the model (8.39) as opposed to (8.38), the resulting MI-smoking odds ratios would be estimated as $\hat{\psi}_1 = 2.80$ and $\hat{\psi}_2 = 7.86$ (0/188 deleted) or $\hat{\psi}_1 = 2.87$ and $\hat{\psi}_2 = 8.22$ ($\frac{1}{2}$ added to all cells).

Using data from a matched case-control study, Holford, White, and Kelsey (1978) discuss an analysis of linear and quadratic trend relating length of oral contraceptive use to the risk of fibroadenoma. Berry (1980) presents analyses of dose response in matched and unmatched case-control studies using a model in which the *relative risk* is assumed to be a linear function of the exposure variable.

Prospective vs. Retrospective Models

Taking the presence ($d = 1$) or absence ($d = 0$) of disease as the dependent variable in a logistic model, Section 8.2 showed that, except for β_0, the logistic parameters were equivalent for case-control and cohort studies. This result applies whether or not interactions are included in the model, and is true irrespective of the particular functional form used to represent the effect of the variables in the logistic equation. Thus, unless there were study bias, one expects equivalent estimates of the logistic parameters (except β_0) from either study design.

Prentice (1976) has given an alternative specification of the logistic model for case-control studies in which the presence or absence of *exposure* is taken to be the dependent variable. This approach assumes that one is interested in the effect of one factor in particular. Suppose that the study factor of interest is a dichotomous variable, say x_1, where $x_1 = 1$ (exposed) and $x_1 = 0$ (not exposed). Corresponding to the "prospective" logistic model with interactions (8.10), a "retrospective" logistic model may be specified as

$$p(x_1 = 1 \mid d, \mathbf{x}_2) =$$

$$1/\{1 + \exp[-(\beta_0^* + \beta_1 d + \sum_{i=2}^{p} \beta_i^* x_i + \sum_{i=2}^{p} \gamma_i(dx_i)]\}. \quad (8.41)$$

The relative odds of *exposure* among diseased individuals as compared with nondiseased individuals may be written as

$$\psi = \frac{p(x_1 = 1 \mid d = 1, \mathbf{x}_2)\, p(x_1 = 0 \mid d = 0, \mathbf{x}_2)}{p(x_1 = 0 \mid d = 1, \mathbf{x}_2)\, p(x_1 = 1 \mid d = 0, \mathbf{x}_2)} \quad (8.42)$$

This odds ratio is mathematically equivalent to the relative odds of *disease* among exposed individuals as compared with unexposed individuals

$$\psi = \frac{p(d = 1 \mid x_1 = 1, \mathbf{x}_2)\, p(d = 0 \mid x_1 = 0, \mathbf{x}_2)}{p(d = 0 \mid x_1 = 1, \mathbf{x}_2)\, p(d = 1 \mid x_1 = 0, \mathbf{x}_2)} \quad (8.43)$$

(Cornfield 1951, Prentice 1976). Substitution of (8.41) into (8.42) results in a log odds ratio

$$\ln \psi = \beta_1 + \sum_{i=2}^{p} \gamma_i x_i. \quad (8.44)$$

Equation (8.44) has the same functional form as equation (8.11). This indicates that irrespective of whether the prospective (8.10) or retrospective (8.41) formulations are used for the logistic model, the log odds ratio shows the same dependence on the variables $x_2, \ldots, x_p$. Breslow (1976) has used the model equation (8.44) as the point of departure for a regression analysis of $\ln \psi$.

One interprets the parameters β_1 and $\gamma_2, \ldots, \gamma_p$ in the retrospective model (8.41) in exactly the same way as one interprets the parameters β_1 and $\gamma_2, \ldots, \gamma_p$ in the prospective model (8.10). Despite this fact, the maximum likelihood estimates $\hat{\beta}_1, \hat{\gamma}_2, \ldots, \hat{\gamma}_p$ derived from fitting the model (8.10), which takes the presence or absence of *disease* as the dependent variable, will generally differ from the maximum likelihood estimates derived from fitting the model (8.41), which takes the presence or absence of *exposure* as the dependent variable. The two models yield increasingly similar estimates of these parameters, however, with increasing degrees of adjustment through the terms $\Sigma\beta_i x_i$ and $\Sigma\beta_i^* x_i$ in the two model equations. When the variables $x_2, \ldots, x_p$ are discrete, the maximum likelihood estimates of the parameters $\beta_1, \gamma_2, \ldots, \gamma_p$ will be identical for the two models when the number of parameters in the terms $\Sigma\beta_i x_i$ and $\Sigma\beta_i^* x_i$ is equal to the number of cells formed by the multiple cross-classification of the variables $x_2, \ldots, x_p$ (Breslow and Powers 1978).

The parameters β_0 and $\beta_2, \ldots, \beta_p$ in the prospective model (8.10) relate a set of variables to the occurrence of *disease*, whereas β_0^* and β_2^*, $\ldots, \beta_p^*$ in the retrospective model (8.41) relate the variables to the occurrence of *exposure*. As a consequence, these two sets of parameters have different interpretations, and their estimates will not be equal.

There are two advantages to using the "prospective" model (8.10) or (8.1) for the analysis of a case-control study. First, all of the parameters may be interpreted in terms of associations between the variables and the study disease. This is usually of greater interest than an association of the variables with the study exposure. A second advantage of using the prospective formulation occurs when one has a continuous risk factor or when several risk factors are being considered simultaneously. One models their effects and interactions in a case-control study using equations (8.1) or (8.10) exactly as one would for a cohort study. Using the retrospective formulation of equation (8.41), one would have to categorize the individual and joint "exposures" to the risk factors into a relatively few categories representing differing levels of exposure. One would then need to fit a logistic model for each level of exposure relative to some designated reference level. [See Breslow and Powers (1978) for details.] The retrospective formulation is more convenient for assessing the effect of a single dichotomous exposure when there are several case and/or control types. In this circumstance, one may use a model such as (8.41), introducing a set of indicator variables for the disease and control categories in place of the variable d. Cox (1966, 1970) describes the corresponding analysis for the prospective model in which the response variable has multiple categories.

8.8 MATCHED ANALYSIS

Estimation of Logistic Parameters

Logistic regression can be applied to the analysis of matched case-control studies with either a single control per case (Prentice 1976, Holford 1978, Holford, White, and Kelsey 1978) or multiple controls per case (Thomas 1977, Breslow et al. 1978). The logistic model is specified precisely as in equations (8.1) or (8.10), except that the term β_0 is allowed to vary among the pairs or matched sets.

Suppose that controls are matched to cases on the basis of a set of variables $z_1, \ldots, z_k$. The risk of disease associated with the unmatched variables $x_1, \ldots, x_p$ for each member of the jth pair (or matched set) may be represented as

$$p_x = p(d = 1 | x) = 1/\{1 + \exp[-(\alpha_j + \sum_{i=1}^{p} \beta_i x_i)]\}. \quad (8.45)$$

The term α_j represents the effect of the particular configuration of matching variables for the jth pair or matched set, whereas the coefficient β_i represents the additional effect of the variable x_i. One sees from (8.45) that the relationship between each variable x_i and the risk of disease is assumed to be the same for all pairs or matched sets.

From (8.45), the logit of risk as a function of the variables $x_1, \ldots, x_p$ is

$$\ln p_x/q_x = \alpha_j + \sum_{i=1}^{p} \beta_i x_i. \quad (8.46)$$

Thus, for two individuals who are identical on the matching variables $z_1, \ldots, z_k$, the relative odds of disease for an individual with values $x_1^*, \ldots, x_p^*$ as compared with an individual with values $x_1', \ldots, x_p'$ is given by

$$\ln \psi(x^* : x') = \sum_{i=1}^{p} \beta_i(x_i^* - x_i'). \quad (8.47)$$

By referring to equation (8.23), one sees that the estimated logistic parameters $\hat{\beta}_1, \ldots, \hat{\beta}_p$ are interpreted identically for matched and unmatched analyses. Matched logistic regression extends the analysis of Miettinen (1970b), which applies to a single dichotomous exposure.

Suppose that one has matched c controls to each of n cases, and that for each individual one has information on a set of unmatched variables $x_1, \ldots, x_p$. Within the jth matched set, let the value of x_i for a case be denoted by x_{j0i} and let the value of x_i for the kth matched control be x_{jki}. Breslow et al. (1978) have shown that the mle's of the logistic parameters β_i in equation (8.45) are determined by maximizing the following conditional log likelihood function:

$$L(\beta) = -\sum_{j=1}^{n} \ln \left\{ 1 + \sum_{k=1}^{c} \exp\left[\sum_{i=1}^{p} \beta_k (x_{jki} - x_{j0i}) \right] \right\}. \quad (8.48)$$

The computations require a high-speed computer. Breslow and Day (1980) give listings of the requisite computer programs.

In the special case of $1:1$ pair matching, ordinary logistic regression can be applied to the within-pair differences on the variables x_i, so that widely available programs for fitting logistic models to unmatched data can be applied in this situation (Holford, White, and Kelsey 1978). Breslow and Day (1980) also provide computer programs for analyses of more generally matched designs, including frequency matching and variable numbers of controls per case.

Any variable used for matching cannot be studied as a risk factor, since cases and controls are constrained to be "equal" with respect to variables that are matched. From the log likelihood function (8.48), one sees that if controls were exactly matched to cases on a particular variable, say x_m, then $(x_{jkm} - x_{j0m}) = 0$ for all values of j and k. The terms involving β_m would therefore drop out of equation (8.48), so that one could not obtain an estimate of β_m, which represents the effect of the variable x_m.

With cases and controls matched on a set of variables $z_1, \ldots, z_k$, one cannot obtain unbiased estimates of their effects on the risk of disease. One may, however, investigate whether the odds ratio involving the study disease and any unmatched variable depends on a variable used for matching. This is done by performing a paired analysis within strata of the matching variable, or by incorporating interaction terms in the logistic model (Prentice 1976, Breslow et al. 1978). By introducing an interaction term such as $\gamma_i(z_i x_m)$ in the logistic model, one can determine whether the effect of the unmatched variable x_m depends on the value of the matched variable z_i. Although this may seem peculiar at first glance, one can give an intuitive explanation for its correctness.

Consider, for example, controls matched exactly on age to cases. Then one could not discriminate a case from a control on this basis; age would appear to have no association with disease. The effect (if any) of age was "matched out." Now consider some other variable, say, use of oral contraceptives, for which there was no case-control matching. One could estimate an overall association between oral contraceptive use and disease by using the paired estimate of the odds ratio $\hat{\psi} = B/C$ (Chapter 7). Furthermore, one could stratify cases on the basis of the matching variable age. Since the controls are assumed to be exactly matched on age to the cases, one could retain the pairing across the age strata, and obtain a paired estimate of the odds ratio, in the jth stratum $\hat{\psi}_j = B_j/C_j$, for each of the age strata. If $\hat{\psi}_j$ varied significantly across the strata, then one would have evidence for an interaction on a multiplicative scale between the effects of age and oral contraceptive use.

Unmatched Analysis of Matched Data

If cases and controls have been matched on a variable that is associated with the study exposure, then an analysis that does not account for the matching will result in an estimate of the odds ratio that is biased toward unity (Chapter 4). On the other hand, if matching were done on the basis of variables that were not associated with exposure, an analysis that accounted for the matching would be unnecessary and would increase the variance of the estimated logistic parameters $\hat{\beta}_i$. As a consequence, the odds ratio would be less precisely estimated (Chase 1968, Breslow et al. 1978). Thus an important issue concerns the extent to which it is necessry to account for the matching in the analysis.

With variables such as sex, race, age, or socioeconomic status, matching is somewhat arbitrary in the sense that any two individuals may be paired, provided they are similar on all of the matching variables. This situation differs from that in which siblings, relatives, or associates of cases are used as pair-matched controls, since this basis of pairing generally distinguishes each pair uniquely.

In situations where pairing is done on the basis of factors that have a quantitative or qualitative dimension that can be used for grouping, one may consider a stratified analysis as an alternative to a fully paired analysis. For example, suppose that controls were matched to cases on the basis of sex (male, female), ethnic group (white, black, Asian) and age ($\pm$ 2 years). If the target population of interest has an age range of 30–49 years, one might stratify the age variable into four groups (30–34, 35–39, 40–44, 45–49). One would then have a total of 24 subgroups ($2 \times 3 \times 4$) resulting from the multiple cross-classification of the three matching variables. To control for the effect of the matching variables by means of the preceding stratification, one designates one of the subgroups as a reference (e.g., white females 30–34 years of age) and introduces indicator variables I_j for each of the remaining subgroups. One may then fit the following logistic model:

$$p_x = p(d = 1 \,|\, x) = 1/\{1 + \exp[-(\alpha_0 + \sum_{j=1}^{23} \alpha_j I_j + \sum_{i=1}^{p} \beta_i x_i)]\} \cdot$$

The parameters of substantive interest are the βs, which represent the effects of the variables $x_1, \ldots, x_p$ adjusted for the joint effects of the matching factors. The terms $\alpha_1, \ldots, \alpha_{23}$ represent the effects of each subgroup relative to the reference.

In some instances one or more subgroups will have cases but no controls, or vice versa. In this situation, the maximum likelihood estimates of the parameters α_j corresponding to these strata are undefined, and the algorithm for calculating the estimates will not converge. One approach to handling this problem is to omit the data from these subgroups. Anderson (1974) gives a heuristic argument for an alternative procedure that retains all of the data.

Related to the problem of subgroups that lack either cases or controls is the question of whether all of the matching factors need to be considered in forming the strata. Thus, if age could be dropped from the preceding analysis, one would have only six strata instead of the original 24. The problem of subgroups containing only cases or controls would accordingly diminish. Another possibility is a coarser grouping on age, perhaps using two strata (30–39, 40–49) instead of four. A weakness of the stratified approach becomes apparent when one considers subgroup boundaries. Thus, a white male who is 29 years old is grouped with one who is 25 years old, rather than with one who is 30 years old, etc.

In practice, the only unequivocal way of determining whether the matching can be eliminated, or whether one or more matching factors may be deleted in a stratified analysis, is to compare a fully matched analysis with an unmatched analysis and with alternative stratified analyses that incorporate the matching factors in various combinations. This approach is illustrated by an analysis of a case-control study of oesophageal cancer in Iran (Breslow et al. 1978). Since cancer incidence and many environmental variables showed marked geographic variation, controls were matched to cases by village of residence as well as by age and sex. The analysis focused on the effects of social class, garden ownership, and the consumption of cucumbers and raw, green vegetables. These represented the best available indicators of socioeconomic and dietary status.

The first column of Table 8.7 shows the estimated effects $(\hat{\beta}_i)$ of the socioeconomic and dietary variables in a logistic analysis that retained the individual case-control matching. The last column shows the estimated coefficients from the logistic analysis that ignored the matching. All of the coefficients are biased toward zero (odds ratios are thus biased toward unity), indicating smaller effects on risk. The remaining columns show the estimated coefficients when one replaces the pairing by various levels of stratification. This is accomplished by performing an unmatched analysis with indicator variables for each of the strata formed by the matching variables. As the degree of stratification increases, from 4 to 6 to 28 strata, the coefficients $\hat{\beta}_i$ converge to the estimates based on the fully paired analysis, which involved 80 strata (80 cases, each matched to 4 controls).

Table 8.7. Case-Control Study of Oesophageal Cancer in Iran: Coefficients (± Standard Errors) of Variables in the Multiple Relative Risk Function, Using a Variety of Analyses

	Type of analysis					
		Stratified into:				
Variables in equation	Fully matched	7 regions, 4 age groups	4 regions, 4 age groups	4 regions	4 age groups	Unmatched
	Coeff. ± SE	Coeff. ± SE	Coeff. ± SE	Coeff. ± SE	Coeff. ± SE	Coeff. ± SE
Social class	−1.125 ± 0.254	−0.808 ± 0.212	−0.782 ± 0.206	−0.745 ± 0.201	−0.684 ± 0.180	−0.682 ± 0.179
Ownership of garden	−0.815 ± 0.250	−0.614 ± 0.222	−0.602 ± 0.219	−0.592 ± 0.218	−0.326 ± 0.191	−0.307 ± 0.190
Consumption of raw green vegetables	−0.552 ± 0.220	−0.459 ± 0.203	−0.439 ± 0.199	−0.432 ± 0.198	−0.429 ± 0.188	−0.440 ± 0.187
Consumption of cucumbers	−0.640 ± 0.217	−0.539 ± 0.196	−0.548 ± 0.192	−0.562 ± 0.192	−0.466 ± 0.182	−0.449 ± 0.181
Log likelihood	−187.69	−388.27	−388.80	−390.40	−393.52	−394.78

Source: Breslow et al. 1978.

Compared with the fully matched estimates, the coefficients $\hat{\beta}_i$ resulting from an analysis using 4 strata for region show less bias than those based on an analysis using 4 age strata. This suggests that region is a more important matching variable. Also note the increase in the standard errors of the estimates the more finely one incorporates the matching. The trade-off between matched, unmatched, and stratified analyses is thus one of reducing the variance of an estimate at the risk of increasing its bias.

8.9 CONFOUNDER SCORE

A technique that simplifies the explanation and reporting of results of a multivariate analysis, and is intuitively appealing, is the use of a *confounder score* (Miettinen 1976b). Each case and control is assigned a score that indicates how "caselike" that person is estimated to be in the absence of exposure to the study factor. The score is based on variables that either are risk factors for the disease or are related to exposure. These are potential confounders for the disease-exposure association under study. On the basis of the confounder score, each individual is assigned to one of several (usually 5) strata. This allows one to compute stratum-specific odds ratios and a combined estimate by the Mantel-Haenszel method. One may also assess whether the odds ratios vary across the strata.

For this technique to be of any use, the score function must be carefully chosen. There are numerous possibilities, but the most appropriate scoring method is generally based on logistic regression. Let $x_1, \ldots, x_p$ be a set of variables in which x_1 represents the study factor of primary interest, where $x_1 = 1$ (exposed) and $x_1 = 0$ (unexposed). Taking case-control status as the dependent variable in a logistic regression analysis, the estimated log odds for the jth individual (either a case or a control), with values $x_{j1}, \ldots, x_{jp}$ for the variables $x_1, \ldots, x_p$, is given by

$$\ln p_j/q_j = \hat{\beta}_0 + \hat{\beta}_1 x_{j1} + \ldots + \hat{\beta}_p x_{jp}.$$

For each case and control, one sets $x_{j1} = 0$ and computes the score

$$\hat{s}_j = \hat{\beta}_0 + \hat{\beta}_2 x_{j2} + \ldots + \hat{\beta}_p x_{jp}. \tag{8.45}$$

Based on data from a case-control study, the score $\hat{s}_j$ estimates the log odds of "disease" for the jth individual, had he not been exposed to the study factor x_1. If the score function were derived from cohort study data, then $\hat{s}_j$ would represent the estimated logit of risk in the absence of exposure. Thus, grouping individuals on the basis of their scores $\hat{s}_j$ provides a means of forming strata in which cases and controls were presumably at equal risk of disease, apart from their respective exposures to the study factor x_1.

Next, the scores need to be partitioned into groups. A rule of thumb (Miettinen 1976b) suggests that one compare the scores for the cases with those for the controls and exclude any individuals with scores that are far beyond the common range. One then examines the deciles of the remaining set of scores, and combines adjacent strata until only five remain. Essentially one wants to group the scores into strata of approximately equal size, while minimizing within-strata differences and maximizing the differences between strata. Disease-exposure odds ratios may then be computed separately for each of the strata, tested for variation across strata, and combined by the Mantel-Haenszel technique to form a summary estimate that is adjusted for the joint potential confounding effect of the variables $x_2, \ldots, x_p$. In practice, the resulting estimate $\hat{\psi}_{mh}$ is likely to be close to the estimate $\hat{\psi} = \exp(\hat{\beta}_1)$ based directly on the fitted logistic regression model.

As an example of the confounder score technique, consider again the data in Table 7.6. Suppose that one wants to assess the effect of recent oral contraceptive use on the risk of a myocardial infarction. Table 8.2 gives the maximum likelihood estimates of the linear logistic model involving OC use (x_1), age (x_2) and smoking (x_3, x_4). The corresponding score function is given by

$$\hat{s} = -9.2834 + 0.1521x_2 + 1.1246x_3 + 2.1371x_4.$$

Table 8.8 shows the scores for each level of the variables x_2 (age), x_3 (1–24 cigarettes per day), and x_4 (25 or more cigarettes per day), along with the number of cases and controls from Table 7.6. Since age and smoking are grouped, there are only 15 distinct values of $\hat{s}_j$, corresponding to the 15 subgroups resulting from the cross-classification of age and smoking. Had these variables been treated as continuous factors, the score function could have taken a possible 1976 values (234 cases + 1742 controls).

Table 8.9 shows a grouping of the scores and demonstrates a definite trend in the odds ratio. Compared with individuals with the lowest scores (Group I), the relative odds of disease increase with increasing values of the confounder score. This table highlights the usefulness of communicating results of a multivariate analysis in terms of a confounder score.

Table 8.8. Confounder Score ($\hat{s}_j$) and Corresponding Rank for Each Level of Variables x_2 (Age), x_3 (1-24 Cig/Day) and x_4 (≥ 25 Cig/Day)[1]

x_2	x_3	x_4	$\hat{s}_j$	Rank	No. cases	No. controls
27	0	0	-5.18	1	1	131
32	0	0	-4.42	2	0	188
37	0	0	-3.66	4	3	161
42	0	0	-2.90	7	11	169
47	0	0	-2.14	10	23	157
27	1	0	-4.05	3	1	104
32	1	0	-3.29	5	6	152
37	1	0	-2.53	8	12	130
42	1	0	-1.77	11	21	134
47	1	0	-1.01	13	42	97
27	0	1	-3.04	6	4	51
32	0	1	-2.28	9	15	83
37	0	1	-1.52	12	22	65
42	0	1	-0.76	14	39	68
47	0	1	$+0.00$	15	34	52

1. $\hat{s}_j = -9.2834 + 0.1521x_2 + 2.1371x_3 + 1.1246x_4$, based on logistic regression analysis (Table 8.2) of data in Table 7.6.

Table 8.9. Stratification Based on Confounder Score

Score	Group	No. cases	(%)	No. controls	(%)	Odds ratio
-5.18 -4.42 -4.05	I	2	(0.9)	423	(24.3)	1.0[1]
-3.66 -3.29	II	9	(3.8)	313	(18.0)	6.1
-3.04 -2.90 -2.53	III	27	(11.5)	350	(20.1)	16.3
-2.28 -2.14 -1.77 -1.52	IV	81	(34.6)	439	(25.2)	39.0
-1.01 -0.76 0.00	V	115	(49.1)	217	(12.5)	112.1
	Total	234	(99.9)	1742	(100.1)	

1. Reference group.

Table 8.10. Relation of Oral Contraceptive Use to
Myocardial Infarction within Confounder Score Subgroups

Group	OC use	MI	Control	Group-specific odds ratio
I	Yes	1	63	5.71
	No	1	360	
II	Yes	1	18	2.05
	No	8	295	
III	Yes	5	27	2.72
	No	22	323	
IV	Yes	14	23	3.78
	No	67	416	
V	Yes	8	4	3.98
	No	107	213	
Total	Yes	29	135	1.68
	No	205	1607	

The score combines the individual effects of all of the variables $x_2, \ldots,$ x_p, excluding the primary study factor, into a single index of susceptibility to the study disease.

In relative terms, the odds of disease for individuals in Group V is 112 times greater than the odds of disease in Group I. However, this tells us nothing about the effect of recent use of oral contraceptives on the risk of myocardial infarction, which is the association of primary interest. Table 8.10 pursues this issue by showing oral contraceptive use for cases and controls within each of the five strata of the confounder score, along with the stratum-specific estimates of the MI-OC odds ratio. The Mantel-Haenszel combined estimate of the MI-OC odds ratio is $\hat{\psi}_{mh} = 3.48$ with an approximate 95 percent confidence interval (2.02, 5.79). Thus, adjusted for differences in susceptibility to MI due to smoking and age, the risk of an MI is 3.5 times higher among women who recently used oral contraceptives. The result is very similar to the estimate based directly on logistic regression. From Table 8.2, the estimated relative odds of an MI associated with oral contraceptive use, adjusted for smoking and age, is $\hat{\psi} = \exp(1.1883) = 3.28$, with an approximate 95 percent confidence interval (1.97, 5.47). [The Mantel-Haenszel estimate of the MI-OC odds ratio, adjusted for age and smoking by direct stratification on these factors, is $\hat{\psi}_{mh} = 3.33$ (Chapter 7, Section 7.2).]

The fact that the crude estimate of the MI-OC odds ratio $\hat{\psi} = 1.68$ is smaller than all of the stratum-specific estimates in Table 8.10 is noteworthy, and is explained by making further calculations from this table. Whereas the preponderance of cases (196 of 234) occur in Groups IV and V, only a small fraction of the controls (656 of 1742) occur in these strata. Furthermore, oral contraceptive use is least common in Groups IV and V. Among the 852 individuals in these groups, 49 were recent users. By contrast, there were 115 users of OCs among the 1124 individuals in Groups I–III. Failure to control for confounding by age and smoking thus effectively overestimates the OC exposure rate among controls. As a result, the crude MI-OC odds ratio is spuriously low.

The confounder score technique should be used judiciously. The possibility of important interactions between the study factor and one or more of the variables included in the score function should not be ignored. One cannot determine from the preceding analysis, for example, whether or not there is an interactive effect of smoking and oral contraceptive use on the risk of myocardial infarction. The confounder score technique can be applied to answer questions of interaction, however. For example, suppose that one is interested in assessing the individual and joint effects of two variables, say x_1 and x_2, with adjustment for the effects of a set of other variables $x_3, \ldots, x_p$. One can fit the logistic model

$$\ln p_x/q_x = \beta_0 + \beta_1 x_1 + \beta_2 x_2 + \gamma(x_1 x_2) + \beta_3 x_3 + \ldots + \beta_p x_p,$$

and estimate the following score function for the jth individual:

$$\hat{s}_j = \hat{\beta}_3 x_{3j} + \ldots + \hat{\beta}_p x_{pj}.$$

For each stratum of the confounder score, one may then look at the distribution of cases and controls within subgroups formed by the cross-classification of variables x_1 and x_2. Estimates of the individual and joint effects of x_1 and x_2, which are adjusted for the effects of variables x_3, $\ldots$, x_p, are then derived by the approach of Section 7.3 in Chapter 7. As the number and complexity of potential interactions increase, a confounder score approach is best replaced by an analysis using logistic regression or loglinear models.

As a general precaution, one should review the profiles of cases and controls on each of the confounding factors within strata of the confounder score. This provides a check that cases and controls, although falling in the same stratum, are not greatly different on the confounders, which may also prove to be unsuspected effect modifiers. If there are large differences, one may want to choose alternative stratum boundaries. The exposure factor x_1 need not be dichotomous. Miettinen (1976b) gives an example in which the exposure is taken to be daily consumption of coffee, expressed in cups per day and represented by three strata (0, 1–5, 6 or more).

If the logistic model that is used to construct the confounder score correctly represents the relationship between the variables $x_1, \ldots, x_p$ and the risk of disease, then the estimated disease-exposure odds ratio based on either logistic regression or the confounder score technique will agree. The confounder score approach, however, may yield an exaggerated significance level (Pike, Anderson, and Day 1979).

The confounder score technique is closely related to the use of matching based on a linear discriminant function, suggested by Cochran and Rubin (1973) as a method for controlling bias in observational studies. Table 1.3 (Chapter 1) shows an application of the confounder score technique to the analysis of a historical cohort study (Neutra et al. 1978). Examples of its use in case-control studies are given by Stasson et al. (1976) and by Jick et al. (1973). The paper by Miettinen (1976b) should be consulted for a more detailed discussion of the method.

8.10 LOGLINEAR MODELS

Loglinear models provide a unified approach to analyzing case-control data when all of the variables of interest are discrete, being either categorical variables or continuous variables that have been stratified. For data arranged in a multidimensional contingency table, a loglinear model represents the logarithm of the expected cell counts in terms of parameters that denote the individual and joint effects of the variables forming the multiple cross-classification. A loglinear model does not distinguish between explanatory (independent) variables and response (dependent) variables. However, when such a distinction is appropriate, a loglinear model can be converted into a logistic or logit model in which the log odds of the response variable is represented as a linear combination of the effects of the explanatory variables (Fienberg 1980).

To fix ideas, refer back to the data in Table 7.9, which derives from a case-control study of lung cancer among male residents of an 11-county area of coastal Georgia (Blot et al. 1978). Employment in shipbuilding (six months or more), cigarette smoking, and case-control status constitute the three dimensions of this contingency table. Let x_{ijk} denote the observed frequencies in the table. The index (i) represents the levels of variable 1, case-control status, with $i = 1$ (case) or 2 (control); the index (j) represents the level of variable 2, employment in shipbuilding, with

$j = 1$ (yes) or 2 (no); the index k represents the levels of variable 3, smoking, with $k = 1$ (minimal), 2 (moderate), or 3 (heavy). Thus $x_{111} = 11$, $x_{121} = 50$, $x_{112} = 70$, ..., $x_{213} = 3$, $x_{223} = 50$.

If one writes m_{ijk} for the expected values of the corresponding observed frequencies x_{ijk}, then the general loglinear model for a three-dimensional table may be written, using notation similar to the analysis of variance, as

$$\ln m_{ijk} = u + u_{1(i)} + u_{2(j)} + u_{3(k)} + u_{12(ij)}$$
$$+ u_{13(ik)} + u_{23(jk)} + u_{123(ijk)}. \qquad (8.46)$$

We shall indicate shortly that the parameters of the loglinear model, the u terms, are best interpreted for our purposes in terms of odds and odds ratios. As in the analysis of variance, the u terms may be regarded as *main effects* $[u_{1(i)}, u_{2(j)}, u_{3(k)}]$, *first order interactions* $[u_{12(ij)}, u_{13(ik)}, u_{23(jk)}]$ and *second order interactions* $[u_{123(ijk)}]$ for the three variables. For example, the parameters $u_{12(11)}$, $u_{12(12)}$, $u_{12(21)}$, and $u_{12(22)}$ are four terms which constitute the first order interaction between variables 1 and 2.

In general, the first variable, corresponding to case-control status, may have $i = 1, \ldots, I$ different categories. For instance, one may have controls deriving from several sources or cases stratified by severity of disease or certainty of diagnosis. Similarly, the second variable, which we shall regard as the exposure or study factor of primary interest, may have $j = 1, \ldots, J$ different categories. Thus, employment in shipbuilding may be categorized by the specific job performed (welder, painter, engineer, etc.) or years of service, rather than simply "yes" or "no" as in Table 7.9. Finally, the third variable, corresponding to some factor that may alter the effect of exposure on the risk of disease, or otherwise confound a disease-exposure association, may have $k = 1, \ldots, K$ different categories. For simplicity of discussion, we shall assume that $I = 2$ and $J = 2$.

The observed odds of "disease" (the odds of being a "case" within a sample of cases and controls) are equal to x_{1jk}/x_{2jk} for any level (j, k) of the other two variables. The expected odds of "disease" are m_{1jk}/m_{2jk}, and the log odds, from equation (8.46), is

$$\ln(m_{1jk}/m_{2jk}) = [u_{1(1)} - u_{1(2)}] + [u_{12(1j)} - u_{12(2j)}]$$
$$+ [u_{13(1k)} - u_{13(2k)}] + [u_{123(1jk)} - u_{123(2jk)}]. \qquad (8.47)$$

The parameters of a loglinear model are subject to the constraint that the summation over any index i, j, or k is equal to zero. Thus $\Sigma_i u_{1(i)} = \Sigma_j u_{2(j)} = \Sigma_k u_{3(k)} = 0$. Similarly $\Sigma_i u_{12(ij)} = \Sigma_j u_{12(ij)} = 0$, and so forth.

As a result of these constraints, equation (8.47) can be written

$$\ln(m_{1jk}/m_{2jk}) = 2[u_{1(1)} + u_{12(1j)} + u_{13(1k)} + u_{123(1jk)}]$$
$$= w + w_{2(j)} + w_{3(k)} + w_{23(jk)}. \qquad (8.48)$$

The w terms represent the effects of a constant term, $w = 2u_{1(1)}$, terms that depend only on the level of the second variable, $w_{2(j)} = 2u_{12(1j)}$, terms that depend only on the level of the third variable, $w_{3(k)} = 2u_{13(1k)}$, and terms that depend on the joint levels of the second and third variables, $w_{23(jk)} = 2u_{123(1jk)}$. The representation of the log odds in (8.48) is called a *logit model*.

The ratio of the odds of "disease" among exposed individuals ($j = 1$) relative to the odds of "disease" among unexposed individuals ($j = 2$) can be expressed as

$$\psi = (m_{11k}/m_{21k}) \div (m_{12k}/m_{22k}) = (m_{11k}\, m_{22k})/(m_{21k}\, m_{12k}). \qquad (8.49)$$

Using equation (8.48), one therefore can write

$$\ln \psi = [w_{2(1)} - w_{2(2)}] + [w_{23(1k)} - w_{23(2k)}] = w^* + w^*_{3(k)}. \qquad (8.50)$$

The disease-exposure odds ratio ψ is thus seen to depend on the level of the third variable:

$$\psi = \exp[w^* + w^*_{3(k)}]. \qquad (8.51)$$

The loglinear model (8.46) includes a three-factor interaction term, $u_{123(ijk)}$. The preceding development indicates that the presence of a three-factor interaction in a loglinear model implies that the odds ratio (involving variables 1 and 2) depends on the level of the third variable. In the absence of a three-factor interaction, that is, $u_{123(ijk)} = 0$ for all values of i, j, and k, the disease-exposure odds ratio ψ is constant:

$$\psi = \exp(w^*).$$

Thus, in a loglinear model involving three variables, the absence of a three-factor interaction implies that the odds ratio involving variables 1 and 2 is constant across the levels of the third variable.

Interaction terms involving variable 1 (case-control status), such as u_{12}, u_{13}, and u_{123} imply that the log odds of "disease" depends respectively on variable 2, on variable 3, and on the joint presence of variables 2 and 3. Similarly, interaction terms involving variable 2 (exposure), such as u_{12}, u_{23}, and u_{123} imply that the log odds of exposure depends respectively on variable 1, on variable 3, and on the joint presence of variables 1 and 3.

If one had a four-dimensional contingency table, the existence of the following three-factor interactions, $u_{123(ijk)}$ and $u_{124(ijl)}$, would imply that the disease-exposure odds ratio (involving variables 1 and 2) depended on variable 3 and on variable 4. Thus, corresponding to the following loglinear model

$$\ln m_{ijkl} = u + u_{1(i)} + u_{2(j)} + u_{3(k)} + u_{4(l)} + u_{12(ij)} \tag{8.52}$$
$$+ u_{13(ik)} + u_{23(jk)} + u_{24(jl)} + u_{123(ijk)} + u_{124(ijl)},$$

the log odds ratio, $\ln \psi = \ln(m_{11kl}m_{22kl})/(m_{12kl}m_{21kl})$, is given by

$$\ln \psi = w^* + w^*_{3(k)} + w^*_{4(l)}. \tag{8.53}$$

The terms w^*, $w^*_{3(k)}$ and $w^*_{4(l)}$ in equation (8.53) may be expressed in terms of the parameters in (8.52):

$$w^* = [u_{12(11)} - u_{12(12)}] - [u_{12(21)} - u_{12(22)}],$$
$$w^*_{3(k)} = [u_{123(11k)} - u_{123(12k)}] - [u_{123(21k)} - u_{123(22k)}],$$

and

$$w^*_{4(l)} = [u_{124(11l)} - u_{124(12l)}] - [u_{124(21l)} - u_{124(22l)}].$$

If a four-factor interaction $u_{1234(ijkl)}$ were included in the loglinear model (8.52), then the odds ratio would not only depend on variables 3 and 4 separately, but also on their joint effect:

$$\ln \psi = w^* + w^*_{3(k)} + w^*_{4(l)} + w^*_{34(kl)}. \tag{8.54}$$

The term $w^*_{34(kl)}$ is given by

$$w^*_{34(kl)} = [u_{1234(11kl)} - u_{1234(12kl)}] - [u_{1234(21kl)} - u_{1234(22kl)}].$$

Similarly, if a fifth variable were included in the analysis, a loglinear model involving interaction terms u_{123}, u_{124}, u_{1234}, and u_{125} would imply that the logarithm of the disease-exposure odds ratio is given by

$$\ln \psi = w^* + w^*_{3(k)} + w^*_{4(l)} + w^*_{34(kl)} + w^*_{5(m)}.$$

The reader undoubtedly sees the generalization to this discussion. Namely, any interaction term that jointly involves one or more variables along with exposure and case-control status implies that the disease-exposure odds ratio depends on those variables specified in the loglinear interaction term.

Transforming the parameters for a loglinear model to those for the corresponding model for logits or log odds ratios can be tedious, unless one has a computer program that will perform the task. More important is understanding the connection between the various representations based on the loglinear, logit, and log odds ratio models. Rarely does one need the parameter estimates (u terms) from a loglinear model, since an analysis focuses on estimates of the expected cell frequencies $\hat{m}_{ijk}$ and the estimated odds ratios. The latter may be calculated directly from the $\hat{m}_{ijk}$.

An Application of Loglinear Models

Details of the procedures by which the parameters of a loglinear model are estimated may be found in Haberman (1978) or Bishop, Fienberg, and Holland (1975). For our purposes, it suffices to know that several computer programs are available that perform the necessary computations. Perhaps the most widely available program is the BMDP program P3F (Dixon and Brown 1979), which we have used for our calculations. This program uses the iterative proportional fitting algorithm given by Haberman (1972).

Using the data in Table 7.9, the expected frequencies based on fitting the following loglinear model

$$\ln m_{ijk} = u + u_{1(i)} + u_{2(j)} + u_{3(k)} + u_{12(ij)} + u_{13(ik)} + u_{23(jk)} \quad (8.55)$$

are given in Table 8.11. Although the data in Table 7.9 suggest a trend in the smoking-specific estimates of the relative odds of lung cancer associated with shipbuilding, the likelihood ratio test (refer to following section on goodness-of-fit) for a three-factor interaction gives a nonsignificant chi-square ($G_2^2 = 0.85$, $p = 0.65$). By comparing observed and expected values in Tables 7.9 and 8.11 respectively, one sees that slight changes in frequency can produce rather large changes in the estimated odds ratios. Cells with small frequencies contribute to instability of the estimates.

The loglinear model (8.55) corresponds to the following logit model

$$\ln p/q = \beta_0 + \beta_1 B + \beta_2 S_1 + \beta_3 S_3, \quad (8.56)$$

where B represents employment in shipbuilding, 1 (yes) or 0 (no), and S_1 and S_2 are indicator variables for smoking. S_1 takes the values 1 (moderate) or 0 (not moderate), and S_2 takes the values 1 (heavy) or 0 (not heavy). Using logistic regression, the estimated equation based on maximum likelihood is

$$\ln p/q = -1.4459 + 0.4892B + 1.4390S_1 + 2.1293S_2. \quad (8.57)$$

Adjusted for smoking, the relative odds of lung cancer associated with employment in shipbuilding is estimated from (8.57) to be $\hat{\psi} = \exp(0.4892) = 1.63$. This is equivalent (see Table 8.11) to the estimate based on the loglinear model in equation (8.55). The estimated standard

Table 8.11. Expected Numbers of Cases and Controls
Based on Fitting the Loglinear Model (8.55) to Table 7.9

Smoking	Shipbuilding	Cancer	Control	$\hat{\psi}_i$
Minimal	Yes	12.8	33.2	1.63
	No	48.2	204.8	
Moderate	Yes	69.2	42.8	1.63
	No	217.8	219.2	
Heavy	Yes	13.0	4.0	1.63
	No	97.0	49.0	

Test of Fit	df	p-value
$\chi^2 = 0.81$	2	0.67
$G^2 = 0.85$	2	0.65

error of $\hat{\beta}_1$ is 0.1780, so that an approximate 95 percent confidence interval for ψ is calculated from equation (8.29) to be (1.15, 2.31). One should consult Haberman (1978) for general formulae and detailed examples of confidence interval calculations for odds-ratio estimates based on loglinear models.

Goodness-of-fit

A test of the goodness-of-fit of a loglinear model is based on a comparison of the observed (O_i) and estimated (E_i) frequencies in each of the cells of the contingency table. Either the Pearson chi-square test

$$\chi^2 = \Sigma(O_i - E_i)^2/E_i \qquad (8.58)$$

or the likelihood ratio test

$$G^2 = 2\Sigma O_i \ln(O_i/E_i) \qquad (8.59)$$

may be used. Summations are taken over all cells in the table. If the fitted model is "correct," then in large samples both χ^2 and G^2 have chi-square distributions with $n - p$ degrees of freedom, where n is the number of cells in the contingency table, and p is the number of independent parameters estimated in the loglinear model. Fienberg (1980) has suggested that as a rule of thumb one might interpret "large samples" to mean that the total sample size is at least ten times the number of cells in the table. The statistics χ^2 and G^2 are commonly used even when the sample size is much smaller (Larntz 1978, Fienberg 1979), although the adequacy of the chi-square approximation to their distributions in small samples is not completely known.

Lack of fit for a given model is indicated by values of χ^2 or G^2 that are "large," in the sense that the associated p-value determined from the chi-square approximation is "small" (for example, $p < 0.05$). Referring to Table 8.11, one sees that the loglinear model (8.55) provides a good fit to the data in Table 7.9, since both χ^2 and G^2 have large p-values.

Model Selection

The observed frequencies in any contingency table can be reproduced exactly by fitting a *saturated model*. This is a model in which the number of independent parameters equals the number of cells in the table. Such models yield values of χ^2 or G^2 equal to zero, indicating perfect fit. Equation (8.46) gives the saturated model for a three-dimensional table.

On grounds of parsimony, one often prefers a simpler model over a more complicated one that provides a better fit. There is a trade-off between model simplicity and goodness-of-fit, and the likelihood ratio statistic G^2 can be used to test whether the improvement in fit of a more complicated model falls within the random variation expected on the basis of the simpler model.

Two loglinear models are *nested* if all of the u terms in one are a subset of the terms included in the other. By comparing a simpler model M_1 that is nested within a more complicated model M_2, the difference in G^2 can be used to test whether the inclusion of the additional terms in M_2 "significantly" improves the fit. This is conceptually equivalent to the likelihood ratio test (8.31) for the logistic regression model. Let E_{1i} and E_{2i} denote the estimated cell frequencies under M_1 and M_2, and let m_1 and $m_2 = m_1 + k$ denote the corresponding number of parameters fitted for the two models. If the expected values in fact satisfy model M_1, then in large samples, the difference

$$G_1^2 - G_2^2 = 2 \, \Sigma O_i \, \ln(E_{2i}/E_{1i}) \qquad (8.60)$$

has an approximate chi-square distribution with $m_2 - m_1 = k$ degrees of freedom. This property does not hold for the Pearson chi-square statistic χ^2 (Fienberg 1980).

Statistical procedures for selecting a particular loglinear model typically use two criteria: (1) that the corresponding value of G^2 (or χ^2) indicates no lack of fit, and (2) that the improvement in fit of a more complicated nested model is not significant by the criterion $G_1^2 - G_2^2$.

Table 8.12. Some Possible Hierarchical Loglinear Models for Three-Dimensional Tables

Model	Bracket Notation
$u + u_1$	[1]
$u + u_2 + u_3$	[2][3]
$u + u_1 + u_2 + u_{12}$	[12]
$u + u_1 + u_2 + u_3 + u_{23}$	[1][23]
$u + u_1 + u_2 + u_3 + u_{12}$	[12][3]
$u + u_1 + u_2 + u_3 + u_{13} + u_{23}$	[13][23]
$u + u_1 + u_2 + u_3 + u_{12} + u_{13} + u_{23}$	[12][13][23]
$u + u_1 + u_2 + u_3 + u_{12} + u_{13} + u_{23} + u_{123}$	[123]

Fienberg (1980) describes several statistical procedures for selecting a loglinear model. Further discussion of this issue, which is beyond our scope, may be found in Goodman (1971), Wermuth (1976a, 1976b), Brown (1976), Whittaker and Aitkin (1978), and Fuchs (1979).

Hierarchical Loglinear Models

Hierarchical loglinear models require that whenever a higher order term is present, all of the possible lower order terms derived from variables making up the higher-order term are included in the model equation. Thus u_{12} can appear in a hierarchical model only if the terms u_1 and u_2 are also included. Inclusion of u_{123} requires that u_{12}, u_{13}, u_{23}, u_1, u_2, and u_3 are all present. We use bracket notation (Fienberg 1980) to conveniently represent hierarchical models. The loglinear model (8.46) is denoted by [123]. This notation represents only the higher order terms in the model equation, and implies that all possible combinations of variables within a pair of brackets appear in the equation (redundancies are omitted). Table 8.12 lists some of the possible hierarchical models for three-dimensional tables and shows the corresponding bracket notation. Models such as

$$\ln m_{ij} = u + u_{1(i)} + u_{12(ij)}$$

and

$$\ln m_{ijk} = u + u_{1(i)} + u_{2(j)} + u_{3(k)} + u_{12(ij)} + u_{123(ijk)}$$

are not hierarchical models. Hierarchical models are important because the constraints imposed by the maximum likelihood estimation procedures, such as the iterative proportional fitting algorithm, require that the fitted models be hierarchical (Bishop 1969, Fienberg 1980). Note that a hierarchical loglinear model requires that a variable included as an effect modifier also be included as a confounder.

Logit Models and Loglinear Models

One should recognize that different loglinear models may give rise to the same form of the logit model. Consider, for example, the following hierarchical loglinear models:

$$\ln m_{ijk} = u + u_{1(i)} + u_{2(j)} + u_{3(k)} + u_{12(ij)} \qquad (8.61)$$

and

$$\ln m_{ijk} = u + u_{1(i)} + u_{2(j)} + u_{3(k)} + u_{12(ij)} + u_{23(jk)}. \qquad (8.62)$$

Taking variable 1 as the response, the log odds ($i = 1$ vs. $i = 2$) for both of these loglinear models is given by

$$\ln(m_{1jk}/m_{2jk}) = [u_{1(1)} - u_{1(2)}] + [u_{12(1j)} - u_{12(2j)}]$$
$$= w + w_{2(j)}. \qquad (8.63)$$

For a set of data, the estimated values of the u terms based on the model (8.61) generally will not be equal to those based on the model (8.62). As a consequence, the estimates of the w terms in the logit model (8.63) will be different, even though both loglinear models give rise to the same logit representation.

Two requirements must be met in order that the estimates of the parameters of a logit model, derived from fitting a logistic regression using indicator variables, be the same as the parameter estimates derived from fitting a loglinear model (Bishop 1969, Fienberg 1980).

(1) Each term included as an explanatory variable in the logit model must be included in the corresponding hierarchical loglinear model as an interaction with the response variable.
(2) All of the explanatory variables in the contingency table must be included with their main effects and all of their higher order interactions in the hierarchical loglinear model.

Requirement (2) corresponds to conditioning on the marginal totals of the explanatory variables, which Cox (1970) has suggested should always be done, irrespective of whether these variables are fixed by the study design (Fienberg 1980).

To elaborate on the points of the previous paragraph, consider again the data in Table 7.6. Let the numbers 1, 2, 3, and 4 designate respectively the variables smoking, case-control status, oral contraceptive use, and age. Taking "disease" (case-control status) as the response variable, one might postulate a variety of models.

Consider first a logit model in which "disease" depends on OC use and age:

$$\ln(m_{i1kl}/m_{i2kl}) = w + w_{3(k)} + w_{4(l)}. \qquad (8.64)$$

The hierarchical loglinear model specified by [23][24][134] will give estimates of the w terms that are identical to the maximum likelihood estimates for the logit regression model (8.64). The terms [23][24] and [134] in the loglinear model derive from conditions (1) and (2) respectively. Although a loglinear model such as [23][24] is formally equivalent to the logit model of equation (8.64), it does not give the same estimates.

As another example, the maximum likelihood estimates for the logit model

$$\ln m_{i1kl}/m_{i2kl} = w + w_{1(i)} + w_{3(k)} + w_{4(l)} \qquad (8.65)$$

corresponds to those based on the loglinear model [21][23][24][134]. Equation (8.65) postulates that the log odds of "disease" depends on cigarette smoking (variable 1), OC use (variable 3), and age (variable 4).

As one more example, the logit model

$$\ln m_{i1kl}/m_{i2kl} = w + w_{1(i)} + w_{3(k)} + w_{4(l)} + w_{13(ik)} \qquad (8.66)$$

corresponds to the loglinear model [24][123][134]. It postulates that the log odds of "disease" depends on age and the separate and joint effects of smoking and oral contraceptive use.

The conditional approach can encounter difficulties with sparse data in a multiway contingency table. If a marginal total contains zero as an entry, and corresponds to an explanatory variable that is fixed by conditioning, then the expected values must be zero for all cells corresponding to the zero marginal. In this case, the corresponding logits and associated parameters are undefined. One way to proceed is to collapse the table over all variables that do not appear in the logit model equation, and fit a loglinear model to the collapsed table.

To continue with the discussion of Table 7.6, suppose that one were interested in the relationship between age and "disease" represented by equation (8.64). Then one could collapse Table 7.6 over smoking and oral contraceptive use, resulting in a two-dimensional contingency table involving only case-control status and age. Fitting either the logit model (8.64) or the loglinear model [24] to the collapsed table would yield identical estimates, because the preceding conditions (1) and (2) for equivalence of the parameter estimates are satisfied. However, the approach of collapsing the table over smoking and oral contraceptive use assumes that these variables neither confound nor modify the association between age and disease. [Fienberg (1980) suggests other approaches to this problem.]

Applications of loglinear models to the analysis of matched case-control studies are discussed by Holford, White, and Kelsey (1978). Holford (1978) gives further details of the theoretical basis for loglinear analyses of pair-matched case-control studies, and discusses models that allow the parameters to vary across pairs. Kullback and Cornfield (1976) use an information theoretic approach to loglinear models in an analysis of Dorn's cohort study of smoking and mortality among American veterans (Kahn 1966). Grizzle, Starmer, and Koch (1969) describe methods based on weighted least squares, which include the loglinear model as a special case. Kullback (1959) and Ku and Kullback (1974) have described the estimation of loglinear models using information theory. Both the weighted least squares and the information theory approach are asymptotically equivalent to estimation based on maximum likelihood (Nelder and Wedderburn 1972, Bishop, Fienberg, and Holland 1975).

Epilogue

Shortly after the initial finding of an association between maternal use of DES and vaginal cancer in daughters, a case-control study confirming the association was reported. Using data from the New York State Cancer Registry, which receives reports of all cancer diagnoses in New York State, exclusive of New York City, Greenwald et al. (1971) identified five women under the age of 30 who were diagnosed with adenocarcinoma of the vagina during the period 1950 through 1970. The five patients, born between the years 1951 and 1953, were 15 through 19 years of age at the time of diagnosis, and all had been exposed to synthetic estrogen therapy (stilbestrol or dienestrol) during their mothers' pregnancies. None of the mothers of eight controls who were matched to the patients on the basis of hospital and date of birth, and maternal age and parity, had a history of stilbestrol exposure.

Assuming that the risk of clear-cell cancer of the vagina or cervix is negligible among young women who were not prenatally exposed to DES, the cumulative risk through age 24 for DES-exposed females has been estimated to be in the range of 0.14 to 1.4 cancers per thousand women exposed (Herbst et al. 1977).

Subsequent experimental studies in rats and mice support an interpretation of the association between DES and vaginal cancer as one of cause and effect. In one study (Vorherr et al. 1979), transplacental and transmammary exposure of rats to DES resulted in the development of vaginal adenosis, endometrial squamous metaplasia, and genital malignancies in 20 to 40 percent of the female offspring. In exposed male offspring, hypospadias, phallic hypoplasia, and inhibition of growth and descent of testes were observed. None of the control animals, which were not exposed to DES, developed a genital malignancy. In another study,

Nomura and Kanzaki (1977) gave pregnant mice a single dose (10g/g body weight) on one of days 7 to 19, which correspond to the first to fifth months of pregnancy in humans. Although adenosis and adenocarcinoma of the vagina were not observed in the female offspring, treatment with DES on days 15 to 19 did result in the induction of persistent urogenital sinus and hypertrophy of the portio vaginalis. Depending on the day of exposure, the percentage of offspring exhibiting such anomalies varied from 0 to 93 percent. Maternal exposure to DES on days 17 to 19 produced hypoplastic undescended testes in approximately 70 percent of the male offspring. None of the control mice (77 female, 46 male) showed any the above abnormalities.

Since the initial report of Herbst, Ulfelder, and Poskanzer (1971), other concerns related to DES exposure in humans have arisen. These include the possibility that use of DES during pregnancy may have increased the maternal risk of breast cancer (Bibbo et al. 1978), that male offspring who were prenatally exposed to DES may be at increased risk of genitourinary abnormalities, abnormal spermatogenesis, and feminizing effects (DES Task Force 1978, Mills and Bongiovanni 1978), and that DES-exposed daughters may have an elevated risk of reproductive problems such as primary infertility, ectopic pregnancy, miscarriage, and premature live births (Bibbo et al. 1978, Barnes et al. 1980, Herbst et al. 1980).

APPENDIX 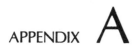A

Case-Control Sample Size

Two quantities pertaining to the study exposure need to be specified: R, the level of relative risk that is regarded as important to detect, and p_0, the exposure rate (proportion exposed) among controls.

The terms α and β represent the Type I and Type II error probabilities respectively. For specified α, β, R, and p_0, these tables give n, the sample size needed in *each* group of cases and controls in an *unmatched* study. Values of R range from .1 to 20, giving table entries that apply to both potential decreases and increases in risk. The tables may also be used for one-sided tests with significance level half the listed α.

CASE-CONTROL SAMPLE SIZE

α=.01(TWO-SIDED)   β=.01

R								P_0						
	.01	.02	.03	.04	.05	.10	.15	.20	.25	.30	.35	.40	.45	.50
0.1	3259	1623	1077	804	640	313	204	150	117	96	81	69	61	54
0.2	4512	2252	1498	1122	896	444	294	219	175	146	125	110	99	91
0.3	6398	3200	2134	1601	1282	643	431	326	264	223	194	174	159	148
0.4	9395	4708	3146	2365	1897	961	651	498	407	348	308	279	259	245
0.5	14520	7288	4878	3674	2951	1509	1032	796	657	568	507	464	435	416
0.6	24236	12184	8167	6160	4956	2554	1760	1368	1139	992	894	826	781	754
0.7	45842	23076	15490	11699	9425	4890	3393	2658	2229	1956	1774	1652	1574	1530
0.8	109345	55111	37039	28008	22593	11795	8236	6491	5479	4838	4417	4141	3971	3888
0.9	462200	233216	156917	118790	95932	50368	35369	28038	23801	21140	19412	18304	17657	17388
1.1	511874	258798	174479	132350	107098	56797	40285	32257	27658	24813	23015	21920	21358	21245
1.2	134184	67903	45821	34788	28176	15010	10694	8604	7408	6675	6219	5949	5822	5816
1.3	62401	31604	21344	16219	13147	7033	5032	4064	3515	3180	2975	2857	2808	2816
1.4	36656	18580	12558	9550	7748	4161	2989	2423	2104	1911	1794	1730	1706	1718
1.5	24456	12405	8391	6386	5184	2795	2015	1640	1429	1302	1227	1188	1175	1188
1.6	17675	8972	6073	4625	3758	2033	1471	1201	1050	961	908	882	876	888
1.7	13494	6855	4643	3538	2877	1562	1134	929	815	748	709	691	688	700
1.8	10721	5450	3694	2817	2292	1248	909	747	657	605	576	562	562	573
1.9	8779	4465	3028	2311	1881	1028	751	619	546	504	481	471	472	483
2.0	7361	3746	2542	1941	1581	866	635	525	464	430	411	404	406	416
2.5	3827	1953	1329	1017	831	461	343	287	257	241	234	232	236	245
3.0	2466	1261	860	660	541	304	228	193	175	166	162	163	167	175
3.5	1779	912	623	479	393	223	169	145	133	127	125	127	131	138
4.0	1376	707	484	373	306	176	134	116	107	103	103	105	109	116
4.5	1114	573	393	304	250	145	112	97	91	88	88	90	95	101
5.0	932	480	330	255	211	123	96	84	79	77	77	80	84	91
6.0	698	361	249	193	160	95	75	66	63	62	64	66	71	77
7.0	556	288	199	155	129	77	62	56	53	53	55	58	62	68
8.0	461	240	166	130	108	66	53	48	47	47	49	52	56	62
9.0	393	205	143	112	93	57	47	43	42	43	45	48	52	57
10.0	343	179	125	98	82	51	42	39	39	40	42	45	49	54
15.0	209	111	78	62	52	34	30	29	29	31	33	36	40	45
20.0	151	81	58	46	40	27	24	24	25	27	29	32	36	41

CASE-CONTROL SAMPLE SIZE

α=.01(TWO-SIDED) β=.01

R	P_0 .50	.55	.60	.65	.70	.75	.80	.85	.90	.95	.96	.97	.98	.99
0.1	54	49	45	42	40	39	39	42	51	82	98	125	179	343
0.2	91	84	80	77	77	79	84	96	123	211	255	330	480	932
0.3	148	141	137	135	137	144	158	185	245	433	529	688	1007	1966
0.4	245	236	232	234	241	257	287	343	461	831	1017	1329	1953	3827
0.5	416	406	404	411	430	464	525	635	866	1581	1941	2542	3746	7361
0.6	754	742	746	766	809	882	1007	1230	1697	3129	3850	5052	7461	14691
0.7	1530	1519	1538	1594	1695	1864	2145	2643	3676	6837	8426	11077	16385	32318
0.8	3888	3883	3960	4131	4425	4900	5678	7044	9867	18482	22810	30030	44484	87867
0.9	17388	17472	17923	18808	20267	22580	26320	32854	46297	87253	107816	142121	210781	416858
1.1	21245	21562	22342	23682	25778	29000	34155	43065	61297	116690	144479	190833	283595	561990
1.2	5816	5929	6170	6568	7180	8115	9595	12150	17367	33201	41142	54387	80892	160435
1.3	2816	2882	3011	3218	3532	4007	4757	6047	8676	16649	20647	27315	40657	80697
1.4	1718	1765	1851	1985	2186	2489	2966	3783	5447	10488	13016	17231	25665	50975
1.5	1188	1224	1288	1386	1532	1750	2092	2677	3866	7468	9274	12285	18309	36388
1.6	888	918	969	1046	1160	1329	1593	2044	2962	5737	7128	9448	14089	28016
1.7	700	726	768	832	925	1063	1277	1644	2388	4639	5766	7647	11409	22699
1.8	573	596	633	687	766	882	1063	1372	1998	3890	4838	6419	9582	19074
1.9	483	504	536	584	652	753	910	1177	1718	3353	4172	5538	8270	16469
2.0	416	435	464	507	568	657	796	1032	1509	2951	3674	4878	7288	14520
2.5	245	259	279	308	348	404	498	651	961	1897	2365	3146	4708	9395
3.0	175	187	203	226	258	304	374	493	732	1454	1815	2418	3623	7239
3.5	138	149	163	182	209	248	308	408	609	1216	1519	2025	3038	6075
4.0	116	126	138	156	180	214	267	355	533	1068	1336	1782	2675	5353
4.5	101	110	122	138	160	191	239	320	481	968	1211	1617	2429	4864
5.0	91	99	110	125	146	175	219	294	444	896	1122	1498	2252	4512
6.0	77	84	95	108	127	153	193	260	395	799	1002	1339	2014	4039
7.0	68	75	85	98	115	139	176	239	363	738	925	1238	1863	3738
8.0	62	69	78	90	107	130	165	224	341	695	872	1168	1758	3529
9.0	57	64	73	85	101	123	156	213	325	664	834	1116	1681	3376
10.0	54	61	69	81	96	117	150	204	313	640	804	1077	1623	3259
15.0	45	51	59	69	83	103	132	181	280	575	722	968	1460	2936
20.0	41	47	55	64	78	96	124	171	264	545	685	919	1386	2788

CASE-CONTROL SAMPLE SIZE

α=.01(TWO-SIDED) β=.05

R	P_0 .01	.02	.03	.04	.05	.10	.15	.20	.25	.30	.35	.40	.45	.50
0.1	2409	1199	796	595	474	232	152	112	88	72	60	52	46	41
0.2	3333	1664	1108	829	662	329	218	163	130	108	93	82	74	68
0.3	4727	2364	1577	1184	947	476	319	242	195	165	144	129	118	110
0.4	6941	3479	2325	1748	1402	711	482	369	302	258	228	207	192	182
0.5	10727	5385	3604	2715	2181	1115	763	589	486	420	375	344	322	308
0.6	17904	9001	6034	4551	3662	1887	1301	1012	842	734	661	611	578	557
0.7	33864	17047	11443	8642	6963	3613	2507	1964	1647	1445	1311	1221	1163	1131
0.8	80773	40711	27361	20690	16690	8714	6084	4796	4048	3575	3264	3060	2934	2873
0.9	341423	172275	115914	87750	70865	37207	26128	20712	17582	15617	14340	13522	13044	12845
1.1	378117	191172	128886	97766	79113	41956	29759	23828	20432	18330	17001	16193	15778	15695
1.2	99121	50160	33848	25699	20814	11088	7900	6354	5473	4932	4594	4395	4301	4297
1.3	46096	23346	15768	11981	9712	5196	3718	3003	2597	2350	2198	2111	2075	2081
1.4	27078	13726	9277	7055	5724	3074	2208	1791	1555	1412	1326	1279	1261	1270
1.5	18066	9164	6199	4718	3830	2065	1489	1212	1056	963	907	878	869	878
1.6	13057	6628	4487	3417	2777	1502	1087	888	776	710	672	652	648	656
1.7	9969	5064	3431	2615	2126	1154	838	687	603	553	525	511	509	518
1.8	7920	4026	2729	2082	1693	923	672	552	486	448	426	416	416	424
1.9	6486	3299	2238	1708	1390	760	555	458	404	373	356	349	350	357
2.0	5438	2768	1879	1435	1169	641	469	388	344	318	305	299	301	308
2.5	2828	1443	982	752	615	342	254	213	191	179	173	172	175	182
3.0	1822	933	636	488	400	225	169	143	130	123	121	121	124	130
3.5	1315	675	461	355	291	166	126	108	99	94	93	94	98	103
4.0	1017	523	358	276	227	131	100	87	80	77	77	78	82	87
4.5	824	424	291	225	185	108	83	73	68	66	66	68	71	76
5.0	689	356	245	189	156	91	71	63	59	58	58	60	63	68
6.0	516	267	185	143	119	71	56	50	47	47	48	50	53	57
7.0	411	214	148	115	96	58	47	42	40	40	41	44	47	51
8.0	341	178	124	97	81	49	40	37	35	36	37	39	42	46
9.0	291	152	106	83	70	43	36	33	32	33	34	36	39	43
10.0	254	133	93	73	61	39	32	30	29	30	32	34	37	41
15.0	155	83	58	47	40	26	23	22	22	23	25	27	30	34
20.0	112	60	43	35	30	21	19	18	19	20	22	25	27	31

CASE-CONTROL SAMPLE SIZE

α=.01 (TWO-SIDED)   β=.05

R	P_0 .50	.55	.60	.65	.70	.75	.80	.85	.90	.95	.96	.97	.98	.99
0.1	41	37	34	32	30	29	30	32	39	61	73	93	133	254
0.2	68	63	60	58	58	59	63	71	91	156	189	245	356	689
0.3	110	105	102	101	102	107	118	138	182	321	391	509	745	1453
0.4	182	175	172	173	179	191	213	254	342	615	752	982	1443	2828
0.5	308	301	299	305	318	344	388	469	641	1169	1435	1879	2768	5438
0.6	557	549	552	567	598	652	744	909	1254	2312	2844	3733	5512	10853
0.7	1131	1122	1137	1178	1253	1378	1585	1953	2716	5051	6225	8183	12104	23874
0.8	2873	2869	2926	3052	3269	3621	4195	5204	7289	13653	16850	22184	32861	64907
0.9	12845	12907	13224	13894	14942	16680	19443	24271	34200	64454	79643	104984	155702	307929
1.1	15695	15929	16505	17495	19042	21429	25231	31812	45280	86198	106726	140967	209489	415137
1.2	4297	4380	4558	4853	5305	5995	7089	8976	12829	24552	30392	40176	59755	118513
1.3	2081	2130	2225	2378	2610	2961	3515	4467	6410	12299	15253	20178	30034	59611
1.4	1270	1304	1368	1467	1616	1840	2191	2795	4024	7748	9615	12729	18959	37655
1.5	878	905	952	1025	1132	1294	1546	1978	2857	5518	6851	9075	13526	26880
1.6	656	679	716	773	857	982	1177	1511	2188	4239	5266	6980	10408	20696
1.7	518	537	568	615	684	786	944	1215	1765	3427	4260	5649	8429	16769
1.8	424	441	468	508	566	652	786	1014	1477	2874	3575	4743	7079	14090
1.9	357	373	397	432	483	557	673	870	1270	2478	3083	4091	6110	12166
2.0	308	322	344	375	420	486	589	763	1115	2181	2715	3604	5385	10727
2.5	182	192	207	228	258	302	369	482	711	1402	1748	2325	3479	6941
3.0	130	139	151	168	191	225	277	365	542	1075	1342	1787	2677	5348
3.5	103	111	121	136	156	184	228	302	451	899	1123	1497	2245	4488
4.0	87	94	103	116	134	159	198	263	394	790	987	1317	1976	3955
4.5	76	82	91	103	119	142	178	237	356	716	895	1195	1795	3594
5.0	68	74	82	93	108	130	163	218	329	662	829	1108	1664	3333
6.0	57	63	71	81	94	114	143	193	292	591	741	990	1489	2984
7.0	51	56	63	73	86	104	131	177	269	546	684	915	1377	2762
8.0	46	52	58	67	79	97	123	166	253	514	645	863	1299	2608
9.0	43	48	55	63	75	91	116	158	241	491	617	825	1243	2495
10.0	41	46	52	60	72	88	112	152	232	474	595	796	1199	2409
15.0	34	39	44	52	62	77	98	135	207	425	534	716	1079	2170
20.0	31	35	41	48	58	72	92	127	196	403	507	679	1025	2061

CASE-CONTROL SAMPLE SIZE

$\alpha = .01$ (TWO-SIDED) $\beta = .10$

R	P_0 = .01	.02	.03	.04	.05	.10	.15	.20	.25	.30	.35	.40	.45	.50
0.1	2016	1004	667	498	397	195	127	94	74	60	51	44	39	35
0.2	2789	1393	927	694	555	276	183	137	109	91	78	69	62	57
0.3	3955	1979	1320	991	793	399	268	203	164	139	121	109	99	93
0.4	5808	2911	1945	1463	1173	595	404	309	253	216	191	174	161	152
0.5	8975	4506	3016	2272	1825	934	639	493	407	352	314	288	270	258
0.6	14980	7531	5049	3808	3064	1579	1089	847	705	614	553	512	484	467
0.7	28333	14263	9574	7231	5826	3023	2098	1644	1378	1210	1097	1022	974	947
0.8	67580	34062	22892	17311	13964	7291	5091	4013	3387	2991	2731	2560	2455	2404
0.9	285656	144136	96981	73417	59290	31130	21860	17329	14711	13066	11998	11314	10913	10748
1.1	316350	159947	107835	81798	66191	35103	24899	19937	17095	15337	14225	13549	13201	13131
1.2	82931	41967	28320	21501	17415	9278	6610	5317	4579	4126	3844	3678	3599	3596
1.3	41967	19534	13193	10025	8126	4348	3111	2513	2173	1966	1840	1767	1736	1742
1.4	22656	11484	7762	5903	4789	2573	1848	1499	1301	1182	1110	1070	1056	1063
1.5	15115	7668	5187	3948	3205	1728	1246	1014	884	806	760	735	728	735
1.6	10925	5546	3751	2860	2323	1257	910	743	650	595	562	546	542	550
1.7	6627	4237	2871	2188	1779	966	702	575	505	463	439	428	426	433
1.8	5427	3369	2284	1742	1417	772	563	463	407	375	357	349	348	355
1.9	4550	2761	1873	1429	1164	636	465	383	339	313	298	292	293	299
2.0	2366	2316	1572	1201	978	536	393	325	288	267	255	251	252	258
2.5	1525	1208	822	630	515	286	213	178	160	150	145	145	147	152
3.0	1101	781	533	409	335	189	142	120	109	104	101	102	104	109
3.5	851	565	386	297	244	139	106	91	83	79	78	79	82	87
4.0	689	438	300	231	190	110	84	73	67	65	65	66	69	73
4.5	577	355	244	189	156	90	70	61	57	55	55	57	60	64
5.0	433	298	205	159	131	77	60	53	50	49	49	51	53	57
6.0	345	224	155	120	100	60	47	42	40	40	40	42	45	48
7.0	286	179	124	97	81	49	39	36	34	34	35	37	39	43
8.0	243	149	104	81	68	42	34	31	30	30	31	33	36	39
10.0	213	128	89	70	59	37	30	28	27	28	29	31	33	37
15.0	130	69	78	62	52	33	27	25	25	26	27	29	31	35
20.0	94	51	37	30	34	22	19	19	19	20	21	23	26	29

CASE-CONTROL SAMPLE SIZE

α=.01(TWO-SIDED)   β=.10

R	.50	.55	.60	.65	.70	.75	.80	.85	.90	.95	.96	.97	.98	.99
0.1	35	31	29	27	26	25	25	27	33	52	62	78	112	213
0.2	57	53	51	49	49	50	53	60	77	131	159	205	298	577
0.3	93	88	86	85	86	90	99	116	153	269	328	426	623	1216
0.4	152	147	145	145	150	160	178	213	286	515	630	822	1208	2366
0.5	258	252	251	255	267	288	325	393	536	978	1201	1572	2316	4550
0.6	467	460	462	475	501	546	623	761	1050	1935	2380	3124	4612	9080
0.7	947	940	952	986	1049	1153	1327	1635	2273	4226	5208	6847	10128	19975
0.8	2404	2401	2449	2554	2736	3030	3510	4355	6099	11424	14098	18561	27494	54306
0.9	10748	10799	11078	11625	12527	13956	16268	20306	28614	53927	66635	87836	130270	257633
1.1	13131	13327	13809	14637	15933	17929	21110	26616	37884	72119	89294	117942	175272	347329
1.2	3596	3665	3814	4060	4439	5016	5931	7510	10734	20520	25428	33614	49995	99155
1.3	1742	1782	1862	1990	2184	2478	2941	3738	5363	10291	12762	16883	25129	49874
1.4	1063	1092	1145	1228	1352	1540	1834	2339	3367	6483	8045	10650	15863	31505
1.5	735	758	797	858	948	1083	1294	1655	2391	4617	5733	7593	11317	22490
1.6	550	568	600	648	718	822	985	1264	1831	3547	4406	5840	8709	17316
1.7	433	450	476	515	573	658	791	1017	1477	2868	3565	4727	7052	14030
1.8	355	369	392	426	474	546	658	849	1236	2405	2991	3968	5923	11789
1.9	299	312	332	362	404	467	564	729	1063	2073	2579	3424	5112	10179
2.0	258	270	288	314	352	407	493	639	934	1825	2272	3016	4506	8975
2.5	152	161	174	191	216	253	309	404	595	1173	1463	1945	2911	5808
3.0	109	116	127	141	160	189	232	306	454	900	1123	1495	2240	4475
3.5	87	93	102	114	131	155	191	253	377	752	940	1253	1878	3756
4.0	73	79	87	97	112	134	166	221	330	661	826	1102	1654	3309
4.5	64	69	76	86	100	119	149	199	299	599	750	1000	1502	3007
5.0	57	62	69	78	91	109	137	183	276	555	694	927	1393	2789
6.0	48	53	60	68	79	96	120	162	245	495	620	829	1246	2497
7.0	43	48	53	61	72	87	110	148	226	457	573	766	1152	2311
8.0	39	44	49	57	67	81	103	139	212	431	540	723	1088	2182
9.0	37	41	46	53	63	77	98	132	202	412	516	691	1040	2088
10.0	35	39	44	51	60	74	94	127	195	397	498	667	1004	2016
15.0	29	33	38	44	53	65	83	113	174	356	447	599	904	1816
20.0	26	30	35	41	49	61	78	107	164	338	424	569	858	1724

CASE-CONTROL SAMPLE SIZE

α=.01(TWO-SIDED)   β=.20

R	P_0 .01	.02	.03	.04	.05	.10	.15	.20	.25	.30	.35	.40	.45	.50
0.1	1583	789	524	391	312	153	100	74	58	48	41	35	31	28
0.2	2190	1094	728	546	436	217	144	108	86	72	62	55	49	45
0.3	3105	1554	1037	778	623	313	217	159	129	109	96	86	79	73
0.4	4560	2286	1528	1149	922	468	317	243	199	170	151	137	127	120
0.5	7046	3537	2368	1784	1433	733	502	387	320	277	247	227	212	203
0.6	11760	5913	3964	2990	2406	1240	855	665	554	483	435	402	380	367
0.7	22242	11197	7517	5677	4574	2374	1648	1291	1083	950	862	803	765	744
0.8	53052	26739	17997	13590	10963	5724	3997	3151	2659	2349	2144	2010	1928	1888
0.9	224344	113149	76132	57634	46544	24438	17161	13604	11549	10258	9419	8882	8568	8438
1.1	248344	125561	84652	64213	51961	27557	19546	15651	13420	12040	11167	10636	10363	10309
1.2	65103	32946	22257	16879	13671	7283	5191	4174	3595	3240	3018	2888	2826	2823
1.3	30276	15335	10357	7870	6380	3414	2443	1973	1706	1544	1445	1388	1363	1368
1.4	17785	9016	6094	4635	3760	2020	1451	1177	1022	928	872	841	829	835
1.5	11866	6020	4072	3100	2517	1357	979	797	694	633	597	578	572	578
1.6	8577	4354	2948	2245	1824	988	715	584	511	467	442	429	426	432
1.7	6548	3327	2254	1718	1397	759	551	452	397	364	345	336	335	341
1.8	5203	2645	1793	1368	1113	607	442	364	320	295	281	274	274	279
1.9	4261	2168	1471	1122	914	500	365	302	266	246	235	230	230	236
2.0	3573	1819	1235	943	768	422	309	256	227	210	201	197	198	203
2.5	1858	949	646	495	404	225	168	141	126	118	115	114	116	120
3.0	1198	613	419	322	264	149	112	95	86	82	80	80	82	86
3.5	865	444	304	234	192	110	84	72	66	62	62	63	65	68
4.0	669	344	236	182	150	87	67	58	53	51	51	52	54	58
4.5	542	279	192	149	123	71	55	48	45	44	44	45	47	50
5.0	453	234	162	125	104	61	48	42	39	39	39	40	42	45
6.0	340	177	122	95	79	47	38	34	32	32	32	34	36	39
7.0	271	141	98	77	64	39	31	28	27	27	28	29	32	34
8.0	225	118	82	64	54	33	27	25	24	24	25	27	29	31
9.0	192	101	71	56	47	29	24	22	22	22	23	25	27	29
10.0	168	88	62	49	41	26	22	20	20	21	22	23	25	28
15.0	103	55	39	31	27	18	16	15	16	16	17	19	21	23
20.0	74	41	29	24	21	15	13	13	13	14	15	17	19	21

CASE-CONTROL SAMPLE SIZE

α=.01(TWO-SIDED)   β=.20

R	P₀ .99	.98	.97	.96	.95	.90	.85	.80	.75	.70	.65	.60	.55	.50
0.1	168	88	62	49	41	26	22	20	20	21	22	23	25	28
0.2	453	234	162	125	104	61	48	42	39	39	39	40	42	45
0.3	955	490	335	258	212	120	91	78	71	68	67	68	70	73
0.4	1858	949	646	495	404	225	168	141	126	118	115	114	116	120
0.5	3573	1819	1235	943	768	422	309	256	227	210	201	197	198	203
0.6	7129	3621	2453	1869	1519	824	598	490	429	394	373	363	361	367
0.7	15681	7951	5376	4089	3318	1785	1284	1042	906	824	774	748	738	744
0.8	42631	21583	14571	11068	8968	4788	3419	2756	2379	2148	2006	1923	1885	1888
0.9	202246	102265	68953	52310	42334	22463	15941	12771	10956	9834	9126	8697	8478	8438
1.1	272659	137592	92587	70097	56615	29740	20895	16572	14075	12508	11491	10841	10463	10309
1.2	77839	39247	26388	19962	16109	8427	5896	4657	3938	3485	3188	2995	2878	2823
1.3	39153	19727	13254	10019	8079	4211	2935	2309	1946	1715	1563	1462	1400	1368
1.4	24732	12453	8361	6316	5090	2644	1837	1440	1209	1062	964	899	858	835
1.5	17655	8884	5962	4501	3625	1877	1300	1016	850	745	674	626	595	578
1.6	13594	6837	4585	3460	2785	1438	993	774	646	564	509	471	447	432
1.7	11014	5537	3716	2799	2252	1160	799	621	517	450	405	374	353	341
1.8	9255	4650	3116	2349	1889	971	667	517	429	373	335	308	290	279
1.9	7991	4014	2688	2025	1628	835	572	443	367	318	284	261	246	236
2.0	7046	3537	2368	1784	1433	733	502	387	320	277	247	227	212	203
2.5	4560	2286	1528	1149	922	468	317	243	199	170	151	137	127	120
3.0	3513	1759	1174	882	707	357	240	183	149	126	111	100	92	86
3.5	2949	1475	984	738	591	297	199	151	122	103	90	80	74	68
4.0	2598	1299	866	649	519	260	174	131	105	89	77	69	62	58
4.5	2361	1180	786	589	471	235	156	117	94	79	68	61	55	50
5.0	2190	1094	728	546	436	217	144	108	86	72	62	55	49	45
6.0	1961	979	651	487	389	193	128	95	76	63	54	47	42	39
7.0	1815	905	602	450	359	178	117	87	69	57	49	42	38	34
8.0	1714	854	568	425	339	167	110	81	64	53	45	39	35	31
9.0	1639	817	543	406	324	159	105	77	61	50	42	37	33	29
10.0	1583	789	524	391	312	153	100	74	58	48	41	35	31	28
15.0	1426	710	471	352	280	137	89	65	51	42	35	30	26	23
20.0	1354	674	447	334	266	130	84	62	48	39	33	28	24	21

CASE-CONTROL SAMPLE SIZE

$\alpha = .05$ (TWO-SIDED) $\beta = .05$

R	P_0 .01	.02	.03	.04	.05	.10	.15	.20	.25	.30	.35	.40	.45	.50
0.1	1752	872	579	432	344	169	110	81	63	52	44	37	33	29
0.2	2425	1211	806	603	482	239	158	118	94	78	67	59	53	49
0.3	3439	1720	1147	861	689	346	232	175	142	120	105	94	86	80
0.4	5051	2531	1691	1272	1020	517	350	268	219	187	166	150	139	132
0.5	7806	3918	2623	1975	1587	811	555	428	353	305	273	250	234	224
0.6	13029	6550	4391	3312	2664	1373	946	736	613	534	480	444	420	405
0.7	24644	12405	8327	6289	5067	2629	1824	1429	1198	1051	954	888	846	823
0.8	58782	29627	19912	15057	12146	6341	4427	3490	2945	2601	2375	2226	2135	2090
0.9	248469	125372	84355	63859	51571	27077	19014	15073	12795	11365	10435	9840	9492	9348
1.1	275173	139124	93796	71149	57573	30533	21656	17341	14869	13339	12372	11784	11482	11421
1.2	72135	36503	24632	18702	15147	8069	5749	4624	3982	3589	3343	3198	3130	3127
1.3	33545	16990	11474	8719	7068	3781	2705	2185	1889	1710	1599	1536	1509	1514
1.4	19706	9988	6751	5134	4165	2237	1607	1303	1131	1027	965	930	917	924
1.5	13147	6669	4511	3433	2787	1503	1083	882	768	700	660	639	632	639
1.6	9502	4823	3265	2487	2020	1090	791	646	565	517	488	474	471	477
1.7	7254	3685	2496	1902	1547	840	609	499	438	402	381	371	370	376
1.8	5764	2930	1986	1514	1232	671	489	402	353	325	310	302	308	308
1.9	4720	2401	1628	1242	1011	553	404	333	294	271	259	253	254	260
2.0	3957	2014	1367	1044	850	466	341	282	250	231	221	217	218	224
2.5	2057	1050	715	547	447	248	184	154	138	130	126	125	127	132
3.0	1326	678	463	355	291	163	123	104	94	89	87	88	90	94
3.5	957	490	335	258	212	120	91	78	71	68	67	68	71	75
4.0	740	380	260	201	165	95	72	63	58	56	55	57	59	63
4.5	599	308	212	163	134	78	60	52	49	47	47	49	51	55
5.0	501	258	178	137	113	66	52	45	42	41	42	43	45	49
6.0	375	194	134	104	86	51	40	36	34	34	34	36	38	41
7.0	299	155	107	84	69	42	33	30	29	29	30	31	34	37
8.0	248	129	90	70	58	35	29	26	26	26	27	28	30	31
9.0	211	110	77	60	50	31	25	23	23	23	23	26	28	28
10.0	184	97	67	53	44	28	23	21	21	21	20	24	26	26
15.0	112	60	42	33	28	19	16	16	16	17	18	20	22	24
20.0	81	44	31	25	21	15	13	13	13	14	16	17	20	22

CASE-CONTROL SAMPLE SIZE

$\alpha=.05$(TWO-SIDED) $\beta=.05$

R	P_0													
	.50	.55	.60	.65	.70	.75	.80	.85	.90	.95	.96	.97	.98	.99
0.1	29	26	24	23	21	21	21	23	28	44	53	67	97	184
0.2	49	45	43	42	41	42	45	52	66	113	137	178	258	501
0.3	80	76	74	73	74	78	85	100	132	233	284	370	541	1057
0.4	132	127	125	126	130	138	154	184	248	447	547	715	1050	2057
0.5	224	218	217	221	231	250	282	341	466	850	1044	1367	2014	3957
0.6	405	399	401	412	435	474	541	661	912	1682	2070	2716	4011	7897
0.7	823	816	827	857	911	1002	1153	1421	1976	3675	4530	5955	8808	17374
0.8	2090	2088	2129	2221	2379	2634	3052	3787	5304	9936	12262	16144	23911	47236
0.9	9348	9392	9635	10111	10895	12138	14149	17662	24888	46906	57960	76401	113311	224014
1.1	11421	11592	12011	12731	13858	15594	18361	23151	32952	62730	77669	102588	152455	302114
1.2	3127	3187	3317	3531	3860	4362	5158	6532	9336	17848	22117	29237	43486	86247
1.3	1514	1550	1619	1730	1899	2154	2557	3251	4664	8950	11100	14684	21857	43381
1.4	924	949	995	1067	1175	1338	1594	2034	2928	5638	6997	9263	13797	27403
1.5	639	658	693	745	824	941	1125	1439	2079	4015	4986	6604	9843	19561
1.6	477	494	521	562	623	714	856	1099	1592	3084	3832	5079	7574	15061
1.7	376	390	413	447	497	571	687	884	1284	2494	3100	4111	6133	12203
1.8	308	320	340	369	412	474	572	738	1074	2091	2601	3451	5151	10254
1.9	260	271	288	314	351	405	489	633	924	1803	2243	2977	4446	8853
2.0	224	234	250	273	305	353	428	555	811	1587	1975	2623	3918	7806
2.5	132	139	150	166	187	219	268	350	517	1020	1272	1691	2531	5051
3.0	94	101	109	122	139	163	201	265	394	782	976	1300	1948	3892
3.5	75	80	88	98	113	134	166	219	328	654	817	1089	1633	3266
4.0	63	68	75	84	97	115	144	191	287	574	718	958	1438	2878
4.5	55	59	66	74	86	103	129	172	259	520	651	869	1306	2615
5.0	49	53	59	67	78	94	118	158	239	482	603	806	1211	2425
6.0	41	45	51	58	68	82	104	140	212	430	539	720	1083	2172
7.0	37	41	46	53	62	75	95	128	195	397	498	666	1002	2009
8.0	33	37	42	49	57	70	89	120	184	374	469	628	945	1897
9.0	31	35	39	46	54	66	84	114	175	357	448	600	904	1815
10.0	29	33	37	44	52	63	81	110	169	344	432	579	872	1752
15.0	24	28	32	37	45	55	71	98	150	309	388	521	785	1579
20.0	22	25	29	35	42	52	67	92	142	293	368	494	745	1499

CASE-CONTROL SAMPLE SIZE

$\alpha = .05$ (TWO-SIDED) $\beta = .10$

R	P_0 .01	.02	.03	.04	.05	.10	.15	.20	.25	.30	.35	.40	.45	.50
0.1	1420	707	469	351	279	137	89	66	52	42	36	31	27	24
0.2	1965	981	653	489	390	194	129	96	77	64	55	48	44	40
0.3	2786	1394	930	698	558	280	188	142	115	97	85	76	70	65
0.4	4092	2051	1370	1030	826	419	284	217	178	152	134	122	113	107
0.5	6323	3174	2125	1600	1286	658	450	347	287	248	221	203	190	182
0.6	10554	5306	3557	2683	2158	1112	767	596	497	433	390	360	340	329
0.7	19962	10049	6745	5094	4105	2130	1478	1158	971	852	773	720	686	667
0.8	47614	23998	16129	12196	9838	5137	3587	2827	2386	2107	1924	1804	1730	1693
0.9	201260	101552	68328	51726	41773	21933	15401	12209	10364	9206	8453	7971	7689	7572
1.1	222890	112691	75975	57631	46635	24732	17542	14046	12044	10805	10022	9545	9300	9251
1.2	58429	29568	19953	15149	12269	6536	4657	3746	3226	2907	2708	2591	2535	2533
1.3	27172	13762	9295	7063	5725	3063	2191	1770	1531	1385	1296	1245	1223	1227
1.4	15962	8091	5469	4159	3374	1812	1302	1056	916	832	782	754	743	749
1.5	10649	5402	3654	2781	2258	1217	878	714	623	568	535	518	512	518
1.6	7697	3907	2645	2014	1637	886	641	523	458	419	396	384	382	387
1.7	5876	2985	2022	1541	1253	680	494	405	355	326	309	301	300	305
1.8	4669	2373	1609	1227	998	544	396	326	287	264	251	245	245	250
1.9	3823	1945	1319	1007	820	448	327	270	238	220	210	206	206	211
2.0	3226	1632	1107	846	689	378	277	229	203	188	180	176	177	182
2.5	1077	851	579	443	362	201	150	125	112	105	102	102	103	107
3.0	775	550	372	288	236	133	100	85	77	73	71	71	73	77
3.5	599	398	272	209	172	98	74	64	58	56	55	56	58	61
4.0	485	308	211	163	134	77	59	51	47	45	45	46	48	51
5.0	406	250	172	133	109	63	49	43	40	39	39	40	42	44
6.0	304	210	144	112	92	54	42	37	35	34	34	35	37	40
7.0	242	158	109	85	70	42	33	29	28	28	28	29	31	34
8.0	201	126	87	68	56	34	27	25	24	24	24	26	27	30
9.0	172	105	73	57	47	29	24	22	21	21	22	23	25	27
10.0	150	90	63	49	41	25	21	18	19	19	20	21	23	25
15.0	91	78	55	43	36	23	19	13	13	14	15	16	18	20
20.0	66	49	34	27	23	15	13	11	11	12	13	14	16	18

CASE-CONTROL SAMPLE SIZE

α=.05(TWO-SIDED)   β=.10

R	P₀ .99	.98	.97	.96	.95	.90	.85	.80	.75	.70	.65	.60	.55	.50
0.1	150	78	55	43	36	23	19	18	17	18	19	20	22	24
0.2	406	210	144	112	92	54	42	37	35	34	34	35	37	40
0.3	856	439	300	231	189	107	81	69	63	60	59	60	62	65
0.4	1667	851	579	443	362	201	150	125	112	105	102	102	103	107
0.5	3206	1632	1107	846	689	378	277	229	203	188	180	176	177	182
0.6	6397	3249	2200	1677	1363	739	536	439	385	353	334	325	324	329
0.7	14073	7135	4824	3669	2977	1601	1151	935	812	739	694	670	662	667
0.8	38261	19370	13077	9933	8048	4297	3068	2473	2134	1927	1799	1725	1691	1693
0.9	181516	91782	61885	46948	37994	20160	14306	11461	9832	8826	8190	7805	7608	7572
1.1	244712	123489	83096	62912	50812	26691	18752	14873	12634	11225	10313	9729	9390	9251
1.2	69860	35224	23683	17915	14457	7563	5291	4179	3534	3127	2860	2687	2582	2533
1.3	35139	17704	11894	8991	7250	3778	2633	2072	1745	1538	1402	1312	1255	1227
1.4	22197	11176	7503	5668	4567	2372	1648	1292	1084	952	865	806	769	769
1.5	15845	7973	5350	4039	3252	1684	1166	911	762	668	604	561	533	518
1.6	12200	6135	4114	3104	2499	1290	891	694	579	505	456	422	400	387
1.7	9885	4968	3330	2511	2020	1040	716	557	463	403	363	335	316	305
1.8	8306	4173	2796	2107	1694	870	598	463	385	334	300	276	260	250
1.9	7172	3602	2412	1817	1460	749	513	397	328	284	255	234	220	211
2.0	6323	3174	2125	1600	1286	658	450	347	287	248	221	203	190	182
2.5	4092	2051	1370	1030	826	419	284	217	178	152	134	122	113	107
3.0	3153	1578	1053	791	634	319	215	163	133	113	99	89	82	77
3.5	2646	1323	882	662	530	266	178	134	109	92	80	71	65	61
4.0	2331	1165	776	582	465	232	155	117	94	79	68	61	55	51
4.5	2118	1058	705	528	422	210	140	105	84	70	60	54	48	44
5.0	1965	981	653	489	390	194	129	96	77	64	55	48	44	40
6.0	1759	877	584	437	348	172	114	85	67	56	48	42	37	34
7.0	1628	812	539	403	322	159	104	77	61	50	43	37	33	30
8.0	1537	766	509	380	303	149	98	72	57	47	40	34	30	27
9.0	1471	732	486	363	290	142	93	69	54	44	37	32	28	25
10.0	1420	707	469	351	279	137	89	66	52	42	36	31	27	24
15.0	1279	636	422	315	251	122	79	58	45	37	31	26	23	20
20.0	1215	604	400	299	238	115	75	54	42	34	28	24	21	18

CASE-CONTROL SAMPLE SIZE

α=.05(TWO-SIDED)   β=.20

R	p_0 .01	.02	.03	.04	.05	.10	.15	.20	.25	.30	.35	.40	.45	.50
0.1	1061	528	351	262	209	103	67	49	39	32	27	23	20	18
0.2	1468	733	488	365	292	145	96	72	58	48	41	37	33	30
0.3	2081	1041	695	521	417	210	141	107	86	73	64	57	52	49
0.4	3056	1532	1024	770	618	313	213	163	133	114	101	91	85	80
0.5	4723	2371	1587	1195	960	491	336	260	214	185	165	152	142	136
0.6	7882	3963	2657	2004	1612	831	573	446	371	323	291	269	255	246
0.7	14908	7505	5038	3805	3066	1591	1104	865	725	637	577	538	512	498
0.8	35560	17923	12046	9109	7348	3837	2679	2112	1782	1574	1437	1347	1292	1265
0.9	150309	75843	51030	38631	31198	16380	11503	9119	7741	6875	6313	5953	5743	5655
1.1	166463	84162	56742	43041	34829	18471	13101	10491	8995	8070	7485	7129	6946	6910
1.2	43638	22083	14902	11314	9164	4882	3478	2798	2410	2171	2023	1935	1894	1892
1.3	20294	10278	6942	5275	4276	2288	1637	1322	1144	1035	968	930	914	917
1.4	11921	6043	4085	3106	2520	1354	973	789	685	622	584	563	556	559
1.5	7954	4035	2729	2077	1687	910	656	534	465	424	400	387	383	387
1.6	5749	2918	1976	1505	1223	662	479	391	342	313	296	287	285	289
1.7	4389	2230	1511	1151	936	509	369	303	266	244	231	225	224	228
1.8	3487	1773	1202	917	746	407	296	244	214	197	188	184	183	187
1.9	2856	1453	986	752	612	335	245	202	178	165	157	154	154	158
2.0	2394	1219	827	632	515	282	207	171	152	140	134	132	133	136
2.5	1245	636	433	332	271	151	112	94	84	79	77	76	77	80
3.0	803	411	280	215	176	99	75	63	58	55	53	54	55	58
3.5	579	297	203	157	129	73	56	48	44	42	41	42	43	46
4.0	448	230	158	122	100	58	44	38	36	34	34	35	36	38
4.5	363	187	129	99	82	48	37	32	30	29	29	30	31	34
5.0	304	157	108	84	69	41	32	28	26	26	26	27	28	30
6.0	228	118	82	63	53	31	25	22	21	21	21	22	24	26
7.0	181	94	66	51	43	26	21	19	18	18	19	20	21	23
8.0	151	79	55	43	36	22	18	16	16	16	17	18	19	21
9.0	129	67	47	37	31	19	16	15	14	15	15	16	18	19
10.0	112	59	41	33	27	17	14	13	13	14	14	15	17	18
15.0	69	37	26	21	18	12	10	10	10	11	11	12	14	15
20.0	50	27	19	16	14	10	9	8	9	9	10	11	12	14

CASE-CONTROL SAMPLE SIZE

α=.05(TWO-SIDED)   β=.20

R	P_0 .50	.55	.60	.65	.70	.75	.80	.85	.90	.95	.96	.97	.98	.99
0.1	18	17	15	14	14	13	13	14	17	27	33	41	59	112
0.2	30	28	27	26	26	26	28	32	41	69	84	108	157	304
0.3	49	47	45	45	45	48	52	61	80	142	173	224	328	640
0.4	80	77	76	77	79	84	94	112	151	271	332	433	636	1245
0.5	136	133	132	134	140	152	171	207	282	515	632	827	1219	2394
0.6	246	242	243	250	264	288	328	401	552	1018	1253	1644	2427	4778
0.7	498	495	501	519	552	607	698	860	1196	2224	2741	3603	5329	10511
0.8	1265	1264	1289	1347	1440	1594	1847	2292	3209	6011	7418	9767	14467	28575
0.9	5655	5682	5829	6117	6592	7344	8560	10685	15056	28376	35063	46219	68547	135564
1.1	6910	7013	7266	7702	8384	9434	11108	14005	19934	37948	46986	62060	92226	182761
1.2	1892	1929	2007	2137	2336	2640	3121	3952	5648	10798	13380	17687	26307	52175
1.3	917	938	980	1047	1149	1304	1548	1967	2822	5415	6715	8884	13222	26244
1.4	559	575	603	646	712	810	965	1231	1772	3411	4233	5604	8347	16578
1.5	387	399	420	452	499	570	681	871	1258	2429	3017	3996	5955	11834
1.6	289	299	316	341	378	433	516	665	964	1866	2319	3073	4582	9112
1.7	228	237	251	271	301	346	416	535	777	1509	1876	2487	3711	7383
1.8	187	194	206	224	250	288	346	447	650	1266	1574	2088	3117	6204
1.9	158	164	175	190	213	246	297	383	559	1091	1357	1802	2690	5356
2.0	136	142	152	165	185	214	260	336	491	960	1195	1587	2371	4723
2.5	80	85	91	101	114	133	163	213	313	618	770	1024	1532	3056
3.0	58	61	67	74	84	99	122	161	239	474	591	787	1179	2355
3.5	46	49	54	60	69	81	101	133	199	396	495	659	989	1976
4.0	38	42	46	51	59	70	87	116	174	348	435	580	870	1742
4.5	34	36	40	46	53	63	78	105	157	315	395	527	790	1582
5.0	30	33	37	41	48	58	72	96	145	292	365	488	733	1468
6.0	26	28	31	36	42	50	63	85	129	261	326	436	656	1314
7.0	23	25	28	32	38	46	58	78	119	241	302	403	606	1216
8.0	21	23	26	30	35	43	54	73	112	227	284	380	572	1148
9.0	19	22	24	28	33	41	52	70	107	217	272	364	547	1099
10.0	18	20	23	27	32	39	49	67	103	209	262	351	528	1061
15.0	15	17	20	23	28	34	44	60	92	188	236	316	476	956
20.0	14	16	18	22	26	32	41	56	87	178	223	299	451	907

CASE-CONTROL SAMPLE SIZE

α = .10 (TWO-SIDED)   β = .10

R	p_0 .01	.02	.03	.04	.05	.10	.15	.20	.25	.30	.35	.40	.45	.50
0.1	1153	574	381	285	227	111	72	53	42	34	29	25	22	19
0.2	1596	796	530	397	317	157	104	78	62	52	44	39	35	32
0.3	2263	1132	755	566	453	228	153	115	93	79	69	62	56	53
0.4	3323	1665	1113	837	671	340	231	176	144	123	109	99	92	87
0.5	5136	2578	1726	1299	1044	534	365	282	233	201	179	164	154	147
0.6	8572	4309	2889	2179	1753	903	622	484	403	351	316	292	276	267
0.7	16213	8162	5479	4138	3334	1730	1200	940	788	692	627	584	557	541
0.8	38673	19491	13100	9906	7991	4172	2913	2296	1938	1711	1562	1465	1405	1375
0.9	163468	82482	55497	42013	33929	17814	12509	9916	8418	7477	6866	6474	6245	6150
1.1	163036	91530	61709	46809	37878	20088	14248	11409	9782	8776	8140	7753	7554	7514
1.2	47458	24016	16206	12304	9965	5309	3782	3042	2620	2361	2199	2104	2059	2057
1.3	22070	11178	7549	5736	4650	2488	1780	1437	1243	1125	1052	1011	993	996
1.4	12964	6571	4442	3378	2740	1472	1057	857	744	676	635	612	604	608
1.5	8649	4388	2968	2259	1834	989	713	580	505	461	434	420	416	420
1.6	6251	3173	2148	1636	1329	719	520	425	372	340	321	312	310	314
1.7	4773	2424	1642	1252	1018	552	401	329	288	265	251	244	243	248
1.8	3792	1928	1307	996	811	442	322	264	233	218	204	192	199	203
1.9	3105	1579	1071	817	665	364	266	219	193	178	170	167	167	171
2.0	2603	1325	899	687	559	306	225	186	164	152	146	143	144	147
2.5	1354	691	470	360	294	163	121	102	91	85	83	82	84	87
3.0	872	446	304	234	191	108	81	68	62	59	58	58	59	62
3.5	629	323	221	170	139	79	60	51	47	45	44	45	47	49
4.0	487	250	171	132	109	62	48	41	38	37	37	37	39	41
4.5	394	203	139	108	89	51	40	35	32	31	31	32	34	36
5.0	330	170	117	90	75	41	34	30	28	27	28	28	30	32
6.0	247	128	88	68	57	34	27	24	22	22	23	24	25	27
7.0	197	102	71	55	46	28	22	20	19	19	20	21	22	24
8.0	163	85	59	46	38	23	19	17	17	17	18	19	20	22
9.0	139	73	51	40	33	20	17	15	15	15	16	17	19	20
10.0	121	64	44	35	29	18	15	14	14	14	15	16	17	19
15.0	74	39	28	22	19	12	11	10	10	11	12	13	14	16
20.0	53	29	21	17	14	10	9	9	9	10	10	12	13	15

CASE-CONTROL SAMPLE SIZE

α=.10(TWO-SIDED)   β=.10

R	P_0 .50	.55	.60	.65	.70	.75	.80	.85	.90	.95	.96	.97	.98	.99
0.1	19	17	16	15	14	14	14	15	18	29	35	44	64	121
0.2	32	30	28	28	27	28	30	34	44	75	90	117	170	330
0.3	53	50	49	48	49	51	56	66	87	153	187	243	356	695
0.4	87	84	82	83	85	91	102	121	163	294	360	470	691	1354
0.5	147	144	143	146	152	164	186	225	306	559	687	899	1325	2603
0.6	267	263	264	271	286	312	356	435	600	1107	1362	1787	2639	5196
0.7	541	537	544	564	600	660	759	935	1300	2418	2980	3918	5795	11477
0.8	1375	1374	1401	1461	1565	1733	2008	2492	3490	6537	8067	10621	15733	31077
0.9	6150	6179	6339	6652	7168	7986	9309	11620	16374	30859	38132	50264	74548	147432
1.1	7514	7626	7902	8376	9117	10260	12020	15231	21679	41270	51099	67493	100300	198761
1.2	2057	2097	2182	2323	2540	2870	3394	4297	6142	11742	14551	19235	28610	56742
1.3	996	1020	1065	1138	1249	1417	1683	2139	3069	5889	7302	9661	14380	28541
1.4	608	624	655	702	773	881	1049	1338	1927	3710	4603	6094	9077	18029
1.5	420	433	456	490	542	619	740	947	1368	2642	3280	4345	6476	12870
1.6	314	325	343	370	410	470	563	723	1048	2029	2521	3342	4983	9909
1.7	248	257	272	294	327	376	452	582	845	1641	2040	2705	4035	8028
1.8	203	211	224	243	271	312	376	485	707	1376	1711	2271	3389	6746
1.9	171	178	190	207	231	267	322	416	608	1186	1476	1959	2925	5825
2.0	147	154	164	179	201	233	282	365	534	1044	1299	1726	2578	5136
2.5	87	92	99	109	123	144	176	231	340	671	837	1113	1665	3323
3.0	62	66	72	80	91	108	132	174	259	514	642	855	1282	2560
3.5	49	53	58	65	74	88	109	144	216	430	537	716	1074	2149
4.0	41	45	49	55	64	76	95	126	189	378	472	630	946	1893
4.5	36	39	43	49	57	68	85	113	170	342	429	572	859	1720
5.0	32	35	39	44	52	62	78	104	157	317	397	530	796	1596
6.0	27	30	34	38	45	54	68	92	140	283	354	474	713	1429
7.0	24	27	30	35	41	49	63	85	129	261	327	438	659	1322
8.0	22	25	28	32	38	46	58	79	121	246	309	413	622	1248
9.0	20	23	26	30	36	44	55	75	115	235	295	395	595	1194
10.0	19	22	25	29	34	42	53	72	111	227	285	381	574	1153
15.0	16	18	21	25	30	37	47	64	99	203	256	343	517	1039
20.0	15	17	19	23	28	34	44	61	94	193	242	325	490	986

CASE-CONTROL SAMPLE SIZE

$\alpha = .10$ (TWO-SIDED) $\beta = .20$

R	P_0 .01	.02	.03	.04	.05	.10	.15	.20	.25	.30	.35	.40	.45	.50
0.1	832	414	275	206	164	80	53	39	30	25	21	18	16	14
0.2	1151	575	383	287	229	114	75	56	45	38	32	29	26	24
0.3	1633	817	545	409	327	164	110	84	68	57	50	45	41	38
0.4	2397	1202	803	604	484	246	167	127	104	89	79	72	66	63
0.5	3705	1860	1245	938	753	385	264	203	168	145	130	119	111	107
0.6	6184	3109	2084	1572	1265	652	449	350	291	254	228	211	200	193
0.7	11695	5888	3952	2985	2405	1248	866	678	569	499	453	422	402	391
0.8	27896	14060	9450	7146	5764	3010	2101	1656	1398	1235	1127	1057	1013	992
0.9	117916	59498	40033	30306	24474	12850	9024	7153	6072	5394	4953	4670	4505	4436
1.1	130588	66024	44513	33765	27323	14490	10278	8230	7056	6331	5872	5593	5449	5420
1.2	34233	17324	11690	8876	7189	3830	2729	2195	1890	1703	1587	1518	1486	1484
1.3	15920	8063	5446	4138	3355	1795	1284	1037	897	812	759	729	717	719
1.4	9352	4740	3204	2437	1977	1062	763	619	537	488	458	442	436	439
1.5	6239	3165	2141	1630	1323	713	514	419	365	333	314	303	300	303
1.6	4510	2289	1550	1180	959	519	376	307	268	245	232	225	224	227
1.7	3443	1749	1185	903	734	399	290	237	208	191	181	177	176	179
1.8	2736	1391	943	719	585	319	232	191	168	155	147	144	144	147
1.9	2240	1140	773	590	480	263	192	158	140	129	123	121	121	124
2.0	1878	956	649	496	404	221	162	134	119	110	105	104	104	107
2.5	977	499	339	260	212	118	88	74	66	62	60	60	61	63
3.0	630	322	220	169	138	78	59	50	45	43	42	42	43	45
3.5	454	233	159	123	101	57	44	37	34	33	32	33	34	36
4.0	351	181	124	96	79	45	35	30	28	27	27	27	28	30
4.5	285	147	101	78	64	37	29	25	23	23	23	23	25	26
5.0	238	123	85	66	54	32	25	22	20	20	20	21	22	24
6.0	179	93	64	50	41	25	19	17	17	16	17	17	18	20
7.0	142	74	51	40	33	20	16	15	14	13	14	15	15	18
8.0	118	62	43	34	28	17	14	13	12	13	13	14	14	16
9.0	101	53	37	29	24	15	12	11	11	11	12	13	13	15
10.0	88	46	32	25	21	13	11	10	10	10	11	12	11	14
15.0	54	29	20	16	14	9	8	8	8	8	9	10	11	12
20.0	39	21	15	12	11	7	7	7	7	7	8	9	10	11

CASE-CONTROL SAMPLE SIZE

α=.10(TWO-SIDED) β=.20

R	.50	.55	.60	.65	.70	.75	.80	.85	.90	.95	.96	.97	.98	.99
p₀ →														
0.1	14	13	12	11	11	10	10	11	13	21	25	32	46	88
0.2	24	22	21	20	20	20	22	25	32	54	66	85	123	238
0.3	38	36	35	35	35	37	41	48	63	111	135	176	257	502
0.4	63	61	60	60	62	66	74	88	118	212	260	339	499	977
0.5	107	104	104	105	110	119	134	162	221	404	496	649	956	1878
0.6	193	190	191	196	207	225	257	314	433	799	983	1289	1904	3748
0.7	391	388	393	407	433	476	548	675	938	1745	2150	2826	4181	8245
0.8	992	991	1011	1054	1129	1251	1449	1798	2518	4716	5820	7662	11349	22417
0.9	4436	4458	4573	4799	5171	5761	6715	8382	11811	22260	27506	36258	53774	106348
1.1	5420	5501	5700	6042	6577	7401	8714	10987	15638	29770	36860	48685	72351	143374
1.2	1484	1513	1574	1676	1832	2071	2448	3100	4431	8471	10496	13876	20637	40930
1.3	719	736	769	821	902	1023	1214	1543	2214	4248	5268	6969	10373	20588
1.4	439	451	473	507	558	636	757	965	1390	2676	3321	4396	6548	13005
1.5	303	313	329	354	391	447	534	683	987	1906	2366	3134	4671	9284
1.6	227	235	248	267	296	339	407	522	756	1464	1819	2411	3595	7148
1.7	179	186	196	213	236	272	326	420	610	1184	1472	1951	2911	5791
1.8	147	152	162	176	196	225	272	350	510	993	1235	1638	2445	4867
1.9	124	129	137	149	167	193	233	301	439	856	1065	1413	2110	4202
2.0	107	111	119	130	145	168	203	264	385	753	938	1245	1860	3705
2.5	63	66	72	79	89	104	127	167	246	484	604	803	1202	2397
3.0	45	48	52	58	66	78	96	126	187	371	464	617	925	1847
3.5	36	38	42	47	54	64	79	104	156	311	388	517	775	1550
4.0	30	32	36	40	47	55	68	91	137	273	341	455	683	1366
4.5	26	28	32	36	41	49	61	82	123	247	309	413	620	1241
5.0	24	26	29	32	38	45	56	75	114	228	287	383	575	1151
6.0	20	22	25	28	33	39	50	67	101	204	256	342	514	1031
7.0	18	20	22	25	30	36	45	61	93	189	236	316	476	954
8.0	16	18	20	23	28	34	42	57	88	178	223	298	449	901
9.0	15	17	19	22	26	32	40	55	83	170	213	285	424	862
10.0	14	16	18	21	25	30	39	53	80	164	206	275	414	832
15.0	12	13	16	18	22	27	34	47	72	147	185	247	373	750
20.0	11	12	14	17	20	25	32	44	68	139	175	235	354	712

CASE-CONTROL SAMPLE SIZE

α = .20 (TWO-SIDED)   β = .20

R / p_0	.01	.02	.03	.04	.05	.10	.15	.20	.25	.30	.35	.40	.45	.50
0.1	608	303	201	150	120	59	38	28	22	18	15	13	12	10
0.2	841	420	279	209	167	83	55	41	33	27	24	21	19	17
0.3	1193	597	398	291	239	120	81	61	49	42	36	33	30	28
0.4	1752	878	587	441	354	179	122	93	76	65	58	52	48	46
0.5	2707	1359	910	685	550	282	192	149	123	106	95	87	81	78
0.6	4518	2272	1523	1149	924	476	328	255	213	185	167	154	146	141
0.7	8546	4302	2888	2181	1757	912	633	496	416	365	331	308	294	286
0.8	20385	10274	6905	5222	4212	2199	1536	1210	1022	902	824	772	740	725
0.9	86167	43478	29254	22146	17885	9390	6594	5227	4437	3941	3619	3413	3292	3242
1.1	95427	48247	32528	24674	19966	10589	7510	6014	5156	4626	4291	4087	3982	3961
1.2	25016	12659	8542	6486	5253	2798	1994	1604	1381	1245	1159	1109	1086	1085
1.3	11633	5892	3979	3024	2451	1311	938	758	655	593	555	533	524	525
1.4	6834	3464	2341	1781	1445	776	557	452	392	356	335	323	318	320
1.5	4559	2313	1564	1191	967	521	376	306	267	243	229	222	219	222
1.6	3295	1673	1132	862	701	379	274	224	196	179	170	165	163	166
1.7	2516	1278	866	660	536	291	211	173	152	140	132	129	128	131
1.8	1997	1016	689	525	427	233	170	139	122	113	107	105	105	107
1.9	1637	833	565	431	351	192	140	116	103	94	90	88	88	78
2.0	1372	699	474	362	295	162	118	98	87	80	77	76	76	46
2.5	714	364	248	190	155	86	64	54	48	45	44	43	44	33
3.0	460	235	161	123	101	57	43	36	33	31	30	31	31	26
3.5	332	170	116	90	73	42	32	27	25	24	24	24	25	22
4.0	257	132	90	70	57	33	25	22	20	19	19	20	21	19
5.0	208	107	73	57	47	27	21	18	17	17	17	17	18	17
6.0	174	90	62	48	39	23	18	16	15	14	15	15	16	14
7.0	130	67	47	36	30	18	14	13	12	12	12	13	13	13
8.0	104	54	37	29	24	15	12	11	10	10	10	11	12	12
9.0	86	45	31	24	20	12	10	9	9	9	9	10	11	11
10.0	73	38	27	21	18	11	9	8	8	8	9	9	10	10
15.0	64	34	23	18	15	7	6	6	6	6	8	8	9	9
20.0	39	21	15	12	10	5	5	5	5	5	6	6	8	8

CASE-CONTROL SAMPLE SIZE

$\alpha = .20$ (TWO-SIDED) $\beta = .20$

R	P_0 = .50	.55	.60	.65	.70	.75	.80	.85	.90	.95	.96	.97	.98	.99
0.1	10	9	9	8	8	7	8	8	10	15	18	23	34	64
0.2	17	16	15	15	14	15	16	18	23	39	48	62	90	174
0.3	28	26	26	25	26	27	30	35	46	81	99	128	188	367
0.4	46	44	43	44	45	48	54	64	86	155	190	248	364	714
0.5	78	76	76	77	80	87	98	118	162	295	362	474	699	1372
0.6	141	139	139	143	151	165	188	230	316	583	718	942	1391	2739
0.7	286	283	287	297	316	348	400	493	685	1275	1571	2065	3055	6025
0.8	725	724	738	770	825	914	1059	1313	1840	3446	4252	5599	8293	16381
0.9	3242	3257	3341	3506	3779	4210	4907	6125	8631	16267	20100	26495	39295	77710
1.1	3961	4020	4165	4415	4806	5408	6368	8029	11428	21754	26935	35577	52870	104770
1.2	1085	1105	1150	1225	1339	1513	1789	2265	3238	6194	7670	10139	15081	29910
1.3	525	538	562	600	659	747	887	1127	1618	3104	3849	5092	7580	15044
1.4	320	329	345	370	408	464	553	705	1016	1955	2427	3212	4785	9503
1.5	222	228	240	259	286	326	390	499	721	1392	1729	2290	3414	6784
1.6	166	171	181	195	216	248	297	381	552	1070	1329	1762	2627	5223
1.7	131	135	143	155	173	198	238	307	445	865	1075	1426	2127	4232
1.8	111	111	118	128	143	165	198	256	373	725	902	1197	1787	3556
1.9	90	94	100	109	122	141	170	220	320	625	778	1033	1542	3070
2.0	78	81	87	95	106	123	149	192	282	550	685	910	1359	2707
2.5	46	48	52	58	65	76	93	122	179	354	441	587	878	1752
3.0	33	35	38	42	48	57	70	92	137	271	339	451	676	1350
3.5	26	28	31	34	39	46	58	76	114	227	283	378	566	1133
4.0	22	24	26	29	34	40	50	66	100	199	249	332	499	998
4.5	19	21	23	26	30	36	45	60	90	181	226	302	453	907
5.0	17	19	21	24	27	33	41	55	83	167	209	279	420	841
6.0	14	16	18	20	24	29	36	49	74	149	187	250	376	753
7.0	13	14	16	18	22	26	33	45	68	138	173	231	347	697
8.0	12	13	15	17	20	24	31	42	64	130	163	218	328	658
9.0	11	12	14	16	19	23	29	40	61	124	156	208	314	630
10.0	10	11	13	15	18	22	28	38	59	120	150	201	303	608
15.0	9	10	11	13	16	19	25	34	52	107	135	181	272	548
20.0	8	9	10	12	15	18	23	32	49	102	128	171	259	520

APPENDIX B

Cumulative Normal Frequency Distribution

CUMULATIVE NORMAL FREQUENCY DISTRIBUTION
(AREA UNDER THE STANDARD NORMAL CURVE FROM $-\infty$ TO Z)

Z	0.0	0.01	0.02	0.03	0.04
0.0	.50000	.50399	.50798	.51197	.51595
0.1	.53983	.54380	.54776	.55172	.55567
0.2	.57926	.58317	.58706	.59095	.59483
0.3	.61791	.62172	.62552	.62930	.63307
0.4	.65542	.65910	.66276	.66640	.67003
0.5	.69146	.69497	.69847	.70194	.70540
0.6	.72575	.72907	.73237	.73565	.73891
0.7	.75804	.76115	.76424	.76731	.77035
0.8	.78814	.79103	.79389	.79673	.79955
0.9	.81594	.81859	.82121	.82381	.82639
1.0	.84134	.84375	.84614	.84850	.85083
1.1	.86433	.86650	.86864	.87076	.87286
1.2	.88493	.88686	.88877	.89065	.89251
1.3	.90320	.90490	.90658	.90824	.90988
1.4	.91924	.92073	.92220	.92364	.92507
1.5	.93319	.93448	.93574	.93699	.93822
1.6	.94520	.94630	.94738	.94845	.94950
1.7	.95543	.95637	.95728	.95818	.95907
1.8	.96407	.96485	.96562	.96638	.96712
1.9	.97128	.97193	.97257	.97320	.97381
2.0	.97725	.97778	.97831	.97882	.97932
2.1	.98214	.98257	.98300	.98341	.98382
2.2	.98610	.98645	.98679	.98713	.98745
2.3	.98928	.98956	.98983	.99010	.99036
2.4	.99180	.99202	.99224	.99245	.99266
2.5	.99379	.99396	.99413	.99430	.99446
2.6	.99534	.99547	.99560	.99573	.99585
2.7	.99653	.99664	.99674	.99683	.99693
2.8	.99744	.99752	.99760	.99767	.99774
2.9	.99813	.99819	.99825	.99831	.99836
3.0	.99865	.99869	.99874	.99878	.99882
3.1	.99903	.99906	.99910	.99913	.99916
3.2	.99931	.99934	.99936	.99938	.99940
3.3	.99952	.99953	.99955	.99957	.99958
3.4	.99966	.99968	.99969	.99970	.99971
3.5	.99977	.99978	.99978	.99979	.99980
3.6	.99984	.99985	.99985	.99986	.99986
3.7	.99989	.99990	.99990	.99990	.99991
3.8	.99993	.99993	.99993	.99994	.99994
3.9	.99995	.99995	.99996	.99996	.99996

0.05	0.06	0.07	0.08	0.09
.51994	.52392	.52790	.53188	.53586
.55962	.56356	.56749	.57142	.57535
.59871	.60257	.60642	.61026	.61409
.63683	.64058	.64431	.64803	.65173
.67364	.67724	.68082	.68439	.68793
.70884	.71226	.71566	.71904	.72240
.74215	.74537	.74857	.75175	.75490
.77337	.77637	.77935	.78230	.78524
.80234	.80511	.80785	.81057	.81327
.82894	.83147	.83398	.83646	.83891
.85314	.85543	.85769	.85993	.86214
.87493	.87698	.87900	.88100	.88298
.89435	.89617	.89796	.89973	.90147
.91149	.91309	.91466	.91621	.91774
.92647	.92786	.92922	.93056	.93189
.93943	.94062	.94179	.94295	.94408
.95053	.95154	.95254	.95352	.95449
.95994	.96080	.96164	.96246	.96327
.96784	.96856	.96926	.96995	.97062
.97441	.97500	.97558	.97615	.97670
.97982	.98030	.98077	.98124	.98169
.98422	.98461	.98500	.98537	.98574
.98778	.98809	.98840	.98870	.98899
.99061	.99086	.99111	.99134	.99158
.99286	.99305	.99324	.99343	.99361
.99461	.99477	.99492	.99506	.99520
.99598	.99609	.99621	.99632	.99643
.99702	.99711	.99720	.99728	.99736
.99781	.99788	.99795	.99801	.99807
.99841	.99846	.99851	.99856	.99861
.99886	.99889	.99893	.99897	.99900
.99918	.99921	.99924	.99926	.99929
.99942	.99944	.99946	.99948	.99950
.99960	.99961	.99962	.99964	.99965
.99972	.99973	.99974	.99975	.99976
.99981	.99981	.99982	.99983	.99983
.99987	.99987	.99988	.99988	.99989
.99991	.99992	.99992	.99992	.99992
.99994	.99994	.99995	.99995	.99995
.99996	.99996	.99996	.99997	.99997

Largest and Smallest Detectable Relative Risks

Largest and Smallest Detectable Relative Risks for Two-Sided Significance Tests[1]

α	p_0	n	β 0.01		0.05		0.10		0.20	
0.05	0.10	25	13.13	0	9.76	0	8.23	0	6.23	0
		50	7.43	0	5.81	0	5.05	0	4.23	0
		100	4.64	0	3.80	0	3.40	0.02	2.96	0.10
		200	3.18	0.06	2.72	0.15	2.49	0.21	2.23	0.29
		500	2.18	0.31	1.95	0.39	1.84	0.44	1.71	0.50
		1000	1.77	0.47	1.63	0.54	1.56	0.58	1.47	0.63
0.05	0.25	25	9.95	0	7.13	0	5.96	0	4.79	0.01
		50	5.37	0	4.22	0.06	3.70	0.11	3.15	0.18
		100	3.43	0.14	2.86	0.22	2.60	0.27	2.30	0.34
		200	2.45	0.30	2.15	0.38	2.00	0.43	1.83	0.49
		500	1.80	0.50	1.64	0.57	1.57	0.60	1.48	0.65
		1000	1.52	0.62	1.43	0.68	1.38	0.70	1.32	0.74
0.05	0.50	25	24.12	0.04	10.57	0.09	7.67	0.13	5.48	0.18
		50	6.49	0.15	4.59	0.22	3.87	0.26	3.17	0.32
		100	3.52	0.28	2.84	0.35	2.55	0.39	2.23	0.45
		200	2.39	0.42	2.07	0.48	1.92	0.52	1.76	0.57
		500	1.73	0.58	1.58	0.63	1.51	0.66	1.43	0.70
		1000	1.47	0.68	1.38	0.72	1.34	0.75	1.29	0.78
0.05	0.75	25	∞	0.10	∞	0.14	∞	0.17	>50	0.21
		50	∞	0.19	17.50	0.24	9.32	0.27	5.64	0.32
		100	7.16	0.29	4.49	0.35	3.66	0.38	2.93	0.43
		200	3.28	0.41	2.61	0.47	2.33	0.50	2.05	0.55
		500	1.99	0.56	1.77	0.61	1.66	0.64	1.54	0.68
		1000	1.60	0.66	1.48	0.70	1.42	0.72	1.35	0.76
0.05	0.90	25	∞	0.08	∞	0.10	∞	0.12	∞	0.15
		50	∞	0.13	∞	0.17	∞	0.20	∞	0.24
		100	∞	0.22	∞	0.26	>50	0.29	9.98	0.34
		200	18.17	0.31	6.50	0.37	4.70	0.40	3.44	0.45
		500	3.25	0.46	2.54	0.51	2.26	0.54	1.98	0.59
		1000	2.12	0.56	1.84	0.61	1.72	0.64	1.58	0.68

α	p_0	n	β							
			0.01		0.05		0.10		0.20	
0.01	0.10	25	16.86	0	12.78	0	10.93	0	8.95	0
		50	9.15	0	7.26	0	6.38	0	5.41	0
		100	5.51	0	4.56	0	4.10	0	3.59	0
		200	3.65	0	3.14	0.06	2.89	0.12	2.60	0.18
		500	2.41	0.24	2.16	0.32	2.04	0.36	1.89	0.42
		1000	1.91	0.41	1.76	0.48	1.68	0.52	1.59	0.56
0.01	0.25	25	13.52	0	9.63	0	8.06	0	6.50	0
		50	6.66	0	5.25	0	4.62	0.03	3.94	0.08
		100	4.01	0.08	3.37	0.15	3.06	0.19	2.72	0.25
		200	2.76	0.24	2.42	0.31	2.26	0.35	2.07	0.41
		500	1.94	0.45	1.78	0.51	1.70	0.54	1.60	0.58
		1000	1.61	0.58	1.51	0.63	1.46	0.66	1.40	0.69
0.01	0.50	25	>50	0.01	21.80	0.05	13.70	0.07	8.90	0.11
		50	9.29	0.11	6.27	0.16	5.20	0.19	4.20	0.24
		100	4.30	0.23	3.44	0.29	3.07	0.33	2.69	0.37
		200	2.73	0.37	2.36	0.42	2.19	0.46	1.99	0.50
		500	1.87	0.54	1.71	0.58	1.63	0.61	1.54	0.65
		1000	1.55	0.64	1.46	0.68	1.41	0.71	1.36	0.74
0.01	0.75	25	∞	0	∞	0.10	∞	0.12	∞	0.15
		50	∞	0.15	∞	0.19	38.90	0.22	12.16	0.25
		100	13.23	0.25	6.81	0.30	5.26	0.33	4.03	0.37
		200	4.14	0.36	3.21	0.41	2.83	0.44	2.46	0.48
		500	2.23	0.51	1.97	0.56	1.85	0.59	1.71	0.62
		1000	1.73	0.62	1.59	0.66	1.52	0.68	1.45	0.71
0.01	0.90	25	∞	0.06	∞	0.08	∞	0.09	∞	0.11
		50	∞	0.11	∞	0.14	∞	0.16	∞	0.18
		100	∞	0.18	∞	0.22	∞	0.24	∞	0.28
		200	∞	0.27	15.66	0.32	8.67	0.35	5.45	0.38
		500	4.22	0.42	3.17	0.46	2.77	0.49	2.39	0.53
		1000	2.43	0.52	2.09	0.57	1.94	0.59	1.78	0.63

1. n = sample size in each group; α, β = type I and II error rates; p_0 = proportion of control group exposed.

Source: Walter 1977.

Largest and Smallest Detectable Relative Risks for One-Sided Significance Tests[1]

α	p_0	n	β 0.01		0.05		0.10		0.20	
0.05	0.10	25	11.48	0	8.43	0	7.06	0	5.62	0
		50	6.64	0	5.15	0	4.45	0	3.70	0
		100	4.24	0	3.45	0.01	3.08	0.08	2.66	0.17
		200	2.96	0.10	2.52	0.20	2.31	0.27	2.06	0.35
		500	2.08	0.35	1.85	0.44	1.74	0.49	1.61	0.55
		1000	1.71	0.50	1.57	0.58	1.50	0.62	1.41	0.67
0.05	0.25	25	8.52	0	6.11	0	5.10	0	4.09	0.07
		50	4.81	0.01	3.77	0.10	3.30	0.16	2.80	0.23
		100	3.16	0.18	2.63	0.27	2.38	0.32	2.11	0.39
		200	2.31	0.34	2.01	0.42	1.88	0.47	1.72	0.53
		500	1.72	0.53	1.58	0.60	1.50	0.63	1.42	0.68
		1000	1.48	0.65	1.39	0.70	1.34	0.73	1.28	0.77
0.05	0.50	25	15.60	0.06	7.98	0.13	6.01	0.17	4.40	0.23
		50	5.50	0.18	3.96	0.25	3.36	0.30	2.77	0.36
		100	3.18	0.31	2.58	0.39	2.32	0.43	2.04	0.49
		200	2.24	0.45	1.94	0.51	1.80	0.55	1.65	0.61
		500	1.66	0.60	1.52	0.66	1.45	0.69	1.37	0.73
		1000	1.43	0.70	1.34	0.74	1.30	0.77	1.25	0.80
0.05	0.75	25	∞	0.12	∞	0.16	∞	0.20	14.54	0.24
		50	>50	0.21	9.97	0.27	6.40	0.30	4.26	0.36
		100	5.67	0.32	3.76	0.38	3.12	0.42	2.54	0.47
		200	2.94	0.43	2.37	0.50	2.12	0.53	1.87	0.58
		500	1.88	0.58	1.67	0.63	1.58	0.67	1.47	0.71
		1000	1.54	0.68	1.43	0.72	1.37	0.75	1.30	0.78
0.05	0.90	25	∞	0.09	∞	0.12	∞	0.14	∞	0.18
		50	∞	0.15	∞	0.19	∞	0.22	∞	0.27
		100	∞	0.24	>50	0.29	13.32	0.33	5.96	0.38
		200	10.11	0.34	4.89	0.40	3.74	0.43	2.85	0.48
		500	2.89	0.48	2.80	0.54	2.06	0.57	1.81	0.62
		1000	1.99	0.56	1.74	0.64	1.62	0.67	1.50	0.71

			β							
α	p_0	n	0.01		0.05		0.10		0.20	
0.01	0.10	25	15.26	0	11.48	0	9.77	0	7.95	0
		50	8.42	0	6.64	0	5.81	0	4.90	0
		100	5.15	0	4.24	0	3.81	0	3.32	0.03
		200	3.45	0.01	2.96	0.10	2.72	0.15	2.45	0.23
		500	2.31	0.27	2.08	0.35	1.69	0.39	1.82	0.45
		1000	1.85	0.44	1.71	0.50	1.63	0.54	1.54	0.59
0.01	0.25	25	11.92	0	8.52	0	7.14	0	5.75	0
		50	6.10	0	4.81	0.01	4.22	0.06	3.60	0.12
		100	3.77	0.10	3.16	0.18	2.87	0.22	2.55	0.28
		200	2.63	0.27	2.31	0.34	2.15	0.38	1.97	0.44
		500	1.88	0.47	1.72	0.53	1.64	0.57	1.55	0.61
		1000	1.58	0.60	1.48	0.65	1.43	0.68	1.37	0.71
0.01	0.50	25	>50	0.02	15.60	0.06	10.60	0.09	7.22	0.14
		50	7.98	0.13	5.50	0.18	4.60	0.22	3.74	0.27
		100	3.96	0.25	3.18	0.31	2.85	0.35	2.49	0.40
		200	2.58	0.39	2.24	0.45	2.08	0.48	1.89	0.53
		500	1.81	0.55	1.66	0.60	1.58	0.63	1.49	0.67
		1000	1.52	0.66	1.43	0.70	1.38	0.72	1.33	0.75
0.01	0.75	25	∞	0.08	∞	0.12	∞	0.14	∞	0.17
		50	∞	0.16	>50	0.21	17.62	0.24	8.45	0.28
		100	9.96	0.27	5.67	0.32	4.50	0.35	3.52	0.39
		200	3.76	0.38	2.94	0.43	2.61	0.47	2.28	0.51
		500	2.13	0.53	1.88	0.58	1.77	0.61	1.64	0.64
		1000	1.67	0.63	1.54	0.67	1.48	0.70	1.41	0.73
0.01	0.90	25	∞	0.07	∞	0.09	∞	0.10	∞	0.13
		50	∞	0.12	∞	0.15	∞	0.17	∞	0.20
		100	∞	0.19	∞	0.24	∞	0.26	33.89	0.30
		200	>50	0.29	10.11	0.34	6.52	0.37	4.44	0.41
		500	3.77	0.43	2.89	0.48	2.55	0.51	2.21	0.55
		1000	2.30	0.54	1.99	0.59	1.85	0.61	1.70	0.65

1. n = sample size in each group; α, β = type I and II error rates; p_0 = proportion of control group exposed.

Source: Walter 1977.

APPENDIX D

Sample Size for Group Sequential Case-Control Studies[1]

R	S	$p_0=0.10$ k	$\bar{n}$	$p_0=0.25$ k	$\bar{n}$	$p_0=0.50$ k	$\bar{n}$	$p_0=0.60$ k	$\bar{n}$
				$\alpha = 0.05, \beta = 0.10$					
2	1	378	378	203	203	182	182	203	203
	2	209	295	113	159	101	142	113	159
	3	146	274	79	149	70	132	79	149
	4	112	264	61	144	54	127	61	144
	5	92	261	49	139	44	125	49	139
3	1	133	133	77	77	77	77	89	89
	2	74	104	43	61	43	61	50	70
	3	52	98	30	56	30	56	35	66
	4	40	94	23	54	23	54	27	64
	5	33	94	19	54	19	54	22	62
4	1	77	77	47	47	51	51	61	61
	2	43	61	27	38	29	41	35	49
	3	30	56	19	36	20	38	24	45
	4	23	54	15	35	16	38	19	45
	5	19	54	12	34	13	37	15	43
				$\alpha = 0.05, \beta = 0.25$					
2	1	250	250	134	134	121	121	134	134
	2	140	221	75	118	68	107	75	118
	3	98	215	53	116	47	103	53	116
	4	76	213	41	115	37	104	41	115
	5	62	211	34	116	30	102	34	116
3	1	88	88	51	51	51	51	59	59
	2	50	79	29	46	29	46	34	54
	3	35	77	20	44	20	44	24	53
	4	27	76	16	45	16	45	18	50
	5	22	75	13	44	13	44	15	51
4	1	51	51	32	32	34	34	41	41
	2	29	46	18	28	20	32	23	36
	3	20	44	13	28	14	31	16	35
	4	16	45	10	28	11	31	13	36
	5	13	44	8	27	9	31	10	34

1. p_0: exposure rate (proportion) among controls; R, relative risk; $\underline{S}$, maximum number of stages; k, number of cases and number of controls per sequential group; $\bar{n}$, average sample size for case and control groups; α, Type I error rate; β, Type II error rate.

Source: Pasternack and Shore 1981.

References

Acheson ED [1967]: Medical Record Linkage. Oxford University Press, New York.

Adatto K, Doebele KG, Galland L, Granowetter L [1979]: Behavioral factors and urinary tract infection. Journal of the American Medical Association 241:2525–2526.

Adour KK, Bell DN, Hilsinger RL [1975]: Herpes simplex virus in idiopathic facial paralysis (Bell palsy). Journal of the American Medical Association 233:527–530.

Althauser RP, Rubin DB [1970]: The computerized construction of a matched sample. American Journal of Sociology 76:325–346.

Anderson JA [1972]: Separate sample logistic discrimination. Biometrika 59:19–35.

Anderson JA [1973]: Logistic discrimination with medical applications. In Discriminant Analysis and Applications, pp. 1–15. Academic Press, New York.

Anderson JA [1974]: Diagnosis by logistic discriminant function: further practical problems and results. Journal of the Royal Statistical Society, Series C 23:397–404.

Anderson TW [1958]: An Introduction to Multivariate Statistical Analysis. Wiley, New York.

Anscombe FJ [1956]: On estimating binomial response relations. Biometrika 43:461–464.

Antunes CMF, Stolley PD, Rosenshein NB, Davies JL, Tonascia JA, Brown C, Burnett L, Rutledge A, Pokempner M, Garcia R [1979]: Endometrial cancer and estrogen use: report of a large case-control study. New England Journal of Medicine 300: 9–13.

Apostol TM [1961]: Calculus. Volume 1. Blaisdell, New York.

Armitage P [1955]: Tests for linear trends in proportions and frequencies. Biometrics 11:375–386.

Armitage P [1967]: Some developments in the theory and practice of sequential medical trials. Proceedings of the Fifth Berkeley Symposium of Mathematical Statistics and Probability. Volume 4:797–804.

Armitage P [1971]: Statistical Methods in Medical Research. Wiley, New York.

Armitage P [1975]: The use of the cross-ratio in aetiological surveys. In Perspectives in Probability and Statistics (Gani J ed.). Academic Press, London.

Armitage P, McPherson CK, Rowe BC [1969]: Repeated significance tests on accumulating data. Journal of the Royal Statistical Society, Series A 132:235–244.

Barnard GA [1979]: In contradiction to J. Berkson's dispraise: conditional tests can be more efficient. Journal of Statistical Planning and Inference 3:181–187.

Barnes AB, Colton T, Gundersen J, Noller KL, Tilley BC, Strama T, Townsend DE, Hatab P, O'Brien PC [1980]: Fertility and outcome of pregnancy in women exposed in utero to diethylstilbestrol. New England Journal of Medicine 302:609–613.

Bayer L, Cox C [1979]: Exact tests of significance in binary regression models. Applied Statistics 28:319–324.

Bean JA, Leeper JD, Wallace RB, Sherman BM, Jagger H [1979]: Variations in the reporting of menstrual histories. American Journal of Epidemiology 109:181–185.

Bennett AE, Ritchie K [1975]: Questionnaires in Medicine—A Guide to their Design and Use. Oxford University Press, London.

Bennett BM [1967]: Tests of hypotheses concerning matched samples. Journal of the Royal Statistical Society, Series B 29: 468–474.

Bennett BM, Kaneshiro C [1974]: On the small-sample properties of the Mantel-Haenszel test for relative risk. Biometrika 61:233–236.

Bennett BM, Underwood RE [1970]: On McNemar's test for the 2 × 2 table and its power function. Biometrics 26:339–343.

Benzer S [1973]: Genetic dissection of behavior. Scientific American 229:24–37.

Berkson J [1946]: Limitations of the application of fourfold table analysis to hospital data. Biometrics Bulletin 2:47–53.

Berkson J [1958]: Smoking and lung cancer: some observations on two recent reports. Journal of the American Statistical Association 53:28–38.

Berry G [1980]: Dose-response in case-control studies. Journal of Epidemiology and Community Health 24:217–222.

Bibbo M, Haenszel WM, Wied GL, Hubby M, Herbst AL [1978]: A twenty-five-year follow-up study of women exposed to diethylstilbestrol during pregnancy. New England Journal of Medicine 298:763–767.

Billewicz WZ [1964]: Matched samples in medical investigations. British Journal of Preventive and Social Medicine 18:167–173.

Billewicz WZ [1965]: The efficiency of matched samples: an empirical investigation. Biometrics 21:623–644.

Birch MW [1963]: Maximum likelihood in three-way contingency tables. Journal of the Royal Statistical Society, Series B 25:220–233.

Birch MW [1964]: The detection of partial association, I: the 2 × 2 case. Journal of the Royal Statistical Society, Series B 26:313–324.

Bishop YMM [1969]: Full contingency tables, logits, and split contingency tables. Biometrics 25:383–399.

Bishop YMM, Fienberg SE, Holland PW [1975]: Discrete Multivariate Analysis. MIT Press, Cambridge, Mass.

Bjerkedal T, Bakketeig LS [1975]: Surveillance of congenital malformations and other conditions of the newborn. International Journal of Epidemiology 4:31–36.

Blot WJ, Day NE [1979]: Synergism and interaction: are they equivalent? American Journal of Epidemiology 110:99–100.

Blot WJ, Harrington JM, Toledo A, Hoover R, Heath CW, Fraumeni JF [1978]: Lung cancer after employment in shipyards during World War II. New England Journal of Medicine 229:620–624.

Boston Collaborative Drug Surveillance Program [1972]: Coffee drinking and acute myocardial infarction. Lancet 2:1278–1281.

Boston Collaborative Drug Surveillance Program [1973]: Oral contraceptives and venous thromboembolic disease, surgically confirmed gallbladder disease, and breast tumors. Lancet 1:1399–1404.

Box GEP [1966]: Use and abuse of regression. Technometrics 8:625–629.

Bracken MB, Holford TR, White C, Kelsey JL [1978]: Role of oral contraception in congenital malformations of offspring. International Journal of Epidemiology 7:309–317.

Breslow N [1975]: Analysis of survival data under the proportional hazards model. International Statistical Review 43:45–57.

Breslow N [1976]: Regression analysis of the log odds ratio: a method for retrospective studies. Biometrics 32:409–416.

Breslow N [1978]: The proportional hazards model: applications in epidemiology. Communications in Statistics A7:315–332.

Breslow N [1981]: Odds ratio estimates when the data are sparse. Biometrika 68:73–84.

Breslow NE, Day NE [1980]: Statistical Methods in Cancer Research. Volume 1. The Analysis of Case-Control Studies. IARC Scientific Publication No. 32. International Agency for Research on Cancer, Lyon.

Breslow NE, Day NE, Halvorsen KT, Prentice RL, Sabai C [1978]: Estimation of multiple relative risk functions in matched case-control studies. American Journal of Epidemiology 108:299–307.

Breslow N, Powers W [1978]: Are there two logistic regressions for retrospective studies? Biometrics 34:100–105.

Brittain E, Schlesselman JJ, Stadel BV [1981]: Cost of case-control studies. American Journal of Epidemiology 114: 234-243.

Broders AC [1920]: Squamous-cell epithelioma of the lip. Journal of the American Medical Association 74:656–664.

Bross IDJ [1954]: Misclassification in 2 × 2 tables. Biometrics 10:478–486.

Bross IDJ [1966]: Spurious effects from an extraneous variable. Journal of Chronic Diseases 19:637–647.

Brown CC [1980]: Logistic regression program. Personal communication.

Brown CC [1981]: The validity of approximation methods for interval estimation of the odds ratio. American Journal of Epidemiology 113:474–480.

Brown MB [1976]: Screening effects in multidimensional contingency tables. Applied Statistics 25:37–46.

Carpenter RG [1977]: Matching when covariables are normally distributed. Biometrika 64:299–307.

Chase GR [1968]: On the efficiency of matched pairs in Bernoulli trials. Biometrika 55:365–369.

Chiang CL [1968]: Introduction to Stochastic Processes in Biostatistics. Wiley, New York.

Cochran WG [1953]: Matching in analytical studies. American Journal of Public Health 43:684–691.

Cochran WG [1954]: Some methods for strengthening the common chi-square tests. Biometrics 10:417–451.

Cochran WG [1965]: The planning of observational studies of human populations (with discussion). Journal of the Royal Statistical Society, Series A 128:234–265.

Cochran WG [1968]: The effectiveness of adjustment by subclassification in removing bias in observational studies. Biometrics 24:295–313.

Cochran WG [1972]: Observational studies. In Statistical Papers in Honor of George W. Snedecor (Bancroft TA, ed.). Iowa State University Press, Ames.

Cochran WG [1977]: Sampling Techniques. Wiley, New York.

Cochran WG, Rubin DB [1973]: Controlling bias in observational studies: a review. Sankhya, Series A 35:417–446.

Code of Federal Regulations 45 CFR 46 [1978]: Protection of Human Subjects. OPPR Reports, Revised 16 November 1978. Department of Health, Education, and Welfare, Washington, D.C.

Cole P [1979]: The evolving case-control study (with comment by ED Acheson and discussion). Journal of Chronic Diseases 32:15-34.

Cole P, MacMahon B [1971]: Attributable risk percent in case-control studies. British Journal of Preventive and Social Medicine 25:242-244.

Cole P, Monson RR, Haning H, Friedell GH [1971]: Smoking and cancer of the lower urinary tract. New England Journal of Medicine 284:129-134.

Conover WJ [1974]: Some reasons for not using the Yates continuity correction on 2 X 2 contingency tables (with comments and a rejoinder). Journal of the American Statistical Association 69:374-382.

Copeland KT, Checkoway H, McMichael AJ, Holbrook RH [1977]: Bias due to misclassification in the estimation of relative risk. American Journal of Epidemiology 105:488-495.

Coppleson LW, Brown B [1974]: Estimation of the screening error rate from the observed detection rates in repeated cervical cytology. American Journal of Obstetrics and Gynecology 119:953-958.

Cornfield J [1951]: A method of estimating comparative rates from clinical data. Applications to cancer of the lung, breast and cervix. Journal of the National Cancer Institute 11:1269-1275.

Cornfield J [1954]: Statistical relationships and proof in medicine. American Statistician 8:19-22.

Cornfield J [1956]: A statistical problem arising from retrospective studies. Proceedings of the Third Berkeley Symposium, Volume IV (Neyman J, ed.). University of California Press, Berkeley, pp. 135-148.

Cornfield J [1962]: Joint dependence of risk of coronary heart disease on serum cholesterol and systolic blood pressure: a discriminant function analysis. Federation Proceedings 21:58-61.

Cornfield J [1969]: Selected risk factors in coronary disease: possible intervention effects (with discussion). Archives of Environmental Health 19:382-394.

Cornfield J, Gordon T, Smith WW [1961]: Quantal response curves for experimentally uncontrolled variables. Bulletin of the International Statistical Institute 38:97-115.

Cornfield J, Haenszel W [1960]: Some aspects of retrospective studies. Journal of Chronic Diseases 11:523-534.

Cornfield J, Haenszel W, Hammond EC, Lilienfeld AM, Shimkin MB, Wynder EL [1959]: Smoking and lung cancer: recent evidence and a discussion of some questions. Journal of the National Cancer Institute 22:173-203.

Cox DR [1957]: Note on grouping. Journal of the American Statistical Association 52:543-547.

Cox DR [1958]: Two further applications of a model for binary regression. Biometrika 45:562-565.

Cox DR [1966]: Some procedures connected with the logistic qualitative response curve. In Research Papers in Statistics: Essays in Honor of J Neyman's 70th Birthday (David FN, ed.). Wiley, London.

Cox DR [1970]: Analysis of Binary Data. Methuen, London.

Cox DR [1972]: Regression models and life-tables (with discussion). Journal of the Royal Statistical Society, Series B 34:187-220.

Cox DR [1977]: The role of significance tests (with discussion). Scandinavian Journal of Statistics 4:49-70.

Cox DR, Hinkley DV [1974]: Theoretical Statistics. Chapman and Hall, London.

Cramer EM [1972]: Significance tests and tests of models in multiple regression. American Statistician 26, No.4:26-29.

Dales LG, Ury HK [1978]: An improper use of statistical significance testing in studying covariables. International Journal of Epidemiology 7:373-375.

Davis JP, Chesney PJ, Wand PJ, LaVenture M and The Investigation and Laboratory Team [1980]: Toxic shock syndrome. Epidemiologic features, recurrence, risk factors and prevention. New England Journal of Medicine 303:1429-1435.

Dawber TR, Kannel WB, Gordon T [1974]: Coffee and cardiovascular disease: observations from the Framingham study. New England Journal of Medicine 291:871-874.

Day NE, Byar DP [1979]: Testing hypotheses in case-control studies—equivalence of Mantel-Haenszel statistics and logit score tests. Biometrics 35:623-630.

Day NE, Byar DP, Green SB [1980]: Overadjustment in case-control studies. American Journal of Epidemiology 112:696-706.

Dayal HH [1978]: On the desirability of the Mantel-Haenszel summary measure in case-control studies of multifactor etiology of disease. American Journal of Epidemiology 108:506-511.

Dayal HH [1980]: Additive excess risk model for epidemiologic interaction in retrospective studies. Journal of Chronic Diseases 33: 653-660.

Denman DW [1980]: Personal communication.

Denman DW, Schlesselman JJ [1981]:Interval estimation of the attributable risk for multiple exposure levels. (submitted for publication).

DES Task Force [1978]: Summary Report. DHEW Publication No. (NIH) 79-1688, National Institutes of Health, Bethesda.

Dixon WJ, Brown MD (eds.) [1979]: BMDP Biomedical Computer Programs, P-Series. University of California Press, Berkeley.

Doll R [1964]: Cancer. In Medical Surveys and Clinical Trials (Witts LJ, ed.), 2nd edition. Oxford University Press, New York.

Doll R, Hill AB [1950]: Smoking and carcinoma of the lung. British Medical Journal 2:739-748.

Doll R, Hill AB [1952]: A study of the aetiology of carcinoma of the lung. British Medical Journal 2:1271-1286.

Doll R, Vessey MP [1970]: Evaluation of rare adverse effects of systemic contraceptives. British Medical Bulletin 26:33-38.

Dorn HF [1951]: Methods of measuring incidence and prevalence of disease. American Journal of Public Health 41:271-278.

Draper N, Smith H [1981]: Applied Regression Analysis, 2nd edition. Wiley, New York.

Edwards AWF [1963]: The measure of association in a 2 × 2 table. Journal of the Royal Statistical Society, Series A 126:109-114.

Efron B [1975]: The efficiency of logistic regression compared to normal discriminant analysis. Journal of the American Statistical Association 70:892-898.

Ejigou A, McHugh R [1977a]: On the factorization of the crude relative risk. American Journal of Epidemiology 106:188-191 [with correction 111:463].

Ejigou A, McHugh R [1977b]: Estimation of relative risk from matched pairs in epidemiologic research. Biometrics 33:552-556.

Ejigou A, McHugh R [1981]: Relative risk estimation under multiple matching. Biometrika 68:85-92.

Elandt-Johnson RC [1975]: Definition of rates: some remarks on their use and misuse. American Journal of Epidemiology 102:267-271.

Evans AS [1976]: Causation and disease: the Henle-Koch postulates revisited. Yale Journal of Biology and Medicine 49:175–195.

Evans AS [1978]: Causation and disease: a chronological journey. American Journal of Epidemiology 108:249–258.

Farewell VT [1979]: Some results on the estimation of logistic models based on retrospective data. Biometrika 66:27–32.

Feinstein AR [1973]: Clinical Biostatistics, XX: The epidemiologic trohoc, the ablative risk ratio, and "retrospective" research. Clinical Pharmacology and Therapeutics 14:291–307.

Feinstein AR [1979]: Methodologic problems and standards in case-control research (with comment by PE Sartwell and discussion). Journal of Chronic Diseases 32:35–50.

Feinstein AR, Horowitz RI [1978]: A critique of the statistical evidence associating estrogens with endometrial cancer. Cancer Research 38:4001–4005.

Feldstein MS [1966]: A binary variable multiple regression method of analyzing factors affecting perinatal mortality and other outcomes of pregnancy. Journal of the Royal Statistical Society, Series A 129:61–73.

Feller W [1968]: An Introduction to Probability Theory and Its Applications, Volume 1. 3rd edition. Wiley, New York.

Fienberg SE [1979]: The use of chi-square statistics for categorical data problems. Journal of the Royal Statistical Society, Series B 41:54–64.

Fienberg SE [1980]: The Analysis of Cross-Classified Data, 2nd edition. MIT Press, Cambridge, Mass.

Finney DJ [1971]: Probit Analysis, 3rd edition. Cambridge University Press, London.

Fisher L, Patil K [1974]: Matching and unrelatedness. American Journal of Epidemiology 100:347–349.

Fisher RA [1935]: Design of Experiments, 1st edition. Oliver and Boyd, Edinburgh.

Fisher RA [1962]: Confidence limits for a cross-product ratio. Australian Journal of Statistics 4:41.

Fleiss JL [1981]: Statistical Methods for Rates and Proportions, 2nd edition. Wiley, New York.

Fleiss JL [1979]: Confidence intervals for the odds ratio in case-control studies: the state of the art (with comment by DJ Finney and O Miettinen). Journal of Chronic Diseases 32:69–82.

Foreman H, Stadel BV, Schlesselman SE, and the Women's Health Study [1982]: The Women's Health Study: IUD usage and fetal loss. Obstetrics and Gynecology (in press).

Fraser DW, McDade JE [1979]: Legionellosis. Scientific American 241 (December):82–101.

Freeman J, Hutchison GB [1980]: Prevalence, incidence and duration. American Journal of Epidemiology 112:707–723.

Fuchs C [1979]: Possible biased inferences in tests for average partial association. American Statistician 33:120–126.

Gail M [1973]: The determination of sample sizes for trials involving several independent 2 × 2 tables. Journal of Chronic Diseases 26:669–673.

Gail M, Williams R, Byar DP, Brown C [1976]: How many controls? Journal of Chronic Diseases 29:723–731.

Garside GR, Mack C [1976]: Actual type 1 error probabilities for various tests in the homogeneity case of the 2 × 2 contingency table. American Statistician 30:18–21.

Gart JJ [1962]: On the combination of relative risks. Biometrics 18:601–610.

Gart JJ [1969]: An exact test for comparing matched proportions in crossover designs. Biometrika 56:75–80.

Gart JJ [1970]: Point and interval estimation of the common odds ratio in the combination of 2 × 2 tables with fixed marginals. Biometrika 57:471–475.

Gart JJ [1971]: The comparison of proportions: a review of significance tests, confidence intervals and adjustments for stratification. Review of the International Statistical Institute 39:148–169.

Gart JJ [1979]: Statistical analyses of the relative risk. Environmental Health Perspectives 32:157–167.

Gart JJ, Thomas DG [1972]: Numerical results on approximate confidence limits for the odds ratio. Journal of the Royal Statistical Society, Series B 34:441–447.

Gart JJ, Thomas DG [1982]: The performance of three approximate confidence limit methods for the odds ratio. American Journal of Epidemiology 115:453–470.

Gart JJ, Zweifel JR [1967]: On the bias of various estimators of the logit and its variance with application to quantal bioassay. Biometrika 54:181–187.

Glass R, Craven RB, Bregman DJ, Stoll BJ, Horowitz N, Kerndt P, Winkle J [1980]: Injuries from the Wichita Falls tornado: implications for prevention. Science 207:734–738.

Glass R, Johnson B, Vessey M [1974]: Accuracy of recall of histories of oral contraceptive use. British Journal of Preventive and Social Medicine 28:273–275.

Goldberg JD [1975]: The effects of misclassification on the bias in the difference between two proportions and the relative odds in the fourfold table. Journal of the American Statistical Association 70:561–567.

Goodman LA [1964]: Simple methods for analyzing three-factor interaction in contingency tables. Journal of the American Statistical Association 59:319–352.

Goodman LA [1969]: On partitioning chi-square and detecting partial association in three-way contingency tables. Journal of the Royal Statistical Society, Series B 31:485–498.

Goodman LA [1971]: The analysis of multidimensional contingency tables: Stepwise procedures and direct estimation methods for building models for multiple classifications. Technometrics 13:33–61.

Gordis L, Gold E [1980]: Privacy, confidentiality and the use of medical records in research. Science 207:153–156.

Gordon GS, Greenberg BG [1976]: Exogenous estrogens and endometrial cancer: an invited review. Postgraduate Medicine 59:66–77.

Gordon T [1972]: Multiple contributors to coronary risk: implications for screening and prevention. Journal of Chronic Diseases 25:561–565.

Gordon T [1974]: Hazards in the use of the logistic function with special reference to data from prospective cardiovascular studies. Journal of Chronic Diseases 27:97–102.

Greenland S [1979]: Limitations of the logistic analysis of epidemiologic data. American Journal of Epidemiology 110:693–698.

Greenland S [1980]: The effect of misclassification in the presence of covariates. American Journal of Epidemiology 112:564–569.

Greenland S [1981]: Multivariate estimation of exposure-specific incidence from case-control studies. Journal of Chronic Diseases (in press).

Greenland S, Neutra R [1980]: Control of confounding in the assessment of medical technology. International Journal of Epidemiology 9:361–367.

Greenwald P, Barlow JJ, Nasca PC, Burnett WS [1971]: Vaginal cancer after maternal treatment with synthetic estrogens. New England Journal of Medicine 285:390–392.

Grizzle J [1967]: Continuity correction in the chi-square test for 2 × 2 tables. American Statistician 21:28–32.

Grizzle JE [1971]: Multivariate logit analysis. Biometrics 27:1057–1062.

Grizzle JE, Starmer CF, Koch GG [1969]: Analysis of categorical data by linear models. Biometrics 25:489–504.

Gross AJ, Clark VA [1975]: Survival Distributions: Reliability Applications in the Biomedical Sciences. Wiley, New York.

Groves RM, Kahn RL [1979]: Surveys by Telephone. A National Comparison with Personal Interviews. Academic Press, New York.

Haberman SJ [1972]: Log-linear fit for contingency tables, algorithm AS 51. Applied Statistics 21:218–224.

Haberman SJ [1978]: Analysis of Qualitative Data. Volume I. Academic Press, New York.

Haldane JBS [1955]: The estimation and significance of the logarithm of a ratio of frequencies. Annals of Human Genetics 20:309–311.

Halperin M [1977]: Re: "Estimability and estimation in case-referent studies." American Journal of Epidemiology 105:496–498.

Halperin M, Blackwelder WC, Verter JI [1971]: Estimation of the multivariate logistic risk function: a comparison of the discriminant function and maximum likelihood approaches. Journal of Chronic Diseases 24:125–158.

Hardy RJ, White C [1971]: Matching in retrospective studies. American Journal of Epidemiology 93:75–76.

Hauck WW [1979]: The large sample variance of the Mantel-Haenszel estimator of a common odds ratio. Biometrics 35:817–819.

Heilbron DC [1981]: The analysis of odds ratios in stratified contingency tables. Biometrics 37: 55-66.

Helwig JT, Council KA (eds.) [1979]: SAS User's Guide, 1979 edition. SAS Institute, Inc., Raleigh, N. C.

Hennekens CH, Drolette ME, Jesse MJ, Davies JE, Hutchison GB [1976]: Coffee drinking and death due to coronary heart disease. New England Journal of Medicine 294:633–636.

Hennekens CH, Rosner B, Jesse MJ, Drolette ME, Speizer FE [1977]: A retrospective study of physical activity and coronary deaths. International Journal of Epidemiology 6:243–246.

Herbst AL, Cole P, Colton T, Robboy SJ, Scully RE [1977]: Age-incidence and risk of diethylstilbestrol-related clear cell adenocarcinoma of the vagina and cervix. American Journal of Obstetrics and Gynecology 128:43–50.

Herbst AL, Hubby MM, Blough RR, Azizi F [1980]: A comparison of pregnancy experience in DES-exposed and DES-unexposed daughters. Journal of Reproductive Medicine 24:62–69.

Herbst AL, Ulfelder H, Poskanzer DC [1971]: Adenocarcinoma of the vagina. Association of maternal stilbestrol therapy with tumor appearance in young women. New England Journal of Medicine 284:878–881.

Hill AB [1953]: Observation and experiment. New England Journal of Medicine 248:995–1001.

Hill AB [1965]: The environment and disease: association or causation? Proceedings of the Royal Society of Medicine 58:295–300.

Hill AB [1971]: Principles of Medical Statistics, 9th edition. Oxford University Press, New York.

Hills M, Armitage P [1979]: The two-period cross-over clinical trial. British Journal of Clinical Pharmacology 8:7–20.

Holford TR [1978]: The analysis of pair-matched case-control studies, a multivariate approach. Biometrics 34:665–672.

Holford TR, White C, Kelsey J [1978]: Multivariate analysis for matched case-control studies. American Journal of Epidemiology 107:245–256.

Hoover RN, Strasser PH [1980]: Artificial sweeteners and human bladder cancer. Lancet 1:837–840.

Hosmer DW, Lemeshow S [1980]: Goodness of fit tests for the multiple logistic regression model. Communications in Statistics A9:1043–1069.

Hosmer DW, Wang CY, Lin IC, Lemeshow S [1978]: A computer program for stepwise logistic regression using maximum likelihood estimation. Computer Programs in Biomedicine 8:121–134.

Hulka BS, Grimson RC, Greenberg BG, Kaufman DG, Fowler WC, Hogue CJR, Berger GS, Pulliam CC [1980]: "Alternative" controls in a case-control study of endometrial cancer and exogenous estrogen. American Journal of Epidemiology 112:376–387.

Hulka BS, Hogue CJR, Greenberg BG [1978]: Methodologic issues in epidemiologic studies of endometrial cancer and exogenous estrogen. American Journal of Epidemiology 107:267–276.

Hutchison GB, Rothman KJ [1978]: Correcting a bias? New England Journal of Medicine 299:1129–1130.

Inman WHW, Vessey MP [1968]: Investigation of deaths from pulmonary, coronary, and cerebral thrombosis and embolism in women of child-bearing age. British Medical Journal 2:193–199.

Jick H, Miettinen OS, Neff RK, Shapiro S, Heinonen OP, Slone D [1973]: Coffee and myocardial infarction. New England Journal of Medicine 289:63–67.

Jick H, Slone D, Westerholm B, Inman WHW, Vessey MP, Shapiro S, Lewis GP, Worchester J [1969]: Venous thromboembolic disease and ABO type: a cooperative study. Lancet 1:539–542.

Jick H, Vessey MP [1978]: Case-control studies in the evaluation of drug-induced illness. American Journal of Epidemiology 107:1–7.

Johnson NL, Kotz S [1969]: Distributions in Statistics. Houghton Mifflin, Boston.

Kahn HA [1966]: The Dorn study of smoking and mortality among U.S. veterans: report on eight and one-half years of observation. In Epidemiologic Approaches to the Study of Cancer and Other Chronic Diseases (Haenszel W, ed.). National Cancer Institute Monograph No. 19, USGPO, Washington.

Kelsey JK, Dwyer T, Holford TR, Bracken MB [1978]: Maternal smoking and congenital malformations: an epidemiological study. Journal of Epidemiology and Community Health 32:102–107.

Kempthorne O [1977]: Why randomize? Journal of Statistical Planning and Inference 1:1–25.

Kempthorne O [1979]: In dispraise of the exact test: reactions. Journal of Statistical Inference and Planning 3:199–213.

Kessler II, Clark JP [1978]: Saccharin, cyclamate, and human bladder cancer: no evidence of an association. Journal of the American Medical Association 240:349–355.

Keys A, Kihlberg JK [1963]: Effect of misclassification on estimated relative prevalence of a characteristic: Part I. Two populations infallibly distinguished. Part II. Errors in two variables. American Journal of Public Health 53:1656–1665.

Kish L [1965]: Survey Sampling. Wiley, New York.

Klatsky AL, Friedman GD, Siegelaub AB [1973]: Coffee drinking prior to acute myocardial infarction. Results from the Kaiser-Permanente Epidemiologic Study of Myocardial Infarction. Journal of the American Medical Association 5:540–543.

Kline J, Stein Z, Susser M, Warburton D [1978]: Induced abortion and spontaneous abortion: no connection? American Journal of Epidemiology 107:290–298.

Kraus AS [1954]: The use of hospital data in studying the association between a characteristic and a disease. Public Health Reports 69:1211–1214.

Kraus AS [1960]: Comparison of a group with a disease and a control group from the same families, in the search for possible etiologic factors. American Journal of Public Health 50:303–311.

Ku HH, Kullback S [1974]: Loglinear models in contingency table analysis. American Statistician 28:115–122.

Kullback S [1959]: Information Theory and Statistics. Wiley, New York. (Dover, New York, 1968).

Kullback S, Cornfield J [1976]: An information theoretic contingency table analysis of the Dorn study of smoking and mortality. Computers and Biomedical Research 9:409–437.

Kupper LL, Hogan MD [1978]: Interaction in epidemiologic studies. American Journal of Epidemiology 108:447–453.

Kurland LT, Elveback LR, Nobrega FT [1970]: Population studies in Rochester and Olmsted County, Minnesota, 1900–1968. In The Community as an Epidemiologic Laboratory: a Casebook of Community Studies (Kessler II & Levin ML eds.). Johns Hopkins, Baltimore.

Laird NM, Weinstein MC, Stason WB [1979]: Sample-size estimation: a sensitivity analysis in the context of a clinical trial for treatment of mild hypertension. American Journal of Epidemiology 109:408–419.

Land CE [1980]: Estimating cancer risks from low doses of ionizing radiation. Science 209:1197–1203.

Lane-Claypon JE [1926]: A further report on cancer of the breast. Reports on Public Health and Medical Subjects 32: Ministry of Health, H.M.S.O., London.

Larntz K [1978]: Small sample comparisons of exact levels for chi-square goodness-of-fit statistics. Journal of the American Statistical Association 73:253–263.

Leung HM, Kupper LL [1981]: Comparisons of confidence intervals for attributable risk. Biometrics 37: 293-302.

Levin AA, Schoenbaum SC, Monson RR, Stubblefield PG, Ryan KJ [1980]: Association of induced abortion with subsequent pregnancy loss. Journal of the American Medical Association 243:2495–2499.

Levin ML [1953]: The occurrence of lung cancer in man. Acta Unio International Contra Cancrum 9:531–541.

Levin ML, Goldstein H, Gerhardt PR [1950]: Cancer and tobacco smoking. A preliminary report. Journal of the American Medical Association 143:336–338.

Leviton A [1973]: Definitions of attributable risk. American Journal of Epidemiology 98:231.

Li S, Simon RM, Gart JJ [1979]: Small sample properties of the Mantel-Haenszel test. Biometrika 66:181–183.

Lilienfeld AM [1959]: "On the methodology of investigations of etiologic factors in chronic diseases"—some comments. Journal of Chronic Diseases 10:41–46.

Lilienfeld AM [1973]: Epidemiology of infectious and non-infectious disease: some comparisons. American Journal of Epidemiology 97:135–147.

Lilienfeld AM, Graham S [1958]: Validity of determining circumcision status by questionnaire as related to epidemiological studies of cancer of the cervix. Journal of the National Cancer Institute 21:713–720.

Lilienfeld AM, Lilienfeld DE [1979]: A century of case-control studies: progress? Journal of Chronic Diseases 32:5–13.

Lilienfeld AM, Lilienfield DE [1980]: Foundations of Epidemiology. Oxford University Press, New York.

Linos A, Gray JE, Orvis AL, Kyle RA, O'Fallon WH, Kurland LT [1980]: Low-dose radiation and leukemia. New England Journal of Medicine 302:1101–1105.

Mack TM, Pike MC, Henderson BE, Pfeffer RI, Gerkins VR, Arthur M, Brown SE [1976]: Estrogens and endometrial cancer in a retirement community. New England Journal of Medicine 294:1262–1267.

MacMahon B [1972]: Concepts of multiple factors. In Multiple Factors in the Causation of Environmentally Induced Disease (Lee DH, Kotin P, eds.). Academic Press, New York.

MacMahon B, Pugh TF [1970]: Epidemiology: Principles and Methods. Little, Brown, Boston.

Mann JI, Vessey MP, Thorogood M, Doll R [1975]: Myocardial infarction in young women with special reference to oral contraceptive practice. British Medical Journal 2:241–245.

Mantel N [1963]: Chi-square tests with one degree of freedom; extensions of the Mantel-Haenszel procedure. Journal of the American Statistical Association 58:690–700.

Mantel N [1973]: Synthetic retrospective studies and related topics. Biometrics 29:479–486.

Mantel N [1977]: Tests and limits for the common odds ratio of several 2 × 2 contingency tables: methods in analogy with the Mantel-Haenszel procedure. Journal of Statistical Planning and Inference 1:179–189.

Mantel N [1980]: Biased inferences in tests for average partial associations. American Statistician 34:190–191.

Mantel N, Brown C, Byar DP [1977]: Tests for homogeneity of effect in an epidemiologic investigation. American Journal of Epidemiology 106:125–129.

Mantel N, Fleiss JL [1980]: Minimum expected cell size requirements for the Mantel-Haenszel one-degree-of-freedom chi-square test and a related rapid procedure. American Journal of Epidemiology 112:129–134.

Mantel N, Greenhouse SW [1968]: What is the continuity correction? American Statistician 22:27–30.

Mantel N, Haenszel W [1959]: Statistical aspects of the analysis of data from retrospective studies of disease. Journal of the National Cancer Institute 22:719–748.

Mantel N, Hankey BF [1975]: The odds ratios of a 2 × 2 contigency table. American Statistician 29:143–145.

Markush RE [1977]: Levin's attributable risk statistic for analytic studies and vital statistics. American Journal of Epidemiology 105:401–406.

Marshall J, Priore R, Haughey B, Rzepka T, Graham S [1980]: Spouse-subject interviews and the reliability of diet studies. American Journal of Epidemiology 112:675–683.

Marshall JR, Priore R, Graham S, Brasure J [1981]: On the distortion of risk estimates in multiple esposure level case-control studies. American Journal of Epidemiology 113:464–473.

Martin-Bouyer G, LeBreton R, Toga M, Stolley PD, Lockhart J [1982]: Report of a large outbreak of hexachlorophene poisoning in France. Lancet, i:91–95.

Mausner JS, Bahn AK [1974]: Epidemiology: An Introductory Text. W.B. Saunders, Philadelphia.

McKinlay SM [1974]: The expected number of matches and its variance for matched-pair designs. Applied Statistics 23:372–383.

McKinlay SM [1975a]: The design and analysis of the observational study—a review. Journal of the American Statistical Association 70:503–520.

McKinlay SM [1975b]: The effect of bias on estimators of relative risks for pair-matched and stratified samples. Journal of the American Statistical Association 70:859–864.

McKinlay SM [1975c]: A note on the chi-square test for pair-matched samples. Biometrics 31:731–735.

McKinlay SM[1977]: Pair matching—a reappraisal of a popular technique. Biometrics 33:725–735.

McKinlay SM [1978]: The effect of nonzero second-order interaction on combined estimators of the odds ratio. Biometrika 65:191–202.

McNemar Q [1947]: Note on the sampling error of the differences between correlated proportions or percentages. Psychometrika 12:153–157.

Meisel A, Roth LH [1980]: What we do and do not know about informed consent: an overview of the empirical studies. Paper presented at Annual Meeting of the American Psychiatric Association, San Francisco, May 8.

Merchant JA, Klouda PT, Soutar CA, Parkes WR, Lawler SD, Turner-Warwick M [1975]: The HL-A system in asbestos workers. British Medical Journal 1:189–191.

Meydrech EF, Kupper LL [1978]: Cost considerations and sample size requirements in cohort and case-control studies. American Journal of Epidemiology 107:201–205.

Miettinen OS [1968a]: Under- and overmatching in epidemiologic studies. In Proceedings of the 5th International Congress of Hygiene and Preventive Medicine, pp. 1–13.

Miettinen OS [1968b]: The matched pairs design in the case of all-or-none responses. Biometrics 24:339–352.

Miettinen OS [1969]: Individual matching with multiple controls in the case of all-or-none responses. Biometrics 25:339–355.

Miettinen OS [1970a]: Matching and design efficiency in retrospective studies. American Journal of Epidemiology 91:111–118.

Miettinen OS [1970b]: Estimation of relative risk from individually matched series. Biometrics 26:75–86.

Miettinen OS [1972]: Components of the crude risk ratio. American Journal of Epidemiology 96:168–172.

Miettinen OS [1974a]: Proportion of disease caused or prevented by a given exposure, trait or intervention. American Journal of Epidemiology 99:325–332.

Miettinen OS [1974b]: Simple interval estimation of risk ratio (abstract). American Journal of Epidemiology 100:515–516.

Miettinen OS [1974c]: Confounding and effect-modification. American Journal of Epidemiology 100:350–353.

Miettinen OS [1976a]: Estimability and estimation in case-referent studies. American Journal of Epidemiology 103:226–235.

Miettinen OS [1976b]: Stratification by a multivariate confounder score. American Journal of Epidemiology 104:609–620.

Miettinen OS [1977a]: The author replies [re: "Estimability and estimation in case-referent studies"]. American Journal of Epidemiology 105:498–502.

Miettinen OS [1977b]: On the factorization of the crude relative risk: reply by Dr. Miettinen. American Journal of Epidemiology 106:191–193.

Miettinen OS, Cook EF [1981]: Confounding: essence and detection. American Journal of Epidemiology (in press).

Miller CT, Neutel CI, Nair RC, Marrett LD, Last JM, Collins WE [1978]: Relative importance of risk factors in bladder carcinogenesis. Journal of Chronic Diseases 31:51–56.

Mills JL, Bongiovanni AM [1978]: Effect of prenatal estrogen exposure on male genitalia. Pediatrics (Supplement) 62:1160–1165.

Morgenstern J, Kleinbaum DG, Kupper LL [1980]: Measures of disease incidence used in epidemiologic research. International Journal of Epidemiology 9:97–104.

Multiple Risk Factor Intervention Trial Group [1977]: Statistical design considerations in the NHLI multiple risk factor intervention trial (MRFIT). Journal of Chronic Diseases 30:261–275.

Murray T, Stolley PD, Schinnar R, Hepler-Smith E [1980]: Report of a large case-control study concerning analgesic use and renal failure. Paper presented at the Annual Meeting of the American Public Health Association, October 12–17.

Nagel E [1965]: Types of causal explanation in science. In Cause and Effect (Lerner D, ed.). Free Press, New York.

Nelder JA, Wedderburn RWM [1972]: Generalized linear models. Journal of the Royal Statistical Society, Series A 135:370–384.

Neutra RR, Drolette ME [1978]: Estimating exposure-specific disease rates from case-control studies using Bayes' theorem. American Journal of Epidemiology 108:214–222.

Neutra RR, Fienberg SE, Greenland S, Friedman EA [1978]: Effect of fetal monitoring on neonatal death rates. New England Journal of Medicine 299:324–326.

Newell DJ [1963]: Misclassification in 2 × 2 tables. Biometrics 19:187–188.

Neyman, J [1955]: Statistics—servant of all sciences. Science 122:401–405.

Nic NH, Hull CH, Jenkins JG, Steinbrenner K, Bent DH [1975]: SPSS. Statistical Package for the Social Sciences, 2nd edition. McGraw-Hill, New York.

NIH Clinical Center [1977]: Informed Consent. Medical Administrative Series Issuance No.77-2. National Institutes of Health, Bethesda.

Nomura T, Kanzaki T [1977]: Induction of urogenital anomalies and some tumors in the progeny of mice receiving diethylstilbestrol during pregnancy. Cancer Research 37:1099–1104.

Odoroff CL [1970]: A comparison of minimum logit chi-square estimation and maximum likelihood estimation in 2 × 2 × 2 and 3 ×2 × 2 contingency tables: tests for interaction. Journal of the American Statistical Association 65:1617–1631.

Ogawa J [1951]: Contributions to the theory of systematic statistics. Osaka Mathematical Journal 4:175–213.

O'Neill RT, Anello C [1978]: Case control studies: a sequential approach. American Journal of Epidemiology 108:415–424.

Ory HW [1979]: Final report on Interagency Agreement #1Y01HD8103700 on development of a concurrent case-control study of the effect of oral contraceptive use on the risk of breast, endometrial, and ovarian cancer 10/31/79. Center for Disease Control, Atlanta.

Pasternack BS, Shore RE [1979]: Group sequential methods in the design and analysis of epidemiological studies. In Proceedings of the 10th International Biometric Conference, Guaruja, SP, Brazil, August 6–10.

Pasternack BS, Shore RE [1980]: Group sequential methods for cohort and case-control studies. Journal of Chronic Diseases 33:365–373.

Pasternack BS, Shore RE [1981]: Sample sizes for group sequential cohort and case-control study designs. American Journal of Epidemiology 113:182–191.

Paul O [1968]: Stimulants and coronaries. Postgraduate Medicine 44:196–199.

Peacock PB [1971]: The non-comparability of relative risks from different studies. Biometrics 27:903–907.

Pearson ES, Hartley HO [1966]: Biometrika Tables for Statisticians. Cambridge University Press, Cambridge.

Pike MC, Anderson J, Day N [1979]: Some insights into Miettinen's multivariate confounder score approach to case-control study analysis. Epidemiology and Community Health 33:104–106.

Pike MC, Casagrande J [1979]: re: "Cost considerations and sample size requirements in cohort and case-control studies." American Journal of Epidemiology 110:100–102.

Pike MC, Casagrande J, Smith PG [1975]: Statistical analysis of individually matched case-control studies in Epidemiology: factor under study a discrete variable taking multiple values. British Journal of Preventive and Social Medicine 29:196–201.

Pike MC, Hill AP, Smith PG [1980]: Bias and efficiency in logistic analyses of stratified case-control studies. International Journal of Epidemiology 9:89–95.

Pike MC, Morrow RH [1970]: Statistical analysis of patient-control studies in epidemiology: factor under investigation an all-or-none variable. British Journal of Preventive and Social Medicine 24:42–44.

Pocock SJ [1977]: Group sequential methods in the design and analysis of clinical trials. Biometrika 64:191–199.

Prentice R [1976]: Use of the logistic model in retrospective studies. Biometrics 32:599–606.

Prentice RL, Breslow NE [1978]: Retrospective studies and failure time models. Biometrika 65:153–158.

Prentice RL, Pyke R [1979]: Logistic disease incidence models and case-control studies. Biometrika 66:403–411.

Press SJ, Wilson S [1978]: Choosing between logistic regression and discriminant analysis. Journal of the American Statistical Association 73:699–705.

Roberts RS, Spitzer WO, Delmore T, Sackett DL [1978]: An empirical demonstration of Berkson's bias. Journal of Chronic Diseases 31:119–128.

Robinson G, Merav A [1976]: Informed consent: recall by patients tested postoperative. Annals of Thoracic Surgery 22:209–212.

Rooks JB, Ory HW, Ishak KG, Strauss LT, Greenspan JR, Paganini Hill A, Tyler CW [1979]: The cooperative liver tumor study group. Epidemiology of hepatocellular adenoma: the role of oral contraceptive use. Journal of the American Medical Association 242:644–648.

Ropes MW, Bennett GA, Cobb S, Jacox R, Jessar RA [1959]: 1958 revision of the diagnostic criteria for rheumatoid arthritis by a committee of the American Rheumatism Association. Arthritis and Rheumatism 2:16–20.

Rosenberg L, Slone D, Shapiro S, Kaufman DW, Stolley PD, Miettinen OS [1980]: Coffee drinking and myocardial infarction in young women. American Journal of Epidemiology 111:675–681.

Rothman KJ [1974]: Synergy and antagonism in cause-effect relationships. American Journal of Epidemiology 99:385–388.

Rothman KJ, Boice JD [1979]: Epidemiologic Analysis with a Programmable Calculator. NIH Pub. No. 79–1649, USGPO, Washington, D.C.

Rothman KJ, Greeniand S, Walker AM [1980]: Concepts of interaction. American Journal of Epidemiology 112:467–470.

Royal College of General Practitioners [1967]: Oral contraception and thromboembolic disease. Journal of the Royal College of General Practitioners 13:267–279.

Royal College of General Practitioners [1974]: Oral Contraceptives and Health. An Interim Report from the Oral Contraception Study of the Royal College of General Practitioners. Whitefriars Press, London.

Rubin DB [1973]: The use of matched sampling and regression adjustment to remove bias in observational studies. Biometrics 29:185–203.

Rubin DB [1979]: Using multivariate matched sampling and regression adjustment to control bias in observational studies. Journal of the American Statistical Association 74:318–328.

Sackett DL [1979]: Bias in analytic research (with comment by MP Vessey and discussion). Journal of Chronic Diseases 32:51–68.

Saracci R [1980]: Interaction and synergism. American Journal of Epidemiology 112:465–466.

Sartwell PE [1947]: Infectious hepatitis in relation to blood transfusion. Bulletin of the U.S. Army Medical Department 7:90–100.

Sartwell PE [1971]: Oral contraceptives and thromboembolism: a further report. American Journal of Epidemiology 94:192–201.

Sartwell PE [1974]: Retrospective studies—a review for the clinician. Annals of Internal Medicine 81:381–386.

Sartwell PE [1979]: Comment on "Methodologic problems and standards in case-control research." Journal of Chronic Diseases 32:42–44.

Sartwell PE, Merrell M [1952]: Influence of the dynamic character of chronic diseases on the interpretation of morbidity rates. American Journal of Public Health 42:579–584.

Schlesselman JJ [1974]: Sample size requirements in cohort and case-control studies of disease. American Journal of Epidemiology 99:381–384.

Schlesselman JJ [1977]: The effect of errors of diagnosis and frequency of examination on reported rates of disease. Biometrics 33:635–642.

Schlesselman JJ [1978]: Assessing effects of confounding variables. American Journal of Epidemiology 108:3–8.

Schlesselman JJ [1980]: The author replies [re: "Assessing effects of confounding variables"]. American Journal of Epidemiology 111:128–129.

Schlesselman SE [1980]: Personal communication.

Schreck R, Baker LA, Ballard GP, Dolgoff S [1950]: Tobacco smoking as an etiologic factor in disease. I. Cancer. Cancer Research 10:49–58.

Schreck R, Lenowitz H [1947]: Etiologic factors in carcinoma of the penis. Cancer Research 7:180–187.

SEER Network [1976]: Cancer Surveillance Epidemiology and End Results Reporting. Program Description and Data Format. National Cancer Institute, Biometry Branch, Bethesda.

Seigel DG, Greenhouse SW [1973a]: Validity in estimating relative risk in case-control studies. Journal of Chronic Diseases 26:219–225.

Seigel DG, Greenhouse SW [1973b]: Multiple relative risk functions in case-control studies. American Journal of Epidemiology 97:324–331.

Shapiro S, Kaufman DW, Slone D, Rosenberg L, Miettinen OS, Stolley PD, Rosenshein NB, Watring WG, Leavitt T, Knapp RC [1980]: Recent and past use of conjugated estrogens in relation to adenocarcinoma of the endometrium. New England Journal of Medicine 303:485–489.

Shapiro S, Slone D, Rosenberg L, Kaufman DW, Stolley PD, Miettinen OS [1979]: Oral-contraceptive use in relation to myocardial infarction. Lancet 1:743–747.

Sheehe PR [1962]: Dynamic risk analysis in retrospective matched pair studies of disease. Biometrics 18:323–341.

Simon R [1980]: re: "Assessing effects of confounding variables." American Journal of Epidemiology 3:127–128.

Simpson EH [1951]: The interpretation of interaction in contingency tables. Journal of the Royal Statistical Society, Series B 13:238–241.

Slone D, Shapiro S, Rosenberg L, Kaufman DW, Hartz SC, Rossi AC, Stolley PD, Miettinen OS [1978]: Relation of cigarette smoking to myocardial infarction in young women. New England Journal of Medicine 298:1273–1276.

Slone D, Shapiro S, Kaufman DW, Rosenberg L, Miettinen OS, Stolley PD [1981]: Risk of myocardial infarction in relation to current and discontinued use of oral contraceptives. New England Journal of Medicine. 305: 420–424.

Smith AH, Kark JD, Cassel JC, Spears GFS [1977]: Analysis of prospective epidemiologic studies by minimum distance case-control matching. American Journal of Epidemiology 105:567–574.

Snedecor GW, Cochran WG [1980]: Statistical Methods, 7th edition. Iowa State University Press, Ames.

Spjøtvoll E [1977]: Discussion of "The role of significance tests." Scandinavian Journal of Statistics 4:63–66.

Stason WB, Neff RK, Miettinen OS, Jick H [1976]: Alcohol consumption and nonfatal myocardial infarction. American Journal of Epidemiology 104:603–608.

Stenhouse NS [1963]: Correction to "Confidence limits for a cross-product ratio." Australian Journal of Statistics 5:125–126.

Stolley PD [1980]: Personal communication.

Stolley PD, Tonascia JA, Sartwell PE, Tockman MS, Tonascia S, Rutledge A, Schinnar R [1978]: Agreement rates between oral contraceptive users and prescribers in relation to drug use histories. American Journal of Epidemiology 107:226–235.

Stolley PD, Tonascia JA, Tockman MS, Sartwell PE, Rutledge AH, Jacobs MP [1975]: Thrombosis with low estrogen oral contraceptives. American Journal of Epidemiology 102:197–208.

Suits DB [1957]: Use of dummy variables in regression equations. Journal of the American Statistical Association 52:548–551.

Survey Research Center [1976]: Interviewer's Manual, revised edition. University of Michigan, Institute for Social Research, Ann Arbor.

Susser M [1973]: Causal Thinking in the Health Sciences. Concepts and Strategies in Epidemiology. Oxford University Press, New York.

Tarone RE, Gart JJ [1980]: On the robustness of combined tests for trends in proportions. Journal of the American Statistical Association 75:110–116.

Taube A [1968]: Matching in retrospective studies; sampling via the dependent variable. Acta Societatis Medicorum Upsaliensis 73:187–196.

Taube A, Hedman B [1969]: On the consequences of matching in retrospective studies with special regard to the calculation of relative risks. Acta Societatis Medicorum Upsaliensis 74:1–16.

Temple RJ, Jones JK, Crout JR [1979]: Adverse effects of newly marketed drugs. New England Journal of Medicine 300:1046–1047.

Thomas DC [1977]: Addendum to "Methods of cohort analysis: appraisal by application to asbestos mining." Journal of the Royal Statistical Society, Series A 140:483–485.

Thomas DG [1975]: Exact and asymptotic methods for the combination of 2 × 2 tables. Computers and Biomedical Research 8:423–446.

Thompson WD [1980]: A study of matched and unmatched designs for case-control investigations of disease etiology. Doctoral dissertation, Yale University, July.

Truett J, Cornfield J, Kannel W [1967]: A multivariate analysis of the risk of coronary heart disease in Framingham. Journal of Chronic Diseases 20:511–524.

Tsiatis AA [1980]: A note on a goodness-of-fit test for the logistic regression model. Biometrika 67:250–251.

Turner KJ, Baldo BA, Hilton JMN [1975]: IgE antibodies to Dermatophagoides pteronyssimus (house-dust mite), Aspergillus fumigatus, and beta-lactoglobulin in Sudden Infant Death Syndrome. British Medical Journal 1:357–360.

Ury HK [1975]: Efficiency of case-control studies with multiple controls per case: continuous or dichotomous data. Biometrics 31:643–649.

Vessey MP [1971]: Some methodological problems in the investigation of rare adverse reactions to oral contraceptives. American Journal of Epidemiology 94:202–209.

Vessey MP, Doll R [1968]: Investigation of relation between use of oral contraceptives and thromboembolic disease. British Medical Journal 2:199–205.

Vessey MP, Doll R [1969]: Investigation of relation between use of oral contraceptives and thromboembolic disease. A further report. British Medical Journal 2:651–657.

Vorherr H, Messer RH, Vorherr UF, Jordan SW, Kornfeld M [1979]: Teratogenesis and carcinogenesis in rat offspring after transplacental and transmammary exposure to diethylstilbestrol. Biochemical Pharmacology 28:1865–1877.

Waksberg J [1978]: Sampling methods for random digit dialing. Journal of the American Statistical Association 73:40–46.

Wald N [1979]: Radiation injury. In Cecil Textbook of Medicine (Beeson PB, McDermott W, Wyngaardner JB, eds.). W. B. Saunders, Philadelphia.

Walker SH, Duncan DB [1967]: Estimation of the probability of an event as a function of several independent variables. Biometrika 54:167–179.

Walter SD [1975]: The distribution of Levin's measure of attributable risk. Biometrika 62:371–374.

Walter SD [1976]: The estimation and interpretation of attributable risk in health research. Biometrics 32:829–849.

Walter SD [1977]: Determination of significant relative risks and optimal sampling procedures in prospective and retrospective comparative studies of various sizes. American Journal of Epidemiology 105:387–397.

Walter SD [1977]: The author replies [re: "Optimal sampling ratios for prospective studies"]. American Journal of Epidemiology 106:436–438.

Walter SD [1978]: Calculation of attributable risks from epidemiological data. International Journal of Epidemiology 7:175–182.

Walter SD [1979]: Matched case-control studies with a variable number of controls per case. Biometrika 66:181–183.

Walter SD [1980a]: Large sample formulae for the expected number of matches in a category matched design. Biometrics 36:1–7.

Walter SD [1980b]: Prevention for multifactorial diseases. American Journal of Epidemiology 112:409–416.

Walter SD [1980c]: Berkson's bias and its control in epidemiologic studies. Journal of Chronic Diseases 33:721–725.

Walter SD [1980d]: Matched case-control studies with a variable number of controls per case. Journal of the Royal Statistical Society, Series C 29:172–179.

Walter SD, Holford TR [1978]: Additive, multiplicative, and other models for disease risks. American Journal of Epidemiology 108:341–346.

Weiss NS, Ure CL, Ballard JH, Williams AR, Daling JR [1980]: Decreased risk of fractures of the hip and lower forearm with postmenopausal use of estrogen. New England Journal of Medicine 303:1195–1198.

Wermuth N [1976a]: Analogies between multiplicative models in contingency tables and covariance selection. Biometrics 32:95–108.

Wermuth N [1976b]: Model search among multiplicative models. Biometrics 32:253–263.

Westoff C, Bumpass L [1973]: The revolution in birth control practices of U.S. Roman Catholics. Science 179:41–44.

Wetherill GB [1975]: Sequential Methods in Statistics, 2nd edition. Chapman and Hall, London.

White C, Bailar JC [1956]: Retrospective and prospective methods of studying association in medicine. American Journal of Public Health 46:35–44.

Whittaker J, Aitkin M [1978]: A flexible strategy for fitting complex log-linear models. Biometrics 34:487–495.

Whittemore AS [1981]: Sample size for logistic regression with small response probability. Journal of the American Statistical Association 76:27–32.

Winbush JS, Springer JA, Liu PT [1978]: Optimization of the number of cases and controls in a retrospective study by nonlinear programming. Paper presented at the Annual Meeting of the American Statistical Association, Biometrics Section, August 14–17.

Wold H [1956]: Causal inference from observational data (with discussion). Journal of the Royal Statistical Society, Series A 119:28–61.

Woolf B [1955]: On estimating the relation between blood group and disease. Annals of Human Genetics 19:251–253.

Wynder EL, Cornfield J, Schroff PD, Doraiswami KR [1954]: A study of environmental factors in carcinoma of the cervix. American Journal of Obstetrics and Gynecology 68:1016–1052.

Wynder EL, Graham EA [1950]: Tobacco smoking as a possible etiologic factor in bronchiogenic carcinoma. Journal of the American Medical Association 143:329–338.

Wynder EL, Stellman SD [1980]: Artificial sweetener use and bladder cancer: a case-control study. Science 207:1214–1216.

Yanagawa T [1979]: Designing case-control studies. Environmental Health Perspectives 32:143–156.

Yates F [1948]: The analysis of contingency tables with groupings based on quantitative characteristics. Biometrika 35:176–181.

Yoon J, Austin M, Onodera T, Notkins AL [1979]: Virus-induced diabetes mellitus. New England Journal of Medicine 300:1173–1179.

Youkeles LH [1963]: Loss of power through ineffective pairing of observations in small two-treatment all-or-none experiments. Biometrics 19:175–180.

Index

ABO blood group, 109
Abortion, sequelae, 151–52
Additive model, 63–65
Adjustment
  by confounder score, 13–14, 275–80
  for confounding. *See* Confounding
  by logistic regression, 254–63
  by Mantel-Haenszel method, 254–63
  for misclassification, 139–40
  overfitting, 262–63
  of sample size for confounding, 159–60
  of sample size for nonresponse, 165–66
  in terms of logistic model, 232–33, 239, 251–52
  unnecessary, 190
Admission diagnoses, bias, 134–35
Analytic study, 17
Antagonism, 64
Apparent relative risk. *See* Relative risk
Artificial sweeteners, 38–39, 82–83
Ascertainment, unbiased, 80
Association. *See also* Odds ratio
  apparent, 56–57
  attenuation from misclassification, 138–39
  concept of, 33, 53–55
  negative, 33
  positive, 33
  in relation to log odds ratio, 175
  in relation to odds ratio, 53–54
  in relation to relative risk, 33, 53–54
  spurious, 56–57

statistical test of, 54–55
  strength of, 56–57
Attack rate, 28
Attributable risk. *See also* Etiologic fraction
  definition, 40–41
  estimation from case-control study, 41–43
  relation to relative risk, 41

Baseline inequality, bias from, 140–42
Bayes' Theorem, 43
Benign breast disease, 11–12, 126
Berkson bias, 130
Bias
  admission diagnoses, 134–35
  baseline inequality, 140–43
  Berkson, 130
  compensating, 128–29
  constitutional hypothesis, 142–43
  definition of, 126
  diagnosis, 126–28
  from hospital control series, 134–35
  improper analysis, 137
  interviewer, 136
  length of stay, 133
  nonrepresentative samples, 237–38
  nonresponse, 131–32
  from overadjustment, 190
  from overmatching, 110
  from prevarication, 137
  recall, 135–36
  referral, 128–31

selection, 131
surveillance, 125–26
survival, 133–34
susceptibility, 141–42
unmatched analysis of matched study, 110, 209
Biological gradient, 23. *See also* Dose response
Biological plausibility, 24
Bladder cancer
  and artificial sweeteners, 38–39, 82–83, 153
  and cigarette smoking, 49–52, 84–85, 215–16
Blood group, 109

Cancer
  bladder. *See* Bladder cancer
  endometrial. *See* Endometrial cancer
  lung. *See* Lung cancer
  oesophogeal. *See* Oesophogeal cancer
  vaginal. *See* Vaginal cancer
"Case," 38, 46
Case-control study
  advantages and disadvantages, 17–20
  compared to cohort study, 15
  definition, 14
  exploratory, 15–17
  history of, 25–26
  hospital based, 15, 128–29
  population based, 15
  sequential, 163–65
Cases
  definition, 71–72
  diagnostic criteria, 72–75
  eligibility, 71–75
  exclusions, 71–72, 167–68
  incident, rationale for, 31, 72
  sampling procedures, 80–85
  sources of, 75
Case-history study, implicit use of controls in, 15
Case report, used to establish causation, 21
Category matching, 117–18
Cause
  definition, 20–21
  experimental criteria for, 21–22
  Henle-Koch postulates, 21–22

observational criteria
  biological gradient, 23
  biological plausibility, 24
  consistency, 22–23
  specificity of effect, 23–24
  strength of association, 23
  temporal sequence, 22
probabilistic concept of, 21
proof of, 25
CHD. *See* Coronary heart disease
Checklist for protocol, 101–4
Chi-square test (χ^2)
  for association, 179
  of fit of logistic model, 263–65
  of fit of loglinear model, 285–86
  of logistic parameters, 248–49, 257–59
  of odds ratio based on matched pairs, 210
  for synergy, 197–98
Cholera, 7–8, 22
Cigarette smoking. *See* Smoking
Closed question, 87
Coffee, consumption in relation to myocardial infarction, 79
Cohort study
  compared to case-control study, 15
  current, 12, 40
  definition, 10
  historical, 13, 40
  Royal College of General Practitioners Study, 10–12
  sampling scheme, 34–36
Community controls, 77
Conditional probability, as cumulative incidence rate, 28
Confidence interval
  for etiologic fraction, 221–23
  exact, 180
  for logistic parameters, 247–48
  for odds ratio
    Cornfield's method, 177–79
    exact, 180
    test-based, 206–7
    Woolf's method, 176–77
  for odds ratio, adjusted for confounding
    Cornfield's method, 191–92
    Mantel-Haenszel method, 184
    test-based, 188, 206–7
    Woolf's method, 191

Confidence interval (*Continued*)
  for odds ratio, based on logistic
      regression, 247–48, 257, 260–61
  for odds ratio, matched study
      approximate, 210–11, 215–19
      exact, 211–12
  for ratio of odds ratios, 195
Confidentiality, assurance of, 94
Confounder score, 13–14, 275–80
Confounding
  adjustment for
      by confounder score, 275–80
      in dose-response relationships,
          265–67
      example, 185–90
      by logistic regression, 254–63
      by Mantel-Haenszel method, 183–
          90, 254–63
      by stratification, 181–82, 192–93
      by Woolf's method, 190–91
  from concomitant disease, 133
  definition, 58
  degree of, 61–62
  in terms of logistic model, 238–40
  test for, 62–63, 137–38
Congenital malformations
  and estrogens, 17–19
  and oral contraception, 83, 146–51,
      162
  in relation to maternal cigarette
      smoking, 202
Consistency, of effect, 22–23
Constitutional hypothesis, concerning
      smoking and coronary disease, 142
Continuity correction, 179, 184
Control group. *See* Controls
Controls
  in case history studies, 15
  community, 77
  definition of, 76
  eligibility criteria, 77–80
  exclusion criteria, 77–80, 167–68
  hospital, 76
  neighborhood, 129
  origin of use, 25–26
  population, 77, 129
  population-based, compared with
      hospital, 82
  requirement for, 14–15
  sampling procedures, 80–85
  selection of, in Royal College of
      General Practitioners Study, 11

  sources of, 76–77
  use of, to estimate population
      exposure rate, 43, 48–51, 147
Cornfield
  confidence interval for adjusted odds
      ratio, 191–92
  confidence interval for odds ratio,
      177–79
  point estimate of adjusted odds ratio,
      191
  use of direct standardization to
      control extraneous variables,
      26
Coronary heart disease
  cumulative incidence of, 28–29
  logistic analysis, 230–35, 263–64
Correction factor (½), 175, 219
Cost
  of matching, 117, 121–22, 158
  use of optimal allocation to minimize.
      See Optimal allocation
Covariance, of logistic parameter
      estimates, 246–47
Cumulative incidence rate. *See also*
      Cumulative risk
  definition, 28
  estimate of, 28–29
  as a proportion, 30
  relation to person-time incidence rate,
      30–31, 52–53
Cumulative risk, 52–53. *See also*
      Cumulative incidence rate
Current cohort study
  definition, 12
  compared to historical cohort study,
      40

Data analysis, preparation for, 99–101
DES. *See* Diethylstilbestrol
Diabetes, 8–9
Diagnosis bias, 126–28
Diethylstilbestrol
  and offspring's reproductive capacity,
      3–5, 141, 291–92
  in relation to vaginal cancer in
      offspring, 3–5, 15, 54, 217, 219–
      20, 291–92
Discriminant analysis
  comparison of estimates with
      maximum likelihood, 240–50
  for logistic model, 245

Disease
  classification in relation to relative
    risk, 57
  diagnostic criteria for, 72–75
  measures of occurrence, 27–34
  odds, 33–34, 36
  odds ratio, 33–34, 38
"Disease," odds of, 37–38, 46
Dose response
  adjustment for confounding, 203–6,
    266–67
  analysis in matched study, 213
  analysis of, 166–68
  estimation by logistic model, 265–67
  examples of, 11–12, 45–47
  extended Mantel-Haenszel procedure,
    203–6, 266–67
  Mantel-Haenszel test, 200–206
  sample size, 166–68
  in terms of logistic model, 228
Dummy variables. See Indicator
  variables

Ectopic pregnancy, 129–30
Effect modifier, 240
Efficiency
  of Mantel-Haenszel test, 193, 206,
    219
  reduction due to overmatching, 100–
    11
Eligibility criteria
  for cases, 71–75
  for controls, 77–80
Epsem, 81, 85
Endometrial cancer. See Estrogens
Estrogens
  and congenital heart defects, 17–19
  and endometrial cancer
    etiologic fraction, 221–22
    matched analysis, 209
    misclassification, 138
    odds ratio, 175–76
    severity, 202
    subgroup analysis, 166–68
    surveillance bias, 125
    susceptibility bias, 142
Etiologic fraction
  adjustment for confounding, 224–26
  confidence limits for, 221–23
  definition, 43–44

estimate of, 49, 221
example of calculation, 49–51, 221–
  22
exposure at multiple levels, 222–23
interpretation of, 51, 226
relation to exposure-specific incidence
  rates, 45
standardized estimate of, 224–26
variance of, 221–22
Exact conditional estimate
  of adjusted odds ratio, 191
  of odds ratio, 181
Exact confidence limits, 180
Exact test
  adjustment for confounding, 191–92
  of odds ratio, 180
  of odds ratio in matched study, 211
Excess relative risk, 64–65
Exclusion criteria
  for cases, 71–72
  for controls, 77–80
  for study of fetal monitoring, 13
Experimental study
  advantages, 8–9
  definition, 7
  disadvantages, 9–10
Exploratory case-control study
  of baby talc powder and neurologic
    disease, 16
  characteristics of, 16
Exploratory study, 15–17
Exposure
  biased determination of, 135–37
  discontinuation of, 142
  dose response. See Dose response
  estimation from control series, 43, 48–
    51, 147
  intensity, 45–46
  interpretation of, 45–48
  odds, 34, 36
  odds ratio, 34, 38
Exposure-specific risk. See Exposure-
  specific incidence rate
Exposure-specific incidence rate
  definition, 42
  estimation from case-control study,
    42–43
  example of calculation, 50–52
  relation to etiologic fraction, 43
Extended Mantel-Haenszel test
  of adjusted dose response, 203–6
  applied to matched study, 213

Extended Mantel-Haenszel test
    (*Continued*)
    compared with logistic model for dose
        response, 266–67
    efficiency of, 219

Fetal loss, and use of IUDs, 127
Fetal monitoring, 13–14
Field operations, 97–99
Fisher exact test, 177–80
Follow-up study. *See* Cohort study
Force of morbidity, 29
Frame, 81
Frequency matching, 112–13

Goodness of fit
    of loglinear model, 285–86
    of logistic model, 263–65
Group sequential analysis
    definition, 163
    sample size, 164–65

Hazard, 29
Henle-Koch postulates, 21–22
Hepatocellular adenoma
    and oral contraceptive use, 41–42, 47
Heterogeneity
    of matched estimate of odds ratio, 213
    of odds ratio, 193–95
    Woolf's test for, 194
Hierarchical model, 287–88
Historical cohort study
    approach to study of DES and
        vaginal cancer, 15–16
    compared to current cohort study, 40
    definition, 13
    of fetal monitoring and neonatal
        death, 13–14
Hospital-based case-control study, 15,
    128–29
Hospital controls
    biased, 134–35
    compared with population-based
        controls, 82
    definition, 76
Hypothesis
    definition of, 70
    likelihood ratio test of logistic, 248–49
Hysterectomy
    and uterine cancer, 142

Incidence
    attack rate, 28
    cumulative rate, 28–31
    definition, 27
    density, 29
    exposure-specific. *See* Exposure-
        specific incidence rate
    instantaneous rate, 29
    person-time rate, 29–31
    rate, 27–31, 35
    relation to prevalence, 31
Indicator variables
    definition, 241
    use in stratified analysis, as
        alternative to matched analysis,
        272–75
    use of, in logistic regression, 241–44,
        254, 265–66, 272–75
Informed consent, 92–94
Instantaneous incidence rate, 29
Institutional review, 98
Interaction
    assessment of effects of matched and
        unmatched factors, 271
    definition, 63
    example of assessment by logistic
        regression, 259–63
    logistic model, 240–41, 250–51,
    loglinear model, 281–83
    model dependence, 67
Interviewer
    bias, 136
    training, 98
Intrauterine device
    and ectopic pregnancy, 129–31
    and fetal loss, 127
Ionizing radiation, low-dose, 9
IUD. *See* Intrauterine device

Joint effect
    in additive model, 64
    adjustment for confounding, 198–200
    assessment of two or more variables,
        196–200
    example of assessment by logistic
        regression, 256–63
    in terms of logistic model, 239–41

Legionnaire's Disease, 17
Length-of-stay bias, 133

Likelihood, 246
Likelihood function, 246
Likelihood ratio test
  example of logistic regression
    analysis, 257–59
  of fit of loglinear model, 285–86
  of goodness of fit of logistic model,
    263–65
  of logistic parameters, 248–49
Linear discriminant function, 245
Linear regression model, 228
Logistic model
  definition, 228
  interaction, 240–41, 250–51
  for matched studies, 269–71
  prospective, 267–69
  rationale for use, 229–30
  relation to multiplicative model, 239
  retrospective, 267–69
  stepwise selection, 253–54
  variable selection, 252–54
Logistic parameters
  confidence interval on odds ratio,
    247–48
  covariance matrix of estimates, 246–
    47
  interpretation of, 230–44, 251–52
  likelihood ratio test, 248–49
  maximum likelihood estimates, 245–
    46
  maximum likelihood vs. discriminant
    estimates, 249–50
  in model for matched data, 269–71
  point estimate of odds ratio, 247–48
  prospective vs. retrospective models,
    267–69
  relation to odds of disease, 233
  relation to odds ratio, 233
  scale of measurement, 241
  standard error, 247
Logistic regression
  comparison with loglinear analysis,
    284–85
  comparison with Mantel-Haenszel
    analysis, 254–63
  confounder score, 275–80
  dose response, 265–67
  example of application, 254–63
  goodness of fit, 263–65
  matched analysis, 269–75
  matched analysis of dose response,
    267

maximum likelihood estimation, 245–
  50
overfitting, 262–63
prospective, 267–69
relation to logit and loglinear models,
  288–90
retrospective, 267–69
stepwise, 253–54
unmatched analysis of matched data,
  272–75
Logistic regression coefficients, 234. See
  also Logistic parameters
Logit model
  definition, 282
  relation to logistic regression, 288–90
  relation to loglinear models, 282–83,
    288–90
Logits, 234
Loglinear model
  definition, 280–81
  example of analysis, 284–85
  goodness of fit, 285–86
  hierarchical, 287–88
  interaction, 281–83
  matched analysis, 290
  model selection, 286–87
  nested, 286
  relation to logit model, 288–90
  relation to odds and odds ratio, 282–
    84
  saturated, 286
Log odds, 234
Log odds ratio
  confidence limits for, 176–77
  as measure of association, 174–75
  variance of, 176
Lung cancer
  and cigarette smoking, 134
  and employment in shipbuilding
    loglinear analysis, 284–85
    loglinear model, 280–81
    joint effect with smoking, 194–
      98
    synergy, 197–98

McNemar's test
  efficiency relative to Mantel-Haenszel
    test, 219
  of odds ratio, 210
  power, 162
  sample size determination, 160–62

Mantel-Haenszel
    adjusted test for dose response, 203–6
    application of method compared with
        logistic regression, 254–63
    efficiency of test, 193, 206, 219
    estimate, as weighted average of odds
        ratios, 185, 192–93
    estimate of odds ratio, 183
    example of application of method,
        185–90
    extended procedure compared with
        logistic model for dose-response,
        266–67
    extended test, applied to matched
        study, 213
    large sample variance of estimate, 184
    odds ratio estimate for matched study,
        208, 215–16
    optimality of test statistic, 105, 184
    procedure applied to matched studies
        with variable number of controls
        per case, 217–18
    technique used with confounder score,
        275–80
    test efficiency with multiple controls,
        219
    test for dose response, 200–6
    test in relation to score statistics, 249
    test of odds ratio for matched study,
        213, 215–18
    test of significance of odds ratio, 183–
        84
Matching
    achievement of comparability by,
        212–13
    advantages and disadvantages, 120–
        22
    alternatives to, 111–15
    assessment of interaction between
        matched and unmatched factors,
        271
    closeness of, 118–19
    comparison of matched and stratified
        analyses, 272–75
    costs of, 117, 121–22, 158
    criteria for, 107–9
    definition of, 105
    effectiveness in bias removal, 115–16
    frequency, 112–13
    objectives of, 106–7
    overmatching, 109–11

    removal of effect of factor matched on,
        120–21, 271
    study efficiency, 116–17
    study power, 162
    unnecessary, 108–11
    variance reduction, 116–17
Matched sampling, 81
Maximum likelihood estimates
    comparison of estimates with
        discriminant analysis, 249–50
    for logistic model, 245–46
MI. See Myocardial infarction
Misclassification
    adjustment for, 139–40
    of disease, 137–38
    of exposure, 138
Multiple comparisons, 173–74
Multiplicative model
    definition, 65–66
    relation to linear logistic model, 239
Myocardial infarction
    and coffee consumption, 79
    in relation to smoking
        confounder score, 276–78
        dose response, 204–5, 266–67
        etiologic fraction, 223–26
        logistic regression analysis, 254–63
        loglinear analysis, 289–90
        Mantel-Haenszel analysis, 185–90,
            204–6
        matched vs. unmatched design,
            120–21
    in relation to use of oral
        contraceptives
        confounder score, 276–79
        confounding, 58–61
        dose response, 266–67
        loglinear analysis, 289–90
        logistic regression analysis, 254–63
        Mantel-Haenszel analysis, 185–90,
            204–6
        strength of association, 56
        unnecessary matching, 109

Negative association, 33
Neighborhood controls, 129
Neonatal death, in relation to fetal
        monitoring, 13–14
Nested model, 286
Nonresponse bias, 131–32

Observational study, 7
Odds
    definition, 33
    of disease, 33–34, 36
    of "disease", 37–38, 46
    of exposure, 34, 36
    in terms of loglinear model, 281
Odds ratio. *See also* Cornfield; Mantel-
        Haenszel; Woolf
    adjustment for confounding. *See*
        Confounding
    as approximation to relative risk, 33–
        34
    bias resulting from
        misclassification, 138–40
        surveillance, 125
        unmatched analysis of matched
            study, 110, 209
    comparison across studies, 67–68
    confidence interval for. *See*
        Confidence interval
    confounding, in terms of logistic
        model, 238–40
    definition, 33
    dependence on reference group, 50
    disease, 34, 38
    estimate of
        loglinear model. *See* Loglinear
            model
        logistic regression. *See* Logistic
            regression
        matched, 208, 215–18
        unmatched, 38, 174–76
        unmatched conditional, 181
    exposure 34, 38
    logistic model, 233
    logit model, 282–84
    loglinear model, 282–84
    relation to attributable risk, 41
    relation to exposure-discordant pairs,
        208
    test for heterogeneity, 193–95
    test of significance. *See* Test of
        significance
Oesophogeal cancer, 273–75
Open-ended question, 87–88
Optimal allocation
    equal case-control costs, 154
    to maximize power, 155–57
    to minimize cost, 157
    practical considerations, 157–58

Oral contraceptives
    and benign breast disease, 11–12, 126
    and congenital malformations, 83,
        146–51, 162
    contraindications, 141
    and endometrial cancer, 142
    and hepatocellular adenoma, 41–42,
        47
    and libido, 173
    and myocardial infarction. *See*
        Myocardial infarction
    and phlebitis, 125, 136
    Royal College of General
        Practitioners Study, 10–12
    and thromboembolism, 24, 78, 126–
        27
Overmatching, 109–11

Pair matching, *See* Matching
Path diagram, 58, 107–8
Pilot test, 94–97
Person-time
    at risk, 29–30
    incidence rate, 29–31
Person-time incidence rate
    relation to cumulative incidence rate,
        30–31
    definition, 29
Phlebitis, 125, 136
Population, 80
Population attributable risk percent. *See*
        Etiologic fraction
Population-based case-control study,
        15
Population controls
    compared with hospital controls, 82
    definition, 77
Population exposure rate, estimation
        from control series, 43, 48–51
Positive association, 33
Post-matching, 105
Post-stratification, 113–14
Power
    definition, 144
    of completed study, 149, 151–52
    multiple controls per case, 151–52
    optimal allocation, 155–57
    of pair-matched study, 162
    of unmatched study, 148–50

Prevalence
    definition, 31
    rate, 31
    relation to incidence, 31
Prevalence rate, 31
Prevarication, 137
Primary sampling unit, 85
Probit model, 228
Proportional hazards model, 230
Prospective model, for logistic regression
        267–69
Prospective study. See Cohort study
Protocol, checklist for, 101–4
PSU, 85
p-value, interpretation of, 173–74

Questionnaire
    construction of, 86–90
    pilot test, 94–97
    reliability, 90–91
    self-administered, 90
    validity, 91–92

Radiation
    ionizing, 9
    lack of specificity, 24
Random digit dialing, 85
Random sampling, 34–40, 81. See also
        Sampling
Recall
    bias, 135–36
    errors of, 138
Reference group, in relation to odds
        ratio, 50
Referral bias, 128–31
Regression analysis
    as alternative to matching, 114–15
    of matched data, 114–15
Relative odds. See Odds ratio
Relative risk. See also Odds ratio
    apparent, 56–57
    as approximation to odds ratio, 33–34
    bias from misclassification, 138–40
    compared to attributable risk, 57
    compared to risk difference, 13–14,
        57
    comparison across studies, 67–68

    definition, 32–33
    estimation from a case-control study,
        38
    excess, 64–65
    interpretation of, 40–41, 49–52
    as measure of association, 33
    as measure of strength of association,
        56–57
    as ratio of incidence rates, 15, 32–33
    relation to attributable risk, 41
    relation to etiologic fraction, 44
    smallest detectable, 152–54
Reliability, of questionnaire, 90–91
Repeated significance tests, 163–64
Representative sample, 77, 237
Retrospective model, for logistic
        regression, 267–69
Retrospective study, synthetic, 236–37
Rheumatoid arthritis, 72–73
Risk
    attributable. See Attributable risk
    definition of, 27
    difference. See Risk difference
    exposure-specific. See Exposure-
        specific incidence rate
    relative. See Relative risk
Risk difference. See also Attributable
        risk
    compared to relative risk, 13–14, 57
    definition, 41
Risk factor, relative importance of, 50
Royal College of General Practitioners
        Study, 10–12

Sample size
    adjustment for confounding, 159–60
    adjustment for nonresponse, 165–66
    for experimental study, 9
    multiple controls per case, 150–52,
        168
    optimal allocation. See Optimal
        allocation
    for pair-matched studies, 160–62
    sensitivity of, 146–47, 168–70
    for sequential studies, 163–65
    and study duration, 147
    for study of congenital heart defects,
        17–19, 146–51, 162

for study of low-dose ionizing
  radiation, 9
subgroup analysis, 166–68
for unmatched studies, 145–48
Sampling
  case-control study, 36–40, 80–85
  cohort study, 34–36, 39–40
  epsem, 81
  fraction, 34–35, 46, 235–38
  matched, 81
  nonrepresentative, 237–38
  procedures for, 80–82
  random, 34–40, 81, 237
  ratio, 36–38, 46
  representative, 77, 237
  stratified, 81, 111–12
  systematic, 81
Sampling fraction, 34–35, 46, 235–38
Saturated model, 286
Selection bias, 131
Sequential case-control study, 163–65
Shipbuilding employment. See Lung
  cancer
SIDS, 127–28
Significance, statistical
  interpretation of, 55
  level of, 144
  test of. See Test of significance
Simpson's paradox, 182
Smallest detectable relative risk, 152–
  54
Smoking
  and bladder cancer, 49–52, 84–85,
    215–16
  and congenital malformations, 202
  and lung cancer, 134
  and myocardial infarction
    confounder score, 276–78
    dose response, 266–67
    etiologic fraction, 223–26
    logistic regression analysis, 254–
      63
    loglinear analysis, 289–90
    Mantel-Haenszel analysis, 185–90,
      204–6
    matched vs. unmatched design,
      120–21
Specificity of effect, 23–24
Stable disease process, 31
Standardized coefficient, 234–35

Statistical analysis
  approach to, 99–101, 171–73
  limitations of, 173–74
Statistical significance. See Significance
Stratified sampling
  as alternative to matching, 110–11
  definition, 81
Stratification
  to adjust for confounding, 181–82,
    192–93
  as alternative to matched analysis,
    213, 243–44, 272–75
  closeness of, 118–19
  to remove bias, 185
Strength of association, 23
Study
  analytic, 17
  case-control. See Case-control study
  cohort. See Cohort study
  experimental, 7–10
  exploratory, 15–17
  follow-up. See Cohort study
  observational, 7
  retrospective. See Case-control study
Sudden Infant Death Syndrome, 127–28
Surveillance bias, 125–26
Survival bias, 133–34
Synergy
  as a public health concept, 67
  adjustment for confounding, 198–200
  definition, 64
  test for, 197–98
Synthetic retrospective study, 236
Systematic sampling, 81

Target population, 80
Temporal sequence, 22
Test-based confidence limits, 206–7
Test of significance
  chi-square. See Chi-square
  Cornfield's. See Cornfield
  exact. See Exact test
  likelihood ratio. See Likelihood ratio
    test
  McNemar's. See McNemar's test
  Mantel-Haenszel. See Mantel-
    Haenszel
  repeated, 163–64
  Woolf's. See Woolf

Thromboembolism
    and ABO blood group, 109
    in relation to use of oral
        contraceptives, 24, 78, 127–28
Trend. *See* Dose response

Vaginal cancer
    in relation to diethylstilbestrol, 3–5,
        15, 54, 217, 219–20, 291–92
Validity
    of questionnaire, 91–92
    reduction due to overmatching, 110
Variable
    disturbing, 8
    explanatory, 280
    relative importance of, 234–35
    response, 280

Withdrawals, allowance for, 28–29
Woolf
    confidence interval on odds ratio,
        176–78
    point estimate of adjusted odds ratio,
        174–75
    point estimate of odds ratio, 175
    procedure for matched analysis, 218
    significance test and confidence
        interval for adjusted odds ratio,
        190–91
    test for heterogeneity of odds ratio,
        194–95

Yates continuity correction, 179, 184